PIONEERS AND EARLY YEARS

PIONEERS
AND
EARLY YEARS

A History of British Radiology

E. H. BURROWS

COLOPHON LIMITED

For Anne

First published in Great Britain 1986
by Colophon Limited
39 Victoria Street, St Anne, Alderney,
Channel Islands

© E. H. Burrows 1986

ISBN 0 9511676 0 x

Designed by Sandie Boccacci
Set in Monophoto Bembo and printed by
BAS Printers Limited, Over Wallop, Hampshire, England

CONTENTS

———

PREFACE

Each generation of x-ray workers knows less about the early days of the speciality than its predecessors, and each sees further items of old apparatus and memorabilia destroyed. This book describes the most vulnerable period of all – namely, the birth of the clinical discipline and its growth before 1930, which is already largely beyond recall. The author hopes that *Pioneers and Early Years, A History of British Radiology* will stimulate others to be interested in the beginnings of the profession, and prompt further research. For example, studies of later diagnostic developments, radiotherapy, and local x-ray services will be required to enable British radiologists to celebrate adequately the centenary of Röntgen's discovery of x-rays in 1995.

The warm sun of fortune shone upon the author for this undertaking. While accepting responsibility for errors (which are unavoidable in books with a high biographical content), he wishes to acknowledge the assistance of many persons – pioneers' descendants and biographers, librarians and x-ray colleagues, some of whom provided information that was indispensible for completing the task.

No book could have been produced without the generous support of the three sponsors, Agfa Gevaert Limited, Nycomed (U.K.) Limited and Picker International. All three companies have occupied trusted positions in the x-ray world for many years, and their contribution to this book is accepted as a service to British radiology.

Thanks are offered to the following individuals and institutions – at the risk of forgetting to mention others who contributed no less. Sir Thomas Lodge, doyen of the radiologists, applied his phenomenal memory and his editorial experience to the manuscript which emerged in better shape, being less turgid, more correct grammatically and ready for the printer. Although written largely in Alderney, the research for the manuscript was carried out in Southampton and London, and the librarians in three institutions deserve special thanks: Mrs. E. R. Jones and Mrs. S. Blaker (Wessex Medical Library), Mrs Gunnel Ingham (The British Institute of Radiology), and Miss Jenny Harris (The Royal Society of Medicine); no praise is too high for their help. The reader can verify for himself, by examining the pleasing results obtained from indifferent old prints, the high professional standards of the two photographers responsible for most of the pictures, David Whitcher (Teaching Media Department, University of Southampton) and J. Cook (The Royal Society of Medicine). Claire Styles and my daughter Emma cheerfully typed the manuscript, some parts over and over again. Listed geographically, the following helped: A. F. MacDonald (Aberdeen), F. S. Grebbell and E. M. McIlrath (Belfast), Major-General Sir John Swinton, K.C.V.O., O.B.E. (Berwickshire), E. B. Rolfe (Birmingham), James Toland and J. B. Prendiville (Dublin), Arthur Wightman (Edinburgh), L. J. Ramsey (Essex), J. G. Duncan (Glasgow), Andrew Baster, T. E. Bridgewater,

Maxwell Wright (London), Ian Isherwood (Manchester), Charles Warrick, C.B.E. (Newcastle-upon-Tyne), David Barker and Peter Cook (Southampton), and Professor Kay de Villiers (Cape Town). Finally, thanks are due to my ever-tolerant wife and family including Charlotte who designed the jacket.

E. H. Burrows

Chapter 1

THE GREAT DISCOVERY

———————

November the eighth, 1895, will ever be memorable in the history of Science. On that day a light which, so far as human observation goes, never was on land or sea, was first observed. The observer, Prof. Wilhelm Conrad Roentgen. The place, the Institute of Physics in the University of Würzburg in Bavaria. What he saw with his own eyes, a faint flickering greenish illumination upon a bit of cardboard, painted over with a fluorescent chemical preparation. Upon the faintly luminous surface a line of dark shadow. All this in a carefully darkened room, from which every known kind of ray had been scrupulously excluded. In that room a Crookes's tube, stimulated internally by sparks from an induction coil, but carefully covered by a shield of black cardboard, impervious to every known kind of light, even the most intense. Yet in the darkness, expressly arranged so as to allow the eye to watch for luminous phenomena, nothing visible until the hitherto unrecognized rays, emanating from the Crookes's tube and penetrating the cardboard shield, fell upon the luminescent screen, thus revealing their existence and making darkness visible.

From seeing the illumination by the invisible rays of a fluorescent screen, and the line of shadow across it, the work of tracing back that shadow to the object which caused it, and of verifying the source of the rays to be the Crookes's tube, was to the practised investigator but the work of a few minutes. The invisible rays – for they were invisible save when they fell upon the chemically painted screen – were found to have a penetrative power hitherto unimagined. They penetrated cardboard, wood, and cloth with ease. They would even go through a thick plank, or a book of 2000 pages, lighting up the screen placed on the other side. But metals such as copper, iron, lead, silver and gold were less penetrable, the densest of them being practically opaque. Strangest of all, while flesh was very transparent, bones were fairly opaque. And so the discoverer, interposing his hand between the source of the rays and his bit of luminescent cardboard, *saw* the bones of his living hand projected in silhouette upon the screen. The great discovery was made.

Professor Silvanus Thompson (1897)[1]

The greatest practical importance of these rays is their utility in medicine. So far they seem to serve no useful purpose in any other domain.

Dr. (later Sir) James MacKenzie Davidson (1902)[2]

The new physics may be said to have begun in 1895 with the discovery of x-rays.

Sir William Dampier (1929)[3]

———————

Most explorers tread in the footprints of their predecessors. Röntgen was no exception. He himself admitted that he was building on what had already been done, telling us that he performed the famous experiments with a tube of the type devised by Crookes and Hittorf and energised by an induction coil invented by Rühmkorff. He expected those who came after him to carry on the work.

The glory of a discovery such as Röntgen's is not tarnished or in any way diminished by alluding to the work done before, sometimes spread over several centuries, and which is necessary before the event can happen. To tell the full story of the evolution of the apparatus which Röntgen used – and without which he would not have discovered his rays – would entail reviewing the growth of experimental science in the 19th century. While this task is impossible, this chapter records the milestones of discovery which enabled physicists such as Crookes, Hittorf, Lenard and Röntgen unwittingly to generate x-rays in the course of their experiments[4].

The production of a radiograph depends on the fact when an interrupted current of electricity is passed through a vacuum tube, a stream of rays flow from the cathode. Where this impinges on another body, such as the glass wall of the tube or a specially positioned target, different rays are produced which can penetrate blackened paper, glass, wood and living tissue, and alter an emulsion. These are x- or Röntgen rays, and they have entirely different properties from cathode rays. The three prerequisites for making a radiograph are thus, a vacuum, a source of electricity, and a sensitive emulsion. By the 1890s each of these was a scientific reality.

The first milestone was the discovery of the vacuum in the middle of the 17th century. Otto von Guericke (1602–86) was a citizen of Magdeburg, a practical man of the world who played a part in civic affairs as well as concerning himself with mathematical and mechanical phenomena. He is the father of the air pump. Von Guericke sought to demonstrate the great pressure of the ambient atmosphere, and for this he constructed a great sphere. First he used wooden casks, but later he built a huge hollow copper sphere in two halves – the Magdeburg hemispheres – which he fitted together in an airtight fashion and then pumped out the air. The experiment was performed before the Imperial Court at Ratisbon in 1654, in a manner guaranteed to keep Von Guericke's name fresh to young scientists down the centuries. When the Court assembled, he hitched two teams of horses to the hemispheres and showed that when fully evacuated no fewer than 24 horses were required to pull them apart. A noise like a cannonshot was heard when the hemispheres separated. Yet when the vacuum was abolished by opening the cock of the air pump and admitting the air, the hemispheres fell apart on their own. The air pump was improved by Robert Boyle (1627–91) and Francis Hauksbee (died 1713) in England and by the Abbé Nollet and others in France and elsewhere. Three hundred years were to pass before Röntgen's discovery, but without Von Guericke's air pump he would not have made it.

Through a coincidence of history Von Guericke also fathered the second prerequisite for x-rays, an electrical source. He filled a large glass tube with molten sulphur and then removed the glass on cooling, and rotated the sulphur sphere in his hands. Although the significance of this discovery may have eluded him, Von Guericke had produced a primitive frictional electrical machine.

The next milestone – namely, producing an electrical discharge within a vacuum, was achieved after 1705 by Francis Hauksbee. He showed that mercury when agitated within an evacuated flask produced a luminosity of its glass walls. Hauksbee realised that this phenomenon depended on a vacuum being present, and he probably suspected that it was electrical in nature. Many of his experiments were carried out with a double-cylinder vacuum pump which is still owned by the Royal Society of London. When overhauled in 1926, the 200-year-old pump was found to be still capable of pumping down to about 1 cm of mercury.[5]

Hauksbee's air pump was put to use by the Frenchman, Jean Antoine Nollet (1700–70) who for the first time separated the discharge tube from the electrical generator. Hauksbee had excited his vacuum tube by warming it with his hands or agitating the frictional machine within it. Nollet made his vacuum tube with a sealed-in wire and produced the Hauksbee effects by attaching it with metal chains and hooks to a static machine. Nollet's tubes were called, in his own day, 'electric eggs' – a surprising name, since in all probability they hatched x-rays. Nollet also produced discharges by means of a Leyden jar, which had then recently been discovered. In the presence of the French King and to amuse the Court, he once delivered a simultaneous shock to members of the Royal Guard who were linked together by holding hands. On another occasion he applied a similar discharge to a line of Carthusian monks 180 yards long, which made them all jump together!

The major contributor to this branch of scientific knowledge in the early 19th century was Michael Faraday, the incomparable experimenter, whose discovery of electro-magnetic induction has been said to have altered civilisation more than the wars of Napoleon.[6] Faraday (1791–1867) was the man who established the relationship between moving electricity and moving magnetism, and who in three brief months in the 1830s defined the laws of electro-magnetism and thereby laid the foundation stone of modern electrical industries such as power, lighting, traction and telegraphy. Shortly after Oersted first came upon the connection between electricity and magnetism, Faraday produced the continuous rotation of a wire carrying a current round a magnet and of the magnet round the wire. His discovery of the dynamo and, in principle, the induction coil or transformer which was later to be used by Crookes and Röntgen in their experiments, opened the road to the scientific study of electricity in vacuum tubes later in the 19th century. It took place mostly in Germany.

One of the earliest inventions which enabled this work to commence, was the technique perfected by Heinrich Geissler in 1838. Geissler, a glassblower in Tübingen, succeeded in sealing two platinum wires into a vacuum tube; Hauksbee's tube had no wires and Nollet's had one. Now the electrical current had to pass through the vacuum to complete the circuit, and low-vacuum tubes came to be called Geissler tubes.[6] Another discovery was Rühmkorff's invention of the induction coil, which replaced the frictional machine as a more convenient means of energising vacuum tubes. Thus the major apparatus was assembled for investigating the nature of the discharge.

Julius Plücker, professor of mathematics at Bonn in the middle of the 19th century, studied the greenish fluorescence on the inside walls of an energised vacuum tube, and attributed this phenomenon to electrical currents flowing between the cathode and the tube wall. In 1869 one of his students, J. W. Hittorf, found that an object placed in front of the cathode cast its shadow on the wall of the tube. Hittorf deduced that this was caused by interruption of the radiations passing out at right angles from the surface of the cathode towards the glass wall, and he called this radiation *Kathodestrahlen*. Thus it was Hittorf (1824–1914) who discovered the cathode rays. Goldstein in 1876 introduced the term 'cathode stream'; and thereafter the search was intensified into the true nature of these rays.

This search in the second half of the 19th century was not confined to German academic physicists, and investigators on both sides of the North Sea and the Atlantic contributed. In Britain, Varley and Crookes showed that the cathode stream was deflected in a magnetic field, and Crookes proved that the stream consisted of electrified particles shot out from the cathode which were negatively charged. He had the advantage over his predecessors of utilising more efficient vacuum pumps and he radically improved the design of vacuum tubes. In the 1870s he constructed a tube of his own which was so successful that it superseded earlier designs and thereafter his name – coupled with that of Hittorf and Philipp Lenard – became synonymous with the high-vacuum discharge tube, which to this day is styled 'the Crookes tube' in Britain and *le tube de Crookes* in France.[5]

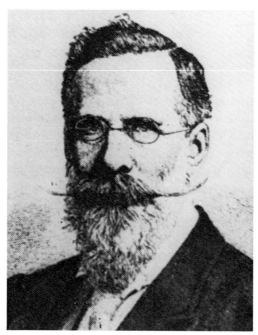

1. *Sir William Crookes*

SIR WILLIAM CROOKES, O.M., K.C.B., F.R.S. (1832–1919) was one of the best-known personalities of Victorian times, the spokesman of science and publicist of the modern physics and electricity. Of relatively humble origin and largely self-taught, he rose to be one of the country's leading teachers and researchers – yet he never attended a university and never held a professorship. Working in his private laboratory in Kensington Park Gardens in London, Crookes in the course of 50 years made countless contributions to chemistry and physics. In 1861 he discovered the element thallium and determined a method of finding its atomic weight – a study which brought him the reward, at the age of 31, of a Fellowship of the Royal Society. Thereafter he investigated the rare earths, and after 1875 devoted 20 years to investigating the passage of electrical discharges through rarefied gases.

Using the high-vacuum tubes which he himself designed, he studied every aspect of matter in the 'ultra-gaseous state', such as the production of colours, the dark space around the cathode, and cathode rays. In his writings he gave a perfect description of an x-ray tube in full action, of all the phenomena occurring within it; but he appeared to ignore, or at least did not mention, what was happening outside it. On turning the pages of Crookes' lectures, it is hard to believe how, during 20 years of experimentation with high-vacuum tubes, these phenomena escaped him. No less surprising is the fact that they went unnoticed by the many thousands of trained workers in universities and schools around the world who operated and lectured upon Crookes tubes.[6]

Honours were showered upon Sir William Crookes throughout his long life – including ironically, those gifts most coveted by university professors. No other Englishman before or since has been: President of the British Association, Royal Society, Institute of Electrical Engineers and the Chemical Society, a Nobel prize winner (chemistry, 1907) and honoured by a knighthood and the Order of Merit. It is a bitter tragedy indeed that Crookes, a prince of science and the inheritor of his countrymen Hauksbee, Boyle and Faraday, should have failed to recognise x-rays when they lay, captured but invisible, in his hands. A biographer characterised him as an excellent experimenter and communicator, who sometimes did not fully interpret the theory.[7] Thus Crookes paved the way for Röntgen to make the Great Discovery and for J. J. Thomson to unveil the subatomic nature of x-rays.

Undoubtedly Crookes, like Hittorf, Lenard and other pioneers, generated x-rays in the course of his experiments. Crookes is known to have accused his suppliers of providing him with defective photographic films and plates after finding some on his laboratory shelf to be unexpectedly fogged. The suppliers denied negligence, but no one could explain the fogging until Röntgen made his discovery. In Philadelphia, the physicist, Arthur Willis Goodspeed (1860–1943) made a 'shadowgraph' using a vacuum tube in 1890, a photograph which he kept – and triumphantly produced six years later. He then asserted, without claiming the credit for any discovery, that his was the first radiograph ever produced.

Another Englishman who unquestionably produced x-rays before Röntgen discovered them was Professor (later Sir) Henry Jackson (1863–1936) of King's College, London.[8] He was a chemist interested in the phenomenon of fluorescence in vacua, and used Crookes tubes for his laboratory experiments. He discovered that a cathode with a dished or concave surface served to restrict the area of phosphorescence on the wall of the tube, which was an advantage in the course of his experiments. In July 1894 he built a tube with a dished cathode made of aluminium and, in addition, inclined

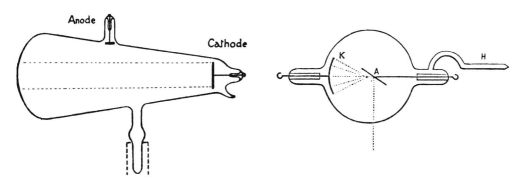

2. *Early vacuum tubes.* Left *Pear-shaped Crookes-Hittorf tube. The cathode stream was directed towards the bulbous end of the tube, and x-rays were generated over a wide area of the wall.* Right *Jackson's focus tube. The dished aluminium cathode K focussed the cathode stream on the platinum anode A. The anode, angled at 45 degrees, deflected the resulting x-rays which were emitted in a more concentrated beam than from the wall of the Crookes tube. The side arm H was used to reverse tube hardness by heating*

the platinum electrode to an angle of 45 degrees in order to deflect the cathode stream at a right angle. This was the original 'focus tube' (*see* 2). Jackson used this tube for another purpose, namely as a source of light for his fluorescence experiments, but he must have generated x-rays with it. Immediately after Röntgen's discovery was announced, this tube was successfully used for radiography.[9] Jackson mistakenly believed that the rays emitted from the cathode were long-wave ultraviolet radiations and, like Crookes and Goodspeed, he at no time advanced any claim to be the discoverer of x-rays. On several occasions he stated expressly that he neither suspected nor discovered the characteristic penetrating power of the radiation emitted by the cathode.[10]

Another contender for the discoverer's palm who was closer geographically to Röntgen was Philipp Lenard, the German physicist whose experiments paralleled Röntgen's. When the Royal Society of London in 1896 awarded its Rumford Medal jointly to the two scientists in recognition of their work, Lenard's name was put first. In February 1896, a meeting in Dublin was announced as a demonstration of the 'New Lenard or Röntgen Rays'.[11] The importance of Lenard's studies of the cathode rays was thus clearly acknowledged, as well as implicitly his contribution to Röntgen's discovery. Lenard, too, must have produced x-rays in the course of his experiments on the absorption of cathode rays in various substances, and he must have noticed some of their properties along with those of the cathode rays. But Lenard used a fluorescent screen coated with pentadecyl-paratolylketone which responds strongly to cathode rays but which is unaffected by x-rays. Consequently he did not identify the x-rays and like Jackson, Crookes and others, failed to establish that x-rays were a different form of radiation from cathode rays.

The third prerequisite for recording x-rays as defined earlier in this chapter, is a sensitive emulsion.[12] The origin of the present-day use of a silver halide for recording x-ray images can be traced to a chance discovery made more than two centuries ago by J. H. Schulze, a German physician. Schulze while experimenting with chalk and nitric acid, happened to use a solution of the acid in which he had previously dissolved silver. He observed that the white mixture turned black on exposure to sunlight, and correctly attributed this change to the actinic effect on silver nitrate. A few years later, Scheele, a Swedish chemist, coated a paper with another halide, chloride of silver, and using a prism to refract the sun's rays, produced an image of the solar spectrum on the paper.

The next photographic milestone was one nearer home at the middle of the 19th century. The famous English potter Josiah Wedgwood had a son Thomas with poor health who was interested in scientific phenomena. Thomas belonged to a group of like-minded persons in London who carried out experiments: one of these was Sir Humphry Davy. Young Wedgwood and Davy repeated Scheele's experiment with silver chloride-coated paper and produced images on it of paintings on glass. They did not know how to 'fix' their images on the paper and so lost their prints, but their experiment revealed the principle of the shadow picture, which is the basis of the modern photograph and radiograph.

Forty years elapsed before the art of 'fixing' photographic images was discovered. Herschel, the great astronomer, discovered the chemical, sodium thiosulphate (hypo) and found that it would dissolve away residual silver chloride. In 1835, the pioneer photographer, Fox Talbot exposed a paper coated with silver chloride in his camera obscura. He obtained only a faint image – until he washed the paper over with a solution containing the weak reducing agents, silver nitrate and gallic acid, and discovered that silver iodide was far more sensitive than silver chloride. More valuable still was the discovery that it was not necessary to expose the paper in the camera until a clear image appeared; an image that was barely visible could be developed further by applying an additional quantity of the reducing agent. An exposure of more than an hour was no longer necessary, a picture could be taken in half a minute! Talbot called his process the Calotype process. Because a latent image was developed to a negative from which any number of prints could be made, this process is the ancestor of modern photography.

Fox Talbot's paper negatives gave way to photography with glass plates using the wet collodion process, which remained a standard method of making photographic negatives for the next 25 years. The glass plate had to be prepared immediately before exposure in the camera while still wet and the development then carried out immediately; a time-consuming and troublesome process which added a folding tent to the equipment of the landscape photographer. In 1871, it was outdated when R. L. Maddox produced the first dry gelatin emulsion for coating plates. When marketed a few years later, these commercially prepared dry plates found immediate acceptance in the photographic world, and soon became part of the bench equipment of physicists and others carrying out experiments with vacuum tubes.

As the 19th century ran its course, the studies of all three groups of scientists – electricians, physicists and chemists, intensified and converged. Answers began to emerge to perennial questions such as why certain chemical combinations produce electrical currents; why such electrical currents decompose certain chemical compounds; and the circumstances controlling the passage of these currents through gases. In the words of the celebrated historian, Sir William Dampier, scientists seemed to be on the point of solving the mystery of the structure of matter in terms of the luminiferous ether.[3] The stage was set for one of the great discoveries in the history of physics, which was to set off a chain reaction of benefits, not only for science but for medicine and for mankind.

In October 1895 there entered the field a German academic physicist with an unorthodox background, W. C. Röntgen. It is necessary to look at the man and his career first, before following the events of that historic autumn.

WILHELM CONRAD RÖNTGEN (1845–1923), the discoverer of x-rays, was born to a German father and a Dutch mother (his parents were cousins) at Lennep-im-Bergishen, near Düsseldorf in the Rhineland. His father was a prosperous cloth merchant in the town. Three years after his birth, the family emigrated to the Netherlands after the February Revolution, renouncing Prussian nationality and becoming Dutch subjects, and settled at Apeldoorn near Utrecht. Here Röntgen spent the next 17 years of his life. He attended the local schools and at the age of 17 was enrolled as a student in the Technical School in Utrecht.

It was here that the incident occurred which blighted Röntgen's educational prospects in the Netherlands. One of his classmates is said to have drawn a caricature of a teacher and failed to own up when challenged, and the blame was pinned on young Röntgen. It appears that he was at times a trouble-maker in the class, and probably the obvious pupil for the teacher to blame. This trivial incident had serious consequences for Röntgen because he was expelled from school without matriculating, and thus preventing him from sitting university examinations. Although he entered the University of Utrecht, he was eventually obliged to go abroad to pursue his studies.[13] All his school reports show him to have been an excellent student: ironically, the only poor marks of the man destined to be the first physicist to win a Nobel Prize were in physics – '*zeer slecht*' (very bad)!

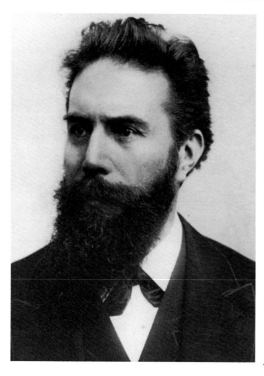

3. Professor W. C. Röntgen

In 1865 he enrolled in the Polytechnikum in Zurich, and three years later at the age of 23 he qualified as a mechanical engineer. But even at this early stage of his adult life, he showed his true vocation by abandoning a career in engineering for one in physical science.

Röntgen's experimental aptitude and unusual qualities were recognised by August Kundt, Professor of Physics in Zurich, who is famous in the physics of sound. Kundt gave him a place in his laboratory and in June 1869 Röntgen received his Ph.D. degree. This launched him upon his career in the German world of academic physics – although even here he was not allowed to forget his Dutch schoolboy prank. When in 1870 Kundt became Professor of Physics at Würzburg in Bavaria and wanted to give his assistant Röntgen academic status, that ancient university refused on the grounds that he had not been properly schooled in Latin and Greek! Thereafter he taught at various German universities, a slowly rising star in the firmament of physics:

1871–2	Kundt's assistant in Würzburg
1872–5	Kundt's assistant in Strasbourg
1875–6	Professor of Physics and Mathematics, Agricultural Academy of Hohenheim, Württemburg
1876–9	Associate Professor to Kundt, Strasbourg
1879–88	Professor of Physics and Director, Physical Institute of Giessen
1888	Appointed Professor of Physics, Würzburg.

Röntgen's appointment to Würzburg at the age of 43 was the highest point of his career; he did not expect to move again. He had repaid the rebuff of his betters in his youth with an exemplary professional career. He wrote his first paper at the age of 20 in his mother's tongue, Dutch. By 1888 he had published over 30 original papers – including one in English, which was published in *Nature*. Of his achievements apart from the discovery of x-rays, especially notable were his experiments with Kundt at Strasbourg on the electro-magnetic rotation of the plane of polarisation of light in gases – a phenomenon which Faraday had tried (and failed) to demonstrate. He also investigated the absorption of heat in water vapour, the compressibility of liquids and solids, and the production of magnetic effects in a dielectric – a study which he ranked as equally important with his discovery of the x-rays. Later he wrote many papers dealing with crystals, which undoubtedly influenced investigators such as Von Laue, Friedrich and Knipping, who in 1912 finally determined the nature of x-rays.

Röntgen's biographer[14] described him as 'a physicist of the old type' – meaning one who built his own apparatus, who verified for himself the findings of others by repeating their experiments, and whose reputation rested on professional integrity. He was certainly clear-headed and dedicated, and he displayed a relentless single-mindedness in the way that he conducted his experiments and ordered his life. In 1894, a year before he decided to investigate Lenard's work, he revealed in the course of a rectorial address at Würzburg the germ of his personal philosophy. Quoting a predecessor of his several centuries before, he made a prophetic utterance: 'Nature often allows amazing miracles to be produced which originate from the most ordinary observations and which are, however, recognised only by those who are equipped with sagacity and research acumen and who consult experience, the teacher of everything. . . . Only gradually has the conviction gained importance, that the experiment is the most powerful and most reliable lever enabling us to extract secrets from nature. . . .'[15]

Röntgen's own study of the passage of electrical currents in discharge tubes was remarkably brief, considering the importance of his discovery. Like all experimental physicists of his day, he had followed the work of Hertz, Lenard and others on electrical discharges in gases. In June 1894 he experimented with a Lenard tube, but it was not until the autumn of 1895 that he set aside all other laboratory work and became engrossed in the problem of these discharges, particularly cathode rays. It may have been his curiosity about the nature of the yellowish-green fluorescence of the surface of the tubes accompanying the production of cathode rays, which drew his interest. He admitted to Mac-Kenzie Davidson, when the latter visited him in Würzburg in July 1896 that he was 'looking for invisible rays'.[14] He was aware that cathode rays showed a fluorescence which extended for only a few centimetres, while their electrical effect could be demonstrated at greater distance from the tube. His choice of a screen made of barium platinocyanide rather than pentadecyl-paratolylketone, the fluorescent substance used by Lenard, is more difficult to explain. Röntgen told Davidson that he thought it a suitable substance because German physicists used it to reveal the invisible rays of the spectrum.

Early in 1896 a London-based journalist, H. J. W. Dam visited Röntgen in his laboratory, and his report provided the world with details of the discovery.[16] The Physical Institute was a modest two-storey building on the Pleischer Ring of the town (*see* 4), and Röntgen demonstrated his discovery to Dam by generating x-rays with apparatus in a room on the ground floor. He used a Rühmkorff coil with a spark of 4–6 inches and a mercury interrupter, energised by a current of 20 amperes (the building had no mains electricity[17]). His tube was an evacuated pear-shaped one of the Hittorf–Crookes type with a flat aluminium cathode at the narrow end and an anode in a side tube, so that the cathode rays struck the broad end. He covered the tube with thin black cardboard to absorb any ultraviolet light that might be emitted. Heavy blinds and curtains were fitted to the laboratory windows to exclude all light, but by the date of Dam's visit Röntgen had fitted up a walk-in tin box as a dark room, and it stood on its end, like a sentry-box in the laboratory. Dam was put inside the box, holding a sheet of photographic paper that had been coated with barium platinocyanide, while Röntgen energised the tube. When the current was passed, the paper screen glowed in the dark. Dam satisfied himself that the rays penetrated not only the aluminium side of the tin box but also a book and a sheet of paper which he held up between the

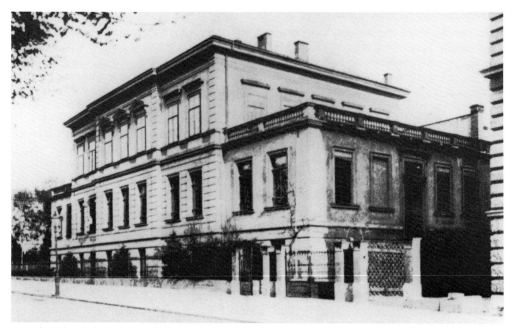

4. *The Physical Institute, Würzburg in 1896. Professor and Mrs. Röntgen lived in the upper apartment*

rays and the screen. 'Then I laid the book and paper down, and put my eyes against the rays. All was blackness and I neither saw nor felt anything. The discharge was in full force and the rays were flying through my head, but they were invisible and impalpable. They gave no sensation whatever. Whatever the mysterious rays may be, they are not to be seen and are to be judged only by their works', concluded Dam.

Then in the next room Röntgen gave Dam details of his discovery. 'I have been for a long time interested in the problems of the cathode rays from a vacuum tube as studied by Hertz and Lenard. I had followed theirs and other researches with great interest and determined as soon as I had time to make some researches of my own. This time I found at the close of last October. I had been at work for some days when I discovered something new. I was working with a Crookes tube covered with a shield of black cardboard. A piece of barium platinocyanide paper lay on the bench there. I had been passing a current through the tube and I noticed a peculiar black line across the paper. The line was the effect of one which only could be produced, in ordinary parlance, by the passage of light. No light could come from the tube, because the shield which covered it was impervious to any light known, even that of the electric arc.'

'And what did you think?' asked Dam.

Röntgen made his famous reply: 'I did not think; I investigated. I assumed that the effect must have come from the tube, since its character indicated that it could come from nowhere else. I tested it. In a few minutes there was no doubt about it. Rays were coming from the tube which had a luminescent effect upon the paper. I tried it successfully at greater and greater distances, even at 2 metres. It seemed at first a new kind of invisible light: It was clearly something new, something unrecorded. Having discovered the existence of a new kind of rays, I of course began to investigate what they would do. It soon appeared from the tests that the rays had penetrative power to a degree hitherto unknown. They penetrated paper, wood and cloth with ease, and the thickness of the substance made no perceptible difference within reasonable limits. The rays passed through all the metals tested with the facility varying, roughly speaking, with the density of the metal. These phenomena I have discussed carefully in my report to the Würzburg Society and you will find all the technical details there. Since the rays had this great penetrative power, it seemed natural that they should penetrate flesh, and so it proved in photographing the hand.'

Röntgen made this crucial observation late on the evening of 8 November in the course of testing the black paper cover of the tube, when none of his assistants was present in the laboratory. The point of discovery came when he realised that the barium platinocyanide screen continued to fluoresce when placed beyond the known range of the cathode rays – namely, up to 2 metres from the tube. After satisfying himself that only the tube could be producing the fluorescence, his next step was to interrupt the rays by various objects known to be opaque to cathode rays. These experiments convinced him that he was dealing with a new kind of radiation, the penetrating power of which varied roughly with the density of the interrupting object. When his hand was the interrupting object, he saw the shadows of the bones on the screen. The next step was to replace the screen by a photographic plate. The first human radiograph was Frau Röntgen's hand with her wedding ring on the middle finger.

Seven weeks of systematic experimentation and verification now commenced. Röntgen applied the formidable experience of his professional life to a detailed evaluation of the physical properties of the new phenomenon. This period must have started early in November and gained momentum as that memorable Friday evening came, and it did not end until he delivered up his completed paper on 28 December. Letters written by his wife at this time testify that he was under obvious stress, being morose and distracted, and spending long hours, all but sleeping in his laboratory. During this period he kept his own counsel, telling neither his staff nor his wife the cause of his preoccupation. He was, in fact, slowly convincing himself by crucial experiments that the phenomenon that he had witnessed on the Friday evening was a new kind of radiation with penetrating powers not known before.

All was revealed on 28 December when, with the remarks to Frau Röntgen that 'Now the devil will be to pay', he released his momentous announcement in the form of a preliminary communication (*Vorläufige Mitteilung*) entitled *Eine neue Art von Strahlen* (On a New Kind of Rays) to his local society, the Physikalisch-Medizinische Gesellschaft of Würzburg. Owing to the Christmas season, there were no meetings, and Röntgen gave no lecture. Instead, he waited upon the President of the Society on that day, and formally presented his communication. Because of its importance, it was accepted for immediate publication in the *Sitzungsberichte* (Proceedings).[18] It was printed a few days later and available to Röntgen by the New Year. He at once posted copies to colleagues and friends. It is known that at least one copy went to Hamburg, two to Berlin, two to Britain – to Lord Kelvin and Arthur Schuster, see Chapter 3 – and one to his friend Franz Exner in Vienna. This last copy was leaked to a newspaper there and then to the international press, and this was the route by which Röntgen's discovery was announced to the world.

Röntgen viewed this famous first paper, consisting of about 3,500 words, as a preliminary or interim scientific report. This was a misconception, because he had already presented the subject in final form. Two points strike the reader of the *Preliminary Communication*. The first is the completeness of Röntgen's investigations. In several weeks he seems to have discovered everything except the ionising property of x-rays and their exact nature. The second point is the absence of all mathematics and formulae – Röntgen was an experimental physicist and, like Faraday, believed in describing what he saw with plain language. Otto Glasser, Röntgen's biographer, stated: 'To scientists (his papers) have become a model for the presenting of results with gravity and simplicity'.

The paper consists of 17 scientific observations carefully described and commented upon. The new radiations – 'I will call the rays, for the sake of brevity, x-rays', he wrote – penetrated many substances opaque to ordinary light during the experiments, apart from the black card with which he surrounded the tube. They cause sensitive surfaces to fluoresce and darken photographic plates. Substances differ in their penetrability according to density and thickness – for example, 3.5 mm of aluminium produces the same effect as 0.1 mm of platinum. Röntgen proved that x-rays are not affected by a prism or a lens, and they are not deviated in a magnetic field. They originate from the place of greatest phosphorescence of the tube walls, and not from the cathode. 'I conclude' – he wrote – 'that the rays are not identical with the cathode rays, but are produced from the cathodic rays at the glass surface of the tube.'

Four weeks later in Würzburg, on 23 January 1896, Röntgen faced his academic colleagues and lectured for the first time. He described his early attempts to take x-rays through the door of his laboratory, and at the end of the lecture, Röntgen demonstrated his discovery by taking an x-ray photograph of the hand of the chairman, Von Köllicker. The latter thereupon proposed that in future the rays should be called 'Röntgen rays'. On 9 March Röntgen's second paper (2,000 words) appeared in the *Sitzungsberichte*.[19] One year later, on 10 March 1897, his third paper (6,500 words) entitled 'Further Observations on the Properties of X-Rays', was printed in the *Proceedings of the Prussian Academy of Sciences*.[20]

After 1897, Röntgen made little further scientific contribution to x-rays although he remained a working physicist and survived another 25 years. Honours and titles now rained on him, but it seems likely that his fame and inherent shyness raised a wall around him in his later years which separated him from wellwishers and the curious. The first political recognition of his great discovery came from the Emperor who summoned him to Potsdam in January 1896, and Röntgen demonstrated x-rays before the Court. In March the University of Würzburg created him an honorary doctor of medicine – the first of many such degrees he received. The same year the Royal Society of London awarded him (with Lenard) the Rumford Medal. In 1901 the first Nobel Prize was awarded to him and he made one of his rare professional visits abroad, travelling to Stockholm to receive it.

In 1900 he became Professor of Physics and Director of the Physical Institute in Munich. There is no clear explanation of his decision to transfer to Munich, but it appears that official pressure was brought to bear by the Bavarian Government who sought his presence to dignify the capital of that State. Earlier he had offended Court circles by accepting the Royal Bavarian Order of the Crown but declining to use the ennobling particle '*von*' which went with it. During the First World War he alienated his British colleagues by sacrificing his Rumford Medal to Germany's demand for gold, although it is said that he later regretted his action.

A question remains over Röntgen's place in the history of science. Glasser, who was his apologist as well as his biographer, concluded 'The salient feature of (his) work, which makes him an excellent representative of classicism, was his persistence and critical honesty in making observations and measurements. . . . (He) was an experimental physicist, in the broadest sense of the word.' On the other hand, some point out that Röntgen's career does not match up to the consistently brilliant achievements of other physicists such as Crookes and Thomson. 'The stage was set for the discovery of x-rays, and Röntgen was the actor chosen by fate to take the cue. Had he failed to do so, the discovery would certainly have been made by another. Even though this is admitted, the value of his work is in no way diminished, and his fame is secure as one of the greatest of mankind's benefactors during the 19th Century.'[8]

MacKenzie Davidson could not have foreseen or perhaps have realised in 1902, when he made the statement quoted at the head of this chapter, that disciplines other than medicine would benefit from Röntgen's work. Already there had been developments in the field of atomic physics which flowed from it, to disprove his prophecy. Science historians such as Dampier view Röntgen's work on x-rays as catalytic, a 'break-through' into new vistas of experimentation, which were to lay the foundation of atomic physics.

The end of the discovery does not lie in Würzburg with Röntgen's three communications. It lies nearer home for Britons – in the Cavendish Laboratories, Cambridge, which became the intellectual powerhouse of atomic physicists at the beginning of this century. The Director, J. J. Thomson, was a man like Faraday, greater than his discoveries.

SIR JOSEPH JOHN THOMSON, O.M., F.R.S. (1856–1940), the discoverer of the electron, was one of the true great pioneers of science.[21]

Born to the wife of a Manchester bookseller, young Joseph was an infant prodigy. He entered Owen's College at the age of 14 and four years later with the aid of Professor Arthur Schuster entered Trinity College, Cambridge as a scholar. At 24 he was a Fellow and at 28 chosen to be Cavendish Professor of Experimental Physics in the University. His 34-year tenure of this post are the Golden Years of British physics. For the last 20 years of his life, Sir Joseph Thomson was Master of Trinity College.

Thomson made his main scientific contribution to the study of the properties of the cathode rays and the conduction of electricity through gases. Röntgen's discovery indicated that the surrounding air, ordinarily an insulator of electricity, becomes a conductor, and Thomson immediately began to investigate the mechanism of conduction. Soon he could support the view of Varley and Crookes that x-rays were generated when rapidly-moving particles of material shot out from the cathode, rather than the undulating rays like light which the German physicists believed them to be. These experiments led Thomson to a fundamental discovery in 1897 when, on measuring the ratio of the charge to the mass, he found that the individual particles had a smaller mass than that of any atom. He concluded that he was dealing with a universal constituent of matter of subatomic size, the particles of which came to be called electrons. He went on to show that not only do electrons striking matter produce x-rays but that, conversely, when x-rays strike matter, they produce electrons. Thus began the path of laying bare the intimate structure of the atom.

Thomson made no practical contribution to medical radiology, unlike his fellow-scientists Schuster and Lodge, who helped doctors to examine patients. But in exploring and revealing the composition of the x-ray beam through a gas, he took up the study abandoned by Röntgen. In completing it, he made a discovery which was perhaps of greater importance to true science.

Chapter 2

THE NEWS RECEIVED

The Roentgen Rays, the Roentgen Rays
What is this craze?
The town's ablaze
With the new phase
Of X-rays's ways.

I'm full of daze,
Shock and amaze,
For nowadays
I hear they'll gaze
Thro' cloak and gown
And even stays,
These naughty, naughty Roentgen rays.

Photography (1896)[6]

The news of the discovery first reached England in the press. Neither of the two British colleagues to whom Röntgen sent copies of the *Preliminary Communication* made public the contents, and nearly three weeks passed before an English translation appeared in *Nature*. Thus it was left to the popular press to exploit the news item from the Continent and to arouse the public's curiosity about the new discovery.[1]

The announcement appeared first in the *Neue Freie Presse* newspaper in Vienna on Sunday, 5 January 1896. The fact that the news broke in the Austrian capital rather than in Berlin, was then less surprising than it would be today. Until the First World War, Vienna was the premier Imperial capital of Europe, culturally and scientifically the metropolis of the Continent. Würzburg, a dreamy provincial town in the then Kingdom of Bavaria, is equidistant from Vienna and Berlin. However, the earlier announcement from Vienna can be explained by two unconnected circumstances.

Franz Exner, Röntgen's friend and former colleague in Kundt's laboratory, lived in Vienna where he was Director of the Physical Institute (and later Professor of Physics) at the University. He and his scientific friends had the habit of meeting informally of an evening to discuss matters of mutual interest. At a meeting in the first week of 1896, Exner described the contents of Röntgen's missive, and it made a profound impression. One of those present was Ernst Lecher, a young physicist and the son of the newspaperman Z. K. Lecher, who was the editor of *Neue Freie Presse*. When Lecher gave his father the news on returning home later that evening, Lecher Senior asked him to prepare a short summary for the morning edition of the paper, observing that a discovery which seemed to have such great potential benefits for mankind should not be ignored. This young Lecher did, and years later he admitted his astonishment at the enormous interest that his short report evoked throughout the world, and he paid tribute to his father's eye for a story.[2]

The second circumstance – why Vienna and not Berlin gave the news to the world – was a coincidence of events. At the beginning of January 1896, the Physical Institute in Berlin was celebrating its 50th anniversary, and although the news of Röntgen's discovery was announced, the members were too preoccupied with the festivities to note or act upon it. The Emperor himself brought them to their senses a week later, when he summoned Röntgen to Berlin to demonstrate his discovery. But by that date radiographs of the human body had been produced in London.

From Vienna after the news broke in the *Neue Freie Presse*, the message was telegraphed to the London newspapers by their correspondents. The first brief announcement appeared in the *Daily Chronicle* on the morning of Monday, 6 January 1896, and it was repeated in the *St. James's Gazette* that evening. The *Manchester Guardian* printed it the following day, close to the letter of Professor Arthur Schuster, which is mentioned below. The London *Evening Standard* of 7 and 8 January carried the first detailed descriptions of Röntgen's experiments, taken from the *Presse*:[3]

A PHOTOGRAPHIC DISCOVERY.

(FROM OUR CORRESPONDENT.)

VIENNA, Monday Night.

A very important scientific discovery has recently been made by Professor Routgen, of Würzburg University, the details of which have already reached Vienna, and are now being carefully examined by several scientific authorities here. Professor Routgen uses the light emitted from one of Crookes' vacuum tubes, through which an electric current is passed, to act upon an ordinary photographic plate. The invisible light rays, of whose existence there is already ample evidence, then show this peculiarity, that to them wood and various other organic substances are transparent, whilst metals and bones, human and animal alike, are opaque to those rays. That is to say, they will, for instance, absorb the rays which have passed through a wooden case in which bones or metals are enclosed. Thus it is possible to photograph in the manner described any bones or metals which may be contained in wooden or woollen coverings. Moreover, as human flesh being organic matter

acts in the same way as such coverings towards the invisible rays from a Crookes' vacuum tube, it has become possible to photograph the bones, say, of a human hand, without the flesh surrounding the bones appearing on the plate. There are photographs of this description already in Vienna. They show the bones of the hand, together with the rings that were worn on the fingers,—metals, as I remarked above, being opaque to these rays—but they show nothing else. They are ghastly enough in appearance, but, from a scientific point of view, they open up a wide field for speculation. Among the practical uses of the new discovery, it is stated that it will henceforth be possible for surgeons to determine by help of this new branch of photography the exact position of any bullet that may be embedded in the human body, or, again, to render visible any fractures there may be in the bones prior to performing any operation on the respective part of the body. And there are various other uses to which the new method may be put, as, for example, in connection with caries and other bone diseases. The *Presse* assures its readers that there is no joke or humbug in the matter. It is a serious discovery by a serious German Professor.

The first news of the discovery to come from Germany did not reach London until 14 January. On that day the Berlin correspondents of the *Daily News* and *Westminster Gazette* described the glittering reception at Potsdam given for Röntgen by the Emperor on the previous evening, at which x-rays were demonstrated. The *Daily News* followed a few days later with a report of a lecture delivered in Berlin by one Doctor Spies before a large audience, but no details were provided of the experiments such as had been sent from Vienna.

The journalistic scoop was responsibly handled and there were few serious errors or omissions. Not all the British newspapers were enthusiastic. The *Morning Post* greeted the discovery with caution, having interviewed Captain W. de W. Abney, a physicist

at the Science Museum in South Kensington, and found that he 'did not see very much
in it'. Others adopted a hesitant or cautious attitude or their reports were confused and
asked more questions than they provided information about the nature of the rays.
Throughout the month of January, *The Times* made no mention of the discovery.

   Punch on 25 January used Röntgen's work to patriotic advantage in a political cartoon
(*see 5*) and gave the news in verse:

THE NEW PHOTOGRAPHY.
[Professor RÖNTGEN, of Würzburg, has discovered how to photograph
through a person's body, giving a picture only of the bones.]

O, RÖNTGEN, then the news is true,
   And not a trick of idle rumour,
That bids us each beware of you,
   And of your grim and graveyard humour.

We do not want, like Dr. SWIFT,
   To take our flesh off and to pose in
Our bones, or show each little rift
   And joint for you to poke your nose in.

We only crave to contemplate
   Each other's usual full-dress photo;
Your worse than "altogether" state
   Of portraiture we bar in *toto!*

The fondest swain would scarcely prize
   A picture of his lady's framework;
To gaze on this with yearning eyes
   Would probably be voted tame work!

The attitude of the popular press had much influence on the future developments and
uses of x-rays. The comments and jokes about the new photography which appeared
in newspapers and periodicals at that time caught the interest of the man in the street.
But Röntgen's discovery did more than that, as J. J. Thomson observed a few months
later:[4] '(It) appeals to the strongest of all human attributes, namely curiosity.' There
was a fear that the rays would be put to wrong use, and especially that they could
be used to intrude upon personal privacy. The public feared that some sort of pocket
apparatus might be developed, and this aroused the imagination of the media further.
A popular seaside postcard showed a bathing machine with a lady inside, and outside
on the sand stood a man manipulating a tiny camera that could 'see through the bathing
machine'.[5] An enterprising London firm advertised the sale of 'x-ray proof under-
clothing for ladies'. This prompted the music-hall jingle, *X-Craze*, which is printed
at the head of this chapter.[6]

   The *Pall Mall Gazette* wrote in 1896: 'We are sick of the Röntgen rays. You can
see other people's bones with the naked eye, and also see through eight inches of solid
wood. On the revolting indecency of this there is no need to dwell.' This misconceived
notoriety of x-rays gave rise to the suggestion that their importation should be banned!

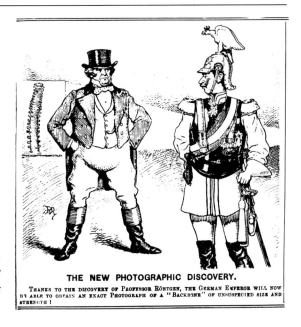

THE NEW PHOTOGRAPHIC DISCOVERY.

Thanks to the discovery of Professor Röntgen, the German Emperor will now be able to obtain an exact Photograph of a "Backbone" of unsuspected size and strength!

5. Punch *cartoon of 25 January 1896, expressing British resentment at the Kaiser's intervention in colonial affairs by alluding to Röntgen's discovery*

It perhaps explains the surprising reaction of the Prince of Wales (later King Edward VII) when shown the radiograph of Campbell Swinton's hand by a peer who was a fellow member of his London club. The Prince remarked, 'How disgusting!'[7]

Alfred Dean recalled that his decision to start building x-ray apparatus in 1896 was made against his father's wishes, because the latter felt that the newspaper cartoons and music-hall jokes had made x-rays a subject of ridicule. Dean Senior was a respectable manufacturer of scientific equipment and glassware in London.[8]

After the journalists of the popular newspapers had had their success, the scientific and medical press considered the implications of the strange new phenomena and their value to medical practice. The first in the field were the craft publications such as the electrical and photographic journals. The broadsheet, *The Electrician*, secured a scoop by reporting the discovery under the title 'A Sensationally Worded Story' as early as 10 January. On the same day the *British Journal of Photography* described the 'Wonder Camera of the Würzburg Professor',[9] and thereafter the photographic journals made the subject of x-rays their own. In February *The Photogram*, another photographic journal published in London, issued a special supplement called 'The New Light and the New Photography', which in the space of a month went to five editions. The March number of *The Photographic Review* was filled with radiographic prints made by Dr. John Hall-Edwards of Birmingham, a keen amateur photographer who was destined to be a pioneer of British radiology.

The commercial photographers' enthusiasm for Röntgen's discovery was not wholly altruistic. A sudden new demand from doctors and patients for clinical radiographs presented an opportunity which they sought to grasp as a branch of their own work. Photographic journals were inundated with enquiries from their readers with the question, 'Is there money in it?' The *British Journal of Photography* replied in July 1896 with a long article entitled 'Röntgen Work for Profit'.[10] This article, which gave an interesting picture of the uncertainties surrounding the use of x-rays at that time, answered readers' questions by pointing out the high cost of installing and operating x-ray equipment, and concluding realistically that, unless the patient could find the fee for the photographs, then 'Röntgen's valuable discovery is as nought to them'.

Several private x-ray laboratories did open in London in 1896. Some of these were operated by commercial photographers who placed advertisements in photographic journals, such as W. E. Gray of 92 Queen's Road, Bayswater.[11] During this period, in the uncertain dawn before the medical profession assumed a monopoly over clinical radiography, other groups also laid their claims. The wellknown electrical engineer, Campbell Swinton, opened his laboratory in Victoria Street in March 1896. It was one of the first and probably the most successful, and Swinton is a distinguished pioneer of British radiology. The physicist, C. E. S. Phillips, another distinguished pioneer, tried a similar venture in South London, but it was an economic failure.

The senior British scientific and medical journals took a more measured view of the news from the Continent. The journal, *Nature*, on 16 January confined itself to a bare announcement of the discovery, then in the next issue on 23 January printed a verbatim translation of Röntgen's *Vorläufige Mitteilung* under the title 'On a New Kind of Rays', which was illustrated by two of his photographs.[12] The translation was sent by Professor Arthur Schuster of Manchester but it was said to have been made by his assistant, Arthur Stanton, whose name appeared in the footnote. Stanton (died 1898) was the son of a sculptor and grew up in Edinburgh in a circle where German and other foreign languages were spoken. He graduated with a B.Sc. degree from Edinburgh University in 1881 and soon after settled in Manchester as Schuster's assistant. Stanton had delicate health but was an expert glass blower and prepared the Crookes tubes required by Schuster for Röntgen photography, see Chapter 3.[13]

The Lancet was the first English-language medical journal in the world to comment on the news. On 11 January it printed an editorial, 'The Searchlight of Photography', which treated Röntgen's findings as a Dickensian joke.[14] A week later, after Campbell Swinton had x-rayed his own hand, it unbent a little and conceded that the application of the discovery, as 'an aid in medical and surgical practice, is a shade nearer probability'.[15] The editors visited Swinton for a demonstration in his laboratory, and thereafter they became enthusiastic. The diagnosis of skeletal abnormalities and the localisation of bullets would be greatly aided, they wrote.[16] The *British Medical Journal* made no reference to the news until 18 January and then published an article by Professor Schuster. By that time Schuster had studied the x-ray photographs which Röntgen had sent him and could affirm that a most important discovery had been made.[17] This was followed on 1 February by a long and enthusiastic leader, announcing the success of Parisian doctors in demonstrating a diseased femur and tuberculous dactylitis by means of x-rays.[18] Thereafter each week for almost a year the subject of x-rays was seldom out of the pages of either *The Lancet* or the *British Medical Journal*, as medical pioneers such as Dawson Turner, MacKenzie Davidson and Hall-Edwards began to report their own first experiences of the new diagnostic method.

On 8 February the *British Medical Journal* secured a scoop when it announced: 'We have commissioned Mr. Sydney Rowland to investigate the application of Roentgen's discovery to medicine and surgery and to study practically its applications'. Rowland pursued his new task with remarkable diligence, and between February and June he contributed 13 weekly reports, comprising descriptions of clinical x-ray experiments, new technical developments and public demonstrations.[19]

SYDNEY DOMVILLE ROWLAND, L.R.C.S., L.R.C.P. (1872–1917) was a 24-year-old undergraduate at St. Batholomew's Hospital in 1896 during his brief career as 'Special Commissioner on the Application of the New Photography to Medicine and Surgery'. He revealed his scientific curiosity while still a student at Downing College, Cambridge, when he served as an assistant demonstrator in physiology and President of the Natural History Society. He was Shuter Scholar at St. Bartholomew's Hospital, where much of his spare time as an undergraduate must have been taken up with x-rays. He played a crucial part as a medical publicist of the new method at an early stage when its protagonists in London were still seeking clinical credibility. He himself produced and demonstrated x-rays before the Medical Society of London early in the year[20] but he made a more important contribution in recording the experiences of other experimenters. Although soon to abandon radiology for another branch of medicine, Rowland ensured a place for himself in the early history of radiology.[21]

For rest of biography, see page 147.

Rowland's contributions to the *British Medical Journal* during this three-month period amounted to a journal of radiology in miniature; it was the ideal form of publicity for the young science. His own experiments and investigations – directed towards improving the reliability of the equipment and the quality of the radiographs – were fully described. The first report was accompanied by a radiographic print of a hand, made in the laboratory of Franz Exner in Vienna, but soon Rowland himself was successful in photographing human limbs and extremities. An illustration appeared on 29 February 1896, showing Rowland taking a radiograph of a patient's ankle (*see* 6). Thereafter he turned his attention to the thicker parts of the body, and a month later a radiograph of the trunk of a three-month-old infant was printed across two pages of the *Journal*; it had been exposed for 14 minutes! The picture was hailed as a scoop for both Rowland and the *Journal*, and the professor of anatomy at St. Thomas's Hospital offered his congratulations: clearly visible were the ossification centres of the vertebral column,

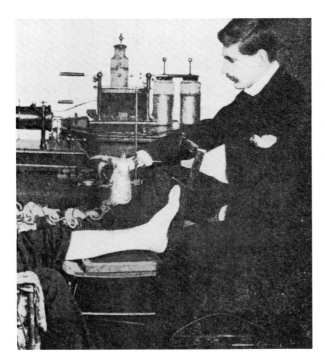

6. Sydney Rowland x-rays an ankle. This illustration appeared in the British Medical Journal *on 29 February 1896 above the caption: 'Photograph of a patient being skiographed (sic) together with the apparatus necessary. On the left is seen the induction coil and on the right the Leyden jars and Tesla transformer. The operator controls the key and passes the current at intervals of a quarter of a minute, so as to give the tube time to cool and to allow the glass to recover from the intense molecular strain'*

gas in the viscera and lungs, and the homogeneous densities of the heart and liver. So great was the interest and the demand for copies from doctors, that Rowland commissioned a commercial company to reprint the negative for sale.

The most dramatic news came on 7 March, when Newton and Company of Fleet Street marketed the first focus tube.[22] The point source of the cathode rays yielded shadows so much sharper that Röntgen's discovery was pushed a major step forward in clinical credibility. Newton and Company's design was copied from the tube of Professor Herbert Jackson, who is usually credited with discovery of the concave cathode. However, it is true that both Crookes and Rowland each independently conceived the idea – and probably also MacKenzie Davidson, who wrote from Aberdeen on 29 February, apropos the difficulty of getting sharp shadows, 'What is required is a tube that will give intense rays coming from a point'.[23]

The majority of the cases reported to Rowland by other experimenters were foreign bodies in the digits and fractures of the limbs. They are interesting, less for the clinical details than for the names of the contributors, who were the first British medical pioneers. Among the names are some of the most respected early radiologists, such as Dawson Turner, John Macintyre and John Hall-Edwards. The first step in each city appears to have been the same: a local doctor or surgeon with a suitable case, usually a needle lodged in the patient's finger or foot, would seek the help of a science professor in the local college or university, and together they would produce a radiograph. The following instances were reported in the *British Medical Journal*:

Sheffield. Professor Hicks, F.R.S. of Firth College after 1 February 1896 produced radiographs of two patients, a boy with a needle in a foot and a man with a needle in the palm of a hand. Both needles were successfully removed. He also photographed several remarkable dissections made by Dr. Christopher Addison, professor of

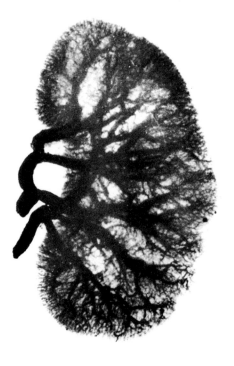

7. Autopsy injection of the blood vessels of a kidney – probably the first human angiogram ever performed. The specimen was prepared and injected by Professor Christopher Addison in Sheffield early in 1896

anatomy at the University College of Sheffield. These were prepared specimens of a human hand and kidney (*see* 7), in which Addison had injected the blood vessels – probably the first human angiograms ever performed.[24] Dr. Addison (1869–1951) later entered politics and served as the country's first Minister of Health under Lloyd George; as Viscount Addison K.G., he was leader of the House of Lords after the Second World War.

Birmingham. Drs. Hall-Edwards and Ratcliffe produced radiographs within a few days of Röntgen's discovery, but after February 1896 Professor Poynting and his colleagues of Mason's College also assisted local doctors, as described in Chapter 3.[25]

Bristol. Charles Morton, a surgeon to the Bristol General Hospital, persuaded Professor Wertheimer, the principal of the Merchant Venturers' Technical College to photograph the foot of a cadaver, in which he had inserted a needle.[26]

Dublin. Professor Barrett of the Royal College of Science on 16 March 1896 successfully demonstrated a needle which had been lodged in a patient's hand for over two years.[27]

Newcastle-upon-Tyne. Mr. G. E. Williamson, a surgeon at the Royal Infirmary, sought the services of Mr. Havelock and Professor Stroud of Newcastle-upon-Tyne College of Science in April 1896.[28]
The parts played by Lord Kelvin and his team in Glasgow, Professor Arthur Schuster in Manchester, and Professor Oliver Lodge in Liverpool are described in Chapter 3.

In this early period when x-rays held the curiosity of the public and before the medical profession had assumed control, many groups such as chemists, engineers and photographers hoped that the taking of x-rays would be their task. The photographers' journals of the period reflect the importance that they attached to Röntgen's discovery and their urge to know more of the 'New Shadow Photography'. This was the title of Campbell Swinton's lecture to the Royal Photographic Society on 11 February 1896, which was the first public demonstration of the art of radiography in England.[29] In the audience was a photographer, Fred Marsh, F.R.P.S., who had had a finger crushed in childhood, and Campbell Swinton was able to produce a picture which showed clearly the deformity of the affected bone.

Lecture-demonstrations thereafter became a popular feature throughout the country, attracting large audiences wishing to verify with their own eyes what they had read in the press. An active publicist who took to the road at this time, was H. Snowden Ward, F.R.P.S., a professional photographer and editor of the magazine *The Photogram* and who with A. W. Isenthal produced in 1898 one of the earliest textbooks, *Practical Radiography*. In the flyleaf of the book, Ward offered his services for 'a popular lecture with full demonstration, prepared in the Spring of 1896, delivered with great success before large audiences in London and many provincial towns'. On 24 March 1896 he was in Southport lecturing on 'The New Light'. He showed a radiograph of a hand of a child with a congenital accessory thumb, which he had made that afternoon with an exposure of less than 1 minute.[30,31] Within a few years the initial excitement about

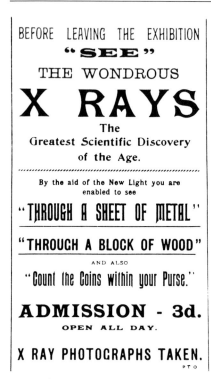

8. Right *Announcement of Snowden Ward's lecture-demonstration in Southport in March 1896*
9. Left *Broadsheet advertising a public demonstration of x-rays at the Crystal Palace Exhibition, 1896*

x-rays died down, and these public demonstrations gradually ceased. They were banished to parochial charitable bazaars where the x-ray fluoroscope became the star turn for people who wished to see the bones of their hand for a few pence.[32]

One lecture-demonstration that had particular medical significance was that of Stanley Kent on 13 February 1896 at St. Thomas's Hospital. The daily press announced this to be the first demonstration to take place in a London hospital.[33] A student's hand was examined using a 6-inch coil and 24-volt accumulators. It may be assumed that the potential diagnostic benefits shown by this demonstration hastened the medical acceptance of x-rays and the introduction of a clinical x-ray service in the Hospital in October of that year.

Eleven days later, it was Rowland's own turn. On 24 February he demonstrated x-rays to members of the Medical Society of London.[34] Starting with a simple electric spark, he was able to show how its nature altered by gradually increasing the vacuum within the tube. He also demonstrated Geissler and Crookes tubes, Tesla and Rühmkorff coils, and various sensitising plates, and explained the uses of the various pieces of apparatus to the audience. Finally, using a vacuum tube and a coil, he produced a radiograph of the bones of the hand in 20 seconds. This successful public demonstration by the 24-year-old undergraduate helped to convince his medical colleagues of the benefits of the x-ray method for their patients. Doubts were rapidly diminishing by this time, and they were finally dispelled by the brilliant lecture-demonstration given on 30 March at 20 Hanover Square by Professor Silvanus Thompson, see Chapter 8.[35]

Much discussion took place in the initial months about what to call the new photographic process. Confusion appears to have arisen because of the misconceptions regarding the nature and uses of the rays. Many early articles use the term 'photography' – strictly a misnomer since, unlike conventional photography, the x-ray picture is not made by reflected light.[36] In March 1896 the *British Medical Journal* printed a leader article 'Wanted a Name: New Photography'.[37] The words 'skiagraphy' and 'actinography' were regarded as vague, 'skiography' was suggested and later 'kathodegraphy', 'shadowgraphy' and several other terms. The question of a name remained unsettled in Britain for many years. Although Rowland's journal used the word 'skiagraphy' in its title, this was altered in 1897 to *Archives of the Roentgen Ray*, in deference to the universal urge at that time to couple Röntgen's name with the rays he discovered, and the formation in London of a Röntgen Society. The word 'radiology' did not appear in the title of the journal until the First World War, when it was introduced purposely to replace the word 'Röntgen'. The discoverer's name was a casualty of the strong anti-German feeling that swept Britain after 1915 and which resulted in all German names and titles being abandoned.

Chapter 3

THE FIRST EXPERIMENTERS

There were of course no x-ray departments at any of the hospitals. There were no experts. There was no literature. No one knew anything about radiographs of the normal, to say nothing of the abnormal. There were no special x-ray plates or films . . . It was only very slowly that knowledge began to accumulate, and yet looking back it seems to me now to be rather astonishing how much was done in those early days.

C. Thurstan Holland (1937)[45]

Of all the readers of the London newspapers, the man perhaps best equipped personally to test the reports from Vienna was a 32-year-old electrical engineer, Alan Campbell Swinton. He was a Scot who had taught himself about photography and electricity and since emigrating to London eight years before, established himself successfully as an installer of electric lights in private houses. He was more practically orientated than most scientists and academics, less interested in the physical properties and nature of the new rays and more likely through his knowledge of photography to be able to verify Röntgen's discovery.

That same day, on the evening of 7 January 1896, Campbell Swinton in his laboratory produced what was probably the first intentional radiograph made in England. He later admitted that the quality was poor, a 'dim shadow of a coin through a thin sheet of aluminium',[1] and this success prompted him to try again.

ALAN ARCHIBALD CAMPBELL SWINTON, F.R.S., M.I.E.E., M.I.C.E., M.I.Mech.E. (1863–1930) was the first of the gifted non-medical experimenters who played a part in the introduction of x-rays into medicine. It is almost certain that he took the first medical radiograph in the British Isles, and it is claimed that in doing so he was the first man in the world after Röntgen to photograph a part of the human body.[2]

Growing up on the family estate in Berwickshire, Campbell Swinton showed an early passion for scientific experimentation. At the age of twelve he mastered the principles of photography, building his own camera and preparing his own light-sensitive paper. His practical instinct also led him to study electricity, and this became his profession. As a schoolboy he built a telephone link that operated over several hundred yards, later when apprenticed to a ship-builder he installed electricity in warships. At the age of 20 he wrote a book called *Elementary Principles of Electric Wiring*. In 1887 he left the shipyard and went into business in London as an electrical contractor and consultant, and installed electric lighting in many large houses.[3]

His seminal contribution to introducing x-rays into medicine in 1896 and 1897 blossomed into a lifelong involvement with the science which Röntgen's discovery created. After 1904 he gave up electrical contracting and devoted more time to his experiments. For the next decade and beyond, his fertile mind devised improvements to x-ray tubes and apparatus aimed at increas-

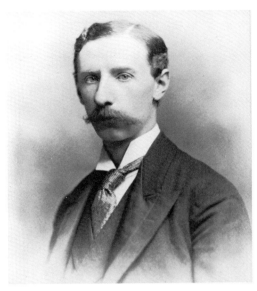

10. A. A. Campbell Swinton

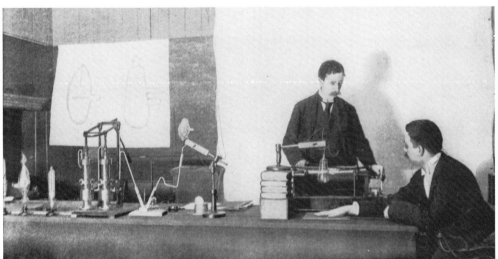

11. A photograph of Campbell Swinton taken during his lecture-demonstration of x-rays before the Royal Photographic Society on 11 February 1896. The man seated may have been Swinton's assistant, J. C. M. Stanton

ing their output, reliability and safety. He also served on several scientific committees, in 1911–12 he was President of the Röntgen Society. The honour which gave him the greatest pleasure, he claimed, was his election to a Fellowship of the Royal Society, a unique achievement for a self-taught man who boasted the fact that he had never passed or tried to pass an examination after the age of 17![4]

On 8 January, the day after the announcement in the *Evening Standard* and Campbell Swinton's first successful radiograph, he produced several more photographs of coins and other objects; these results were more satisfactory. Then on 13 January he did something which was shown by subsequent events to have been his most dramatic contribution, the act for which Campbell Swinton is chiefly remembered: he x-rayed his own

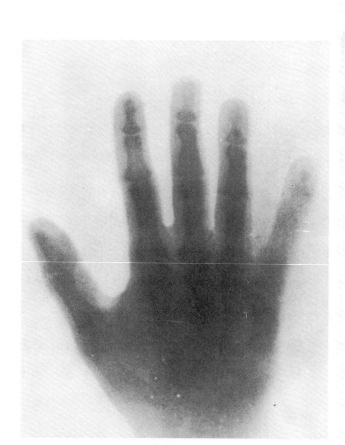 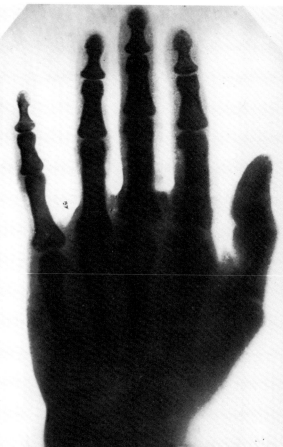

12. Campbell Swinton radiographs his own hand. Left *Radiograph made on 13 January 1896 – his first attempt, exposure time: 20 minutes.* Right *Radiograph made one week later, 18 January 1896 – exposure time: 4 minutes*

hand. The radiograph which he made is the one which is believed to be the first study of the human body in the United Kingdom. On 16 January he exhibited it at a meeting of the Camera Club (*see* 12), and was surprised at the astonishment with which it was received.[1] Next day *The Times* recorded the event.[5] *The Lancet* of that week modified its aloof attitude, no longer dismissing the news from Vienna as unimportant and reporting Campbell Swinton's experiments in full. In the week following, 23 January, the issue of *Nature* which carried Arthur Stanton's translation of Röntgen's paper also contained a letter from Campbell Swinton with an illustration of the 13 January radiograph of his hand.[6]

On 18 January after further attempts Campbell Swinton succeeded in obtaining a better radiograph of his hand, exposing it through a sheet of vulcanised fibre rather than aluminium. This measure enabled him to reduce the exposure time from 20 to four minutes at a focus-film distance of six inches. Five days later when *Nature* appeared, public interest was further aroused and the medical press became interested. The editors of *The Lancet*, after visiting Campbell Swinton to watch him produce radiographs in his laboratory, wrote an enthusiastic editorial.[7]

Campbell Swinton now found himself in demand by the medical profession. He responded by announcing in *The Lancet*[8] that 'I have had so many applications chiefly from medical men for prints of my photograph of the hand that I have arranged for the Swan Electrical Engraving Company to supply photographic prints and printing blocks of this and any other of my subjects to anyone requiring them.' He also opened an x-ray laboratory at 66 Victoria Street, London. At this address, which he described as 'the earliest laboratory in the country',[4] he offered a diagnostic service to doctors and later treated patients with x-rays. He received many visitors, the distinguished and the curious, including the Prime Minister, Lord Salisbury, whose hand he successfully radiographed. On 1 May 1896 the Prime Minister returned with Lady Salisbury, who also wanted a radiograph of her hand.

Apart from Campbell Swinton, at least one other Londoner was ready to exploit Röntgen's discovery when the news reached England – C. E. S. Phillips. He was similar in some ways to Campbell Swinton, being a well-off young man with an inventive turn of mind who had taught himself about science and electricity. In a well-equipped laboratory at Shooters Hill he had made his own vacuum tubes and studied high-tension discharges *in vacuo*. He was acquainted with the physics world and on speaking terms with eminent members of it such as Sir William Crookes and Lord Kelvin, who proposed him for membership of the Royal Institution in 1894. Like Crookes, Phillips almost certainly generated x-rays in his laboratory before the end of 1895.

MAJOR CHARLES EDMUND STANLEY PHILLIPS, O.B.E., F.R.S.Edin., F.Inst.P. (1871–1945) was an early experimenter with x-rays, who became one of the country's first hospital physicists and teachers of medical physics. He helped to create most of the national radiological bodies, and to establish the uniquely British bonds which still link doctors, physicists and manufacturers.

The son of Samuel Phillips, the founder of a well-known firm of electrical marine cable manufacturers, Charles Phillips was privately educated and was aged 24 in 1895. Although fortunate in not being obliged to earn a living, few men worked more purposefully or contributed more to the structure of British radiology.[9]

This contribution was made possible by the two paths along which his experimental work led him. The first was his association with the radiologist Robert Knox, who invited him to be honorary physicist of the Cancer Hospital Fulham. Here he worked until 1927, one of the earliest hospital physicists in the country. His efforts in 1906 to introduce a unit of radiation heralded a lifelong study of radiation control and protection. In 1915 he contributed a chapter, 'The Physics of Radium' to Knox's textbook, *Radiography, X-Ray Therapeutics and Radium Therapy*. The second task he owed to Major (later Sir) Archibald Reid who during the First World War arranged a course of training in practical x-ray work for army medical orderlies to overcome the shortage of radiographers.

Dr. Russell Reynolds gave the medical lectures and Phillips the physics at the Royal Herbert Hospital, Woolwich and at Imperial College. After the War Phillips retained his military association as a member of the War Office X-Ray Advisory Committee until this body was disbanded in 1939, receiving the O.B.E. for his services. He was also elected an Honorary Lecturer in Radiology in University College, London.

Phillips's position and prestige in the early years ensured that he was a founder of most radiological bodies, and a leader of some.[10]

Founder member of the Röntgen Society, President in 1909–10
Founder member of the British Institute of Radiology, President in 1930–1
Founder member, Institute of Physics

Founder member, Society of Radiographers
Honorary Secretary of the Royal Institution, 1929–45.

Cuthbert Andrews once described Phillips as 'the typical English gentleman of the French stage' – meaning that he was tall and distinguished in appearance and always courteous in his manners; and, rarest of attributes in a physicist, that he had a sense of humour.[11] Away from his laboratory he was an accomplished violinist, owning a Stradivarius, and an artist of some ability. He painted the portraits of Robert Knox and Sir Archibald Reid which hang in the house of the British Institute of Radiology.

A month after *The Electrician* published its 'Sensationally Worded Story' on 10 January 1896, Phillips produced his first radiograph, which he called a 'Rontograph'. He used a pear-shaped Lenard tube and gave an exposure of an hour, and recorded in his note-book: 'At first when I excited the tube it glowed with a blueish colour with flickering whiteish flames here and there. This gave no Ronto-effects with $\frac{1}{4}$ hour exposure. The tube then turned greenish after two days' pretty continuous excitation and Ronto-effects with one hour exposure. The tube became bathed in green flames internally licking the glass after another day or two and then the best effects were attained. The best condition lasted about a week and then the resistance of the tube began to increase . . .'[12,13] The Phillips collection of 'Rontographs' in the British Institute of Radiology includes x-ray plates of ordinary objects such as scissors and buttons but also human extremities, some of these with foreign bodies. One unusual radiograph, a hand, is annotated 'hand bitten by tiger'. On one occasion Phillips investigated the effect of x-rays on the growth of mustard seedlings, and failed to demonstrate any effect: apparently he expected the seedlings to bend over towards the x-ray source as they would react to a light source.

Encouraged by the success of Campbell Swinton's laboratory in Victoria Street, Phillips in 1897 tried to establish a consulting room in Woolwich. Although the response from the local doctors was favourable, none thought that it would pay and he abandoned the scheme. A more successful venture was his contribution to the early radiological literature. Within two years of Röntgen's discovery he compiled and published a 68-page book, *Bibliography of X-Ray Literature and Research: Being a Ready Reference Index to the Literature on the subject of Röntgen or X-Rays* (1897). The chapter in this book headed 'Practical Hints' reflects his own experience of generating x-rays at that early date, as well as his interest in solving problems connected with it.[14,15]

Another important reader of the *Evening Standard* on 7 January was a Brixton doctor who pointed out the report from Vienna to his son. The doctor was Dr. John Reynolds, F.R.G.S., a man interested in science and a friend of Sir William Crookes. His son Russell was 15 years old and counted electricity and photography among his hobbies. On reading the reports, son and father decided to build a high-tension induction coil and the other apparatus required to generate x-rays. This coil had a secondary coil wound in 52 sections, and a mercury dipper interrupter activated by an electric motor. The current was supplied by a primary battery of seven chromic acid cells, and the coil gave a 13-inch spark.[16] Reynolds and his father provided a detailed specification of the coil, including diagrams to the editor of the *English Mechanic*, who printed it in 1898.[17] The complete apparatus, which remains in working order and will still produce x-rays, is exhibited in the Science Museum, South Kensington.

RUSSELL J. REYNOLDS, C.B.E., M.R.C.S., M.B., B.S., F.R.C.P., F.F.R., D.M.R.E., M.I.E.E., Hon. F.A.C.R., Hon. F.S.R. (1880–1964) attended Westminster School and qualified in medicine at Guy's Hospital in 1907. After spending two years in general practice he decided to devote himself to radiology, and thus became one of the pioneers of diagnostic and therapeutic radiology in the United Kingdom.[18] In the First World War he served in the Army and spent two years in India as an 'electrical specialist'. On returning to London, he was appointed to the staff of Charing Cross Hospital and the National Hospital for Nervous Diseases, Queen Square. In these two teaching hospitals, he performed his life's work.

Reynolds in 1924 at Charing Cross began to study the possibility of obtaining human ciné films. Abandoning the 'direct' method used originally by John Macintyre in Glasgow, he set about solving the difficulties of the alternative 'indirect' method, in which the x-ray shadows on a fluorescent screen are photographed with a ciné camera. Gradually he overcame them and by 1934 he had built what has since been called 'the first practical cinéradiological unit ever devised'.[19,20]

This work was acclaimed internationally, especially in North America, and brought him many honours. Reynolds was not only a pioneer, but a leader of British radiology:

Secretary of Röntgen Society, elected to membership 1901 when a medical student
Examiner in Radiology, University of Cambridge, the Conjoint Board, and the Faculty of
  Radiologists
Medical Editor, *British Journal of Radiology*
President, British Institute of Radiology, 1937–8
President, Section of Radiology, The Royal Society of Medicine
Hunterian Professor, Royal College of Surgeons, 1936.

When over 75 Reynolds emerged from his retirement to recall the early years of his career, particularly the successful apparatus he had built in his youth.[21] His son, Seymour Reynolds, succeeded him as the radiologist at Charing Cross Hospital.

The schoolboy Russell Reynolds used his primitive coil to activate an early Watson x-ray tube mounted on a wooden retort stand and housed in a cardboard box, in order to repeat some of the experiments described by Röntgen in his paper.[22] Then he made a barium platino-cyanide screen and gave demonstrations for friends in the evening, showing such objects as coins in purses, feet in boots and the bones of his hand and wrist. After a while he noticed that the backs of his hands became red and sore and, attributing the cause to x-rays, tried to protect himself by coating the outside of the cardboard box with lead paint. On one occasion in 1896 Reynolds attended a meeting in London at which x-rays were demonstrated. He took a number of small strips of different metals, each distinctively shaped and stuck down on a photographic plate; the metals included aluminium, copper, nickel, silver and lead. Reynolds handed the plate to the lecturer who exposed it for three minutes at a distance of 12 inches from the source. When developed the plate showed that the lighter metals transmitted x-rays more readily than the heavier ones. This plate is kept in the Science Museum with his home-made x-ray apparatus.

A third pioneer is known to have begun his experiments on the same January evening of the day that Röntgen's discovery became known in London. He was Silvanus Thompson, a professor of physics with an interest in electricity, an academic counterpart of Campbell Swinton. He had an original and brilliant mind and, most important, was a respected figure in academic and electrical engineering circles in London. These qualities, together with the fact that he was already 45 years old, made him a more likely person to gain the ear of the medical profession than most of his scientific colleagues.

PROFESSOR SILVANUS PHILLIPS THOMPSON (1851–1916)
For biography, see page 167.

Within weeks Thompson in his laboratory at Finchley College confirmed the results of Röntgen's experiments and was, he recorded, 'casting shadows of bones and taking photographs'. To a friend he wrote,[23] 'All the world seems to have gone off on two crazes – bicycles and x-rays. With the latter I have myself been badly bitten'. Credit is due to Thompson for realising, even in those early days – perhaps ahead of all his scientific colleagues and the other early enthusiasts – the overriding medical application of Röntgen's discovery and its inevitable control by doctors.

On 30 March he addressed a large and enthusiastic medical audience at a meeting of the Clinical Society of London.[24] Thompson was said to have been the best lecturer of his day in London, and this meeting attracted eminent physicians and surgeons, several of whom wrote later to compliment him. From a medical viewpoint this meeting was a turning point in the process of clinical acceptance of the discovery. Thompson's lecture was the catalyst which also convinced practising doctors to take a lead and form a Röntgen Society, and it was natural that he should have been invited to be the first President, see Chapter 9.

As mentioned earlier, Röntgen is known to have sent copies of his *Preliminary Communication* with photographic prints of radiographs to at least two persons in the British Isles. One of these, Lord Kelvin, was the doyen of British physicists after occupying the chair of natural philosophy in Glasgow for nearly half a century. Röntgen's gesture was probably prompted by respect for the great man, but he may have been aware of the advanced electro-medical research being carried out in Glasgow under Kelvin's supervision. In the world of academic physics, Glasgow in 1896 was the most cultivated soil and the most fertile for Röntgen's seeds. Kelvin was the paternalistic genius, but he had two acolytes who had prepared the ground for a decade already when Röntgen announced his discovery – Lord Blythswood and Dr. John Macintyre. In 1886, soon after Macintyre had been appointed to the staff of the Glasgow Royal Infirmary, the three men were responsible for having the building wired for electricity, probably the first British hospital to be so equipped.[25] In 1887 an Electrical Room was erected and equipped through the munificence of the citizens of Glasgow; and Kelvin contributed batteries and coils, Blythswood a home-made Wimshurst machine and Otto Müller of Hamburg several Crookes tubes. In 1894 a complete electrical plant comprising a gas engine and dynamo was anonymously donated.

WILLIAM THOMPSON, BARON KELVIN OF LARGS, O.M., F.R.S. (1824–1907) was born William Thompson in Belfast, the son of the future professor of mathematics of Glasgow University. He matriculated at the age of ten, and was elected a Fellow of Peterhouse, Cambridge University at 21. He went to Glasgow before he was 30 as the professor of natural philosophy and held that post for 53 years until elected Chancellor of the University in 1904.[26]

Thompson's inventive mind touched all branches of physical science, but his main fields of interest were thermodynamics and electrical conductivity. He defined electrical standards for the British Association and acted as scientific adviser during the laying of submarine telegraphic cables to America and India. For the latter work he received a knighthood, and when Röntgen's letter reached him he had recently been ennobled. In 1896 he was the most distinguished citizen of Glasgow, ageing and ailing.

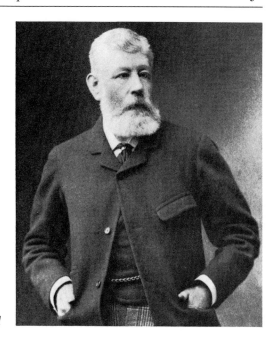

13. Lord Blythswood

SIR CAMPBELL CAMPBELL, BARON BLYTHSWOOD OF BLYTHSWOOD, F.R.S., LL.D. (1835–1908) was the epitome of the gifted Victorian amateur – wealthy enough to be disinterested, brilliant enough to be successful. According to a contributor in the *Dictionary of National Biography*, 'he obtained photographic action through various opaque substances before Röntgen announced his results in 1895, and came near to the discovery of x-rays . . .'.[27] Born in Italy of aristocratic Scottish parents Campbell made a career in the army and politics before settling on his estate in Renfrewshire. He served in the Crimea, being wounded at Sebastopol. After retiring from the army he sat in the House of Commons for a decade or more and was knighted for his services to Conservative Party organisation in Scotland; in 1892 he was created the first Baron Blythswood.

Campbell was a gifted amateur of science and a friend of Lord Kelvin, and he was a familiar and respected patron of the scientific *milieu* of Glasgow. He had a well-equipped laboratory at his country seat where he conducted many scientific experiments and manufactured precision instruments. One of these was a Wimshurst machine which generated 100 kilovolts.[28] Another was a device for exhausting Crookes tubes which enabled Macintyre to make experiments under different vacuum conditions.

Towards the end of his life Blythswood was honoured by election as President of the Röntgen Society. It was a Presidency *in absentia*, for he seldom left his estate and only rarely reached Council meetings in London.[29]

JOHN MACINTYRE, Hon. Ll.D., M.D., F.R.F.P.S.(Glasgow), F.R.S.Edin., M.I.E.E., J.P. (1857–1928) was one of the eight doctors who are recognised as the true medical pioneers of British radiology.[21] He was probably the most vigorous of the early experimenters, publishing seventeen papers in 1896 alone, and he was one of the first doctors in the world to be the head of a department of radiology.

Born in Glasgow to a tailor and his wife, he was early removed from school through ill-health, therefore he was largely self-educated. Before studying medicine, he was apprenticed to an electrical engineer and was involved in some form of electrical work within the Glasgow Royal Infirmary. He qualified M.B., C.M. at the age of 25 and then worked in London and abroad before returning to Glasgow to take up a position as 'Medical Electrician' to the Royal Infirmary in 1885. This post gave him the responsibility for equipping the Hospital with electrical current

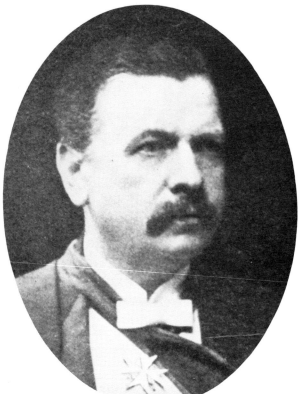

14. John Macintyre

'for medical and surgical purposes'. His innovative ability was then already evident, and in that year the *Glasgow Medical Journal* published his paper entitled 'Some Notes on the Use of Electrical Light in Medicine'.[30] In this paper, he described a variety of ingenious instruments with small electric bulbs powered by batteries, which he had devised for illuminating and examining body cavities. In 1885 also, he was appointed Assistant Surgeon, and seven years later Surgeon in Charge of the Nose and Throat Department. There he spent his entire medical career. In the decade before 1896, Macintyre made his mark as an otolaryngologist – he was President of the British Laryngological and Rhinological Association in 1893. This he combined with his work in the Electrical Pavilion of the Hospital. His activity and large output of papers testified to his thorough preparation and enthusiasm for Röntgen's discovery when it came.

For remainder of biography, see page 118.

Lord Kelvin acknowledged receipt of Röntgen's letter on 6 January. He was ill at the time and did not read it, looking only at the photographs before passing it to his son-in-law, Dr. J. T. Bottomley, of the University Physical Laboratory. Eleven days later on 17 January after Kelvin had studied the letter, he wrote to congratulate Röntgen: 'I need not tell you that when I read the paper I was very much astonished and delighted.' Bottomley meanwhile drafted a note to *Nature* which was published on 23 January.[31] It mentioned Röntgen's 'speculations' but omitted details of the experiments; fortunately his note shared the page with Professor Schuster's more explicit letter referred to below.

Bottomley also passed Röntgen's letter, on his father-in-law's instructions, to John

Macintyre for investigation. It may be assumed that Macintyre soon realised the potential value of x-rays in medical diagnosis and that he was able without delay to verify Röntgen's claims. The Electrical Room was probably better equipped for this purpose than Röntgen's own laboratory. John Scott, the distinguished Glasgow radiographer, once suggested that Macintyre, rather than Campbell Swinton may have produced the first human x-ray in the British Isles.[25]

In January 1896 Macintyre demonstrated 'The New Light – X-Rays' before a large gathering of doctors and scientists at the University of Glasgow. For the practical experiments he used apparatus consisting of batteries, induction coils of 6-inch spark upwards, Crookes tubes and Paget plates. On 5 February he combined with Lord Blythswood and Dr. Bottomley in a similar lecture-demonstration before the Glasgow Philosophical Society, and on 10 March he addressed a well-attended meeting of the Glasgow Medico-Chirurgical Society. These meetings heralded Macintyre's appointment as radiologist to the Royal Infirmary and the opening of an x-ray laboratory – one of the first hospital radiological departments in the world, see Chapter 7.

Macintyre's phenomenal originality and aggressive exploitation of Röntgen's discovery assure him a place as one of the world's pioneer radiologists. He himself in 1907 described his early experiments:[32] 'I began by taking photographs of the hands and feet and passing by degrees into the more difficult parts of the trunk. The latter was completed in March 1896. The picture of the larynx was the first attempt to photograph the soft tissues of the human larynx . . . By experimenting with x-ray tubes at different vacuums and different densities of the body I was convinced that x-rays would be useful to the physician as well as the surgeon by proving that not only could hard tissues of the body be demonstrated, but also soft tissues. The first photographs of the human heart was taken by me two months after Röntgen's discovery and showed the soft tissues within the thoracic cavity. In May 1896 pathological conditions of the heart were recorded.'

Macintyre published his results immediately and they were favourably received. Early in 1896 the *British Medical Journal* printed distinct radiographs which he had produced of a patient's wrist containing a needle.[33] Lord Lister, President of the British Association in that year, referred to Macintyre's successful x-ray identification of an oesophageal foreign body. Also for the first time, Macintyre soon thereafter demonstrated a kidney stone which was verified and removed surgically in the Infirmary. The first issue of *Archives of Clinical Skiagraphy* in April contained three contributions from Macintyre – a radiograph of a chest made with short exposure and one of a pelvis showing a diseased hip joint, and a contribution on cinéradiology.

Cinématography had become a reality in February 1896[34] and Macintyre immediately applied the discovery to his radiographical experiments, searching – he wrote[35] – 'for the best methods of obtaining a rapid exposure with a view to recording the movement of organs within the body'. First he laboriously photographed a succession of x-ray images seen on the fluorescent screen using the ordinary camera, but he soon abandoned this method as being too slow. He then covered the screen in a light-tight box and coupled a cinématograph camera to it, but only very slow movements could be recorded because of the lengthy exposure.

Macintyre then made an important discovery. He found that, by manipulating the mercury interrupter he could obtain instantaneous photographs of his fingers by a single flash of the tube, corresponding to one vibration of the contact breaker. Soon thereafter he produced the famous 40-foot film of the movement of a leg of a frog, which he demonstrated to the Glasgow Philosophical Society and in June 1897 to the Royal Society in London.[36] This was the first cinéradiological series ever made, utilising the technique which was to be perfected by Russell Reynolds in 1934. Copies of this film are still available and sometimes shown at meetings of radiologists.

Another technique to be pioneered by Macintyre was fluoroscopy. Soon after news of Salvioni's cryptoscope reached Britain (see Chapter 4), Macintyre built his own device, using a screen made of potassium platino-cyanide (*see* 15). A few months later, in April 1896, he made a screen of calcium tungstate, the substance chosen for this purpose by the American inventor, Thomas Edison.[37]

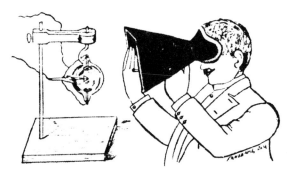

15. *Salvioni's cryptoscope (fluoroscope) in use. This drawing shows the operator testing the hardness of the x-ray tube by screening his own hand – a dangerous practice that was soon condemned. See 29, diagram*

This activity in Glasgow early in 1896 led to a direct correspondence between Macintyre and Röntgen, and in due course Röntgen gifted him one of his original x-ray tubes. This tube was passed to Dr. A. Bruce Maclean, one of Macintyre's successors as radiologist to the Glasgow Royal Infirmary.

Apart from Lord Kelvin, Röntgen sent a copy of his paper to Arthur Schuster, the German-born and educated professor of physics in Manchester. The arrival of this copy was recorded by Schuster's daughter Norah.[38] 'He was so immediately fascinated that he kept his pretty young wife, the cabby and the horse waiting outside in the chill winter evening (on the way from the railway station) while he read the pamphlet twice over in his laboratory. As he came out he excused himself by saying that he had had an extraordinary communication "from that man Röntgen who had been so rude in Pontresina".'

Schuster was sufficiently convinced to act immediately, and he did three things. First he informed his local scientific colleagues. On 7 January 1896 the Manchester Literary and Philosophical Society held an ordinary meeting and according to their records, 'Dr C. E. Lees, on behalf of Dr Schuster, showed photographs by Professor Röntgen of Würzburg by means of radiations of an apparently new kind.' Secondly, Schuster wrote to the *Manchester Guardian*. In his letter which was published on 8 January he gave a concise account of Röntgen's work and offered to show the photographs to anyone interested in the subject. This letter has been claimed to be the first radiological publication in Britain.[39] Schuster's third act was to persuade his assistant, Arthur Stanton to translate Röntgen's paper for *Nature*, and – as mentioned previously – his version appeared in the issue of 23 January.[40]

Experiments followed in the Physical Laboratory of Owen's College, which was already equipped with the apparatus for generating x-rays, because Schuster's interests included optics and the behaviour of electricity in gases. His first patient, examined during February, was a dancing girl from a local pantomime, and the radiograph showed a needle in her foot.[41] Another patient had a fracture-dislocation of the elbow. Schuster's medical collaborator was a fellow countryman of his, Leopold Larmuth, who practised in Manchester as an ear, nose and throat surgeon. On 2 March Schuster gave a lecture-demonstration in Owen's College, successfully x-raying the foot of his 6-year-old son, the exposure taking five minutes. In 1962 the son, 66 years later, could still recall the incident and remember the anxiety of keeping still for that length of time![38]

SIR ARTHUR SCHUSTER, F.R.S., Ph.D. (1851–1934) was born in Frankfurt-am-Main, German to the wife of a banker who emigrated with his family to Manchester in 1870. He had scientific inclinations and entered Owen's College in the following year to study physics and mathematics. He returned to Germany to obtain a Ph.D. at Heidelberg and then spent five years in the newly-created Cavendish Laboratories, Cambridge. He was appointed to the chair of applied mathematics in Manchester, and in 1888 became the Langworthy Professor of Physics in Owen's College – a post which he held for 18 years and voluntarily relinquished to the New Zealander, Ernest (later Lord) Rutherford.

Apart from being a first class scientist, Arthur Schuster excelled at administrative tasks; he was one of the first generation of scientific administrators in Britain. In 1903 he played an important part in ensuring that Owen's College, a constituent of the old Victoria University, became the University of Manchester. Later he left Manchester and immersed himself in the affairs of the Royal Society, of which he had been elected a Fellow in 1879. He served as secretary and Vice-President of the Society and was rewarded by a knighthood in 1920.[42]

A charming footnote: Schuster's daughter confirmed that her father kept the radiograph of the pantomime dancer's foot which he took in February 1896 on his desk for 38 years until the day he died[38] – perhaps an indication of what Schuster considered to be his greatest personal achievement.

After the initial excitement of verifying Röntgen's discovery and proving the practical uses of radiography in medical diagnosis, Schuster bowed out of the picture. He was unwilling to devote too much time to taking photographs and with his laboratory inundated with clinical requests each day, he was prevented from pursuing his own interests. As early as 18 March 1896 he suggested in a lecture to the Manchester Medical Society that, until a suitable place in the hospital could be provided, some rooms nearby should be fitted up for a technical assistant to deal with patients.

Disengagement proved more difficult, and his services were required in a medico-legal *cause célèbre* some months later. A woman, Elizabeth Ann Hartley of Nelson, Lancashire was shot in the head by her husband, Hargreaves Hartley, and she was dying. Schuster's assistants, C. E. Lees and Arthur Stanton, transported the x-ray equipment to Nelson and were able to demonstrate a bullet lodged in the base of her brain. For Stanton this early portable radiograph proved too much: so shattered was he by the experience, according to Schuster's daughter,[38] that he had a nervous breakdown from which he never recovered!

In Liverpool the initiative for introducing x-rays was taken early in 1896 by an up-and-coming orthopaedic surgeon, Robert Jones.[43] The news of Röntgen's discovery first reached him from a German lady in Liverpool, Mrs Wimpfheimer, who had received it in a letter from her relatives. Soon Jones had an occasion to use x-rays – a young boy presented to him who had been shot in the wrist. Jones was unable to detect the position of the pellet by clinical palpation; he guessed that it could best be localised by radiography. Enlisting the help of Oliver Lodge, the professor of physics at the local University College, a diagnostically adequate radiograph was produced on 7 February 1896, as a result of which the boy was successfully treated. Jones and Lodge reported the case in *The Lancet*.[44] The exposure time was 'rather more than two hours'!

SIR ROBERT JONES, Bt., K.B.E., F.R.C.S. (1857–1933) was one of the giants of orthopaedic surgery. In establishing Liverpool as the British home of this branch of surgery, he pioneered in several related directions, and one of them was radiology.

Jones was born in Rhyl to the Welsh wife of a London journalist. An uncle by marriage was Hugh Owen Thomas, the Liverpool bone-setter who was a man of genius and the father of British orthopaedics. When Jones was 13, Thomas offered him a home provided that he read medicine. Jones accepted and he left his parents in 1873 to commence a gruelling part-time apprenticeship as well as attendance on the medical course. Within ten years of qualifying he was established in Liverpool as a surgeon. In 1889 he became the honorary surgeon and dean of the clinical school at the Royal Southern Hospital. The crucial decision of his career came two years later when Thomas died; Robert Jones decided to confine his surgical practice to orthopaedic work and in doing so established orthopaedic surgery as a specialty in the British Isles.

He became a leader of the medical profession and received many honours in later years – a knighthood for War service, a score of honorary degrees and a baronetcy in 1926.[45]

SIR OLIVER LODGE, D.Sc., F.R.S. (1851–1940) served as the professor of physics at Liverpool for nearly 20 years, and first Principal of the University of Birmingham for a similar period. This eminent physicist played a major part in introducing x-rays to Liverpool and Britain.[46]

Born in Staffordshire of a talented family of schoolmasters and clergymen, Oliver Lodge fell early under the spell of science and electro-magnetism, graduating at University College, London in 1877. His most important work was accomplished in Liverpool where, in addition to being a pioneer experimenter, he served radiology in two other respects. He is believed to have been the first physicist to give systematic lectures to medical men on the subject of medical physics. These he repeated in Birmingham at the request of the Dean of the Medical Faculty, and they were published in the *Archives of the Roentgen Ray* in 1904 and 1905.[47]

He served in 1923–4 as President of the Röntgen Society, of which he had been an early supporter and was elected one of its first Honorary Members.[48]

At Robert Jones's instigation and upon his active insistence a doctor was appointed in 1896 as honorary radiologist to the Royal Southern Hospital. He was Charles Thurstan Holland, a 33-year-old general practitioner who for some years had assisted Jones at his free Sunday clinic.

CHARLES THURSTAN HOLLAND, Hon. Ll.D. (Liverpool), Hon. Ch.M., Hon. F.R.C.S., M.R.C.S., L.R.C.P., F.F.R., Hon. F.A.C.R. (1863–1941). A true pioneer and one of the architects of British radiology, Thurstan Holland built up his department until it was regarded as the most advanced in the country between the Wars. After the death of Sir James MacKenzie Davidson he was the leader of British radiology, and in 1925 he was elected President of the first world meeting of radiologists. When he died, it was said that he had done more than any other man to further radiology and to establish it as a department of medicine that could take its place on an equal footing with other special branches.[49]

Born in Bridgwater, Somerset and educated in Bristol and at University College Hospital,

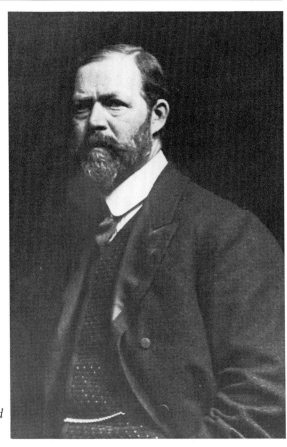

16. Charles Thurstan Holland aged about 40 years

London, Thurstan Holland entered general practice in Liverpool at the end of 1889. Six years later he was persuaded by Robert Jones, the British pathfinder in the field of orthopaedic surgery, to take up and develop radiology as a specialty, which both foresaw would play an important part in surgical and medical diagnosis.

Armed with a small induction coil and a primitive x-ray tube he embarked upon a career which was to lead him to the highest honours. His appointment as honorary radiologist at the Royal Southern Hospital in 1896 was the beginning. The first radiograph for clinical purposes was made on 29 May – a hand showing a fracture deformity of the fifth metacarpal bone. Thereafter and before the end of the year 261 examinations were made, which Holland described in the valedictory paper of his career 40 years later, written shortly before his death, see Chapter 7.[43]

For rest of biography, see page 124.

In Birmingham on the day after the press announcement of Röntgen's discovery, one of the city's general practitioners met Dr. J. R. Ratcliffe in Baynton's photographic shop. He was Dr. J. F. Hall-Edwards, and he and Ratcliffe shared ordinary photography as a hobby. Nearly 50 years later Dr. Ratcliffe recalled this meeting and the subsequent events:[50] 'I asked (Hall-Edwards) what he thought of the discovery and the claim that the rays would penetrate opaque substances. He said there might be something in it and suggested we give it a trial. He had a friend who had made the largest induction coil in the Midlands and he knew he could borrow it and would do so if he got a

Crookes tube. It so happened that Philip Harris had one small tube, sausage-shaped with two straight electrodes. This we got and after evening surgery at his house we coupled up and put a leather purse on a plate. As the break in the coil was the rather close spring one, the exposure was prolonged, but when the plate was developed it showed the contents, some coins and a key plainly. Then I suggested we photograph my hand, which was done, to see if the bones would show – they did, but the definition was not very sharp due to the electrodes, but fairly good considering. Thus my hand was the first to be radiographed in Birmingham. On seeing the result, it occurred to me that it might be of service in detecting foreign bodies such as needles, and to test this I pushed a sterilised needle under the skin of my hand, and on developing the plate it showed well enough.'

Hall-Edwards x-rayed Ratcliffe's hand on the evening of 12 February 1896. He signed the bromide print in the bottom corner, as professional photographers are wont to do, and it was published in the February 1896 issue of a local magazine, *The Moseley Society Journal*.[51] The needle is clearly visible in Ratcliffe's thumb muscles. The radiograph and a portrait of Dr. Hall-Edwards illustrated a biographical article which read: 'There is little necessity to introduce readers to the subject of this month's sketch. His name in the past few weeks has become almost a household word. Moseley had been honoured by having in it a gentleman whose enthusiasm and scientific skill has brought "our village" to prominence throughout the whole of the country.'

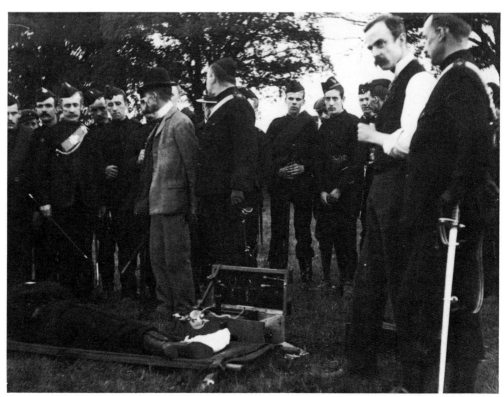

17. Dr. John Hall-Edwards (second right) giving a public demonstration of x-rays on Hodge Hill Common, Birmingham early in 1896

JOHN FRANCIS HALL-EDWARDS, F.R.S.Edin., L.R.C.P.Edin., D.M.R.E. Cantab., Hon. F.R.P.S. (1858–1926), a Birmingham general practitioner, was one of the first British doctors to apply Röntgen's discovery to clinical diagnosis and to be appointed 'Surgeon Radiographer' to a hospital. He lost a hand and a forearm and several fingers of his other hand through radiation injuries, and his is one of the 14 original British names recorded on the Martyrs' Memorial in Hamburg.

Hall-Edwards was born in Moseley, a suburb of Birmingham, and he studied medicine at Mason's College (now the University of Birmingham) and successfully took the Edinburgh diploma at the age of 27. He was the fifth eldest son of his family to qualify in medicine; his great-grandfather practised in Birmingham at the time of the Corn Law Riots. After qualifying he immediately settled in Moseley but, according to his surgeon, Sir Gilbert Barling, his heart was never really in general practice.

Hall-Edwards in his undergraduate days discovered that the scientific side of medicine interested him most; as a student he is said to have been the best mounter of histological material in the Midlands. This interest he early combined with photography and micro-photography, which became his lifelong hobby, and soon he was well known in the local photographic societies. His ability was recognised by his receiving more than 25 gold medals for his photographs which were shown at exhibitions around the world and reproduced in artistic journals. He was a versatile lecturer and by 1890 he was known in Birmingham as the expert on 'the medical side of photography'. In 1895 he was elected an honorary Fellow of the Royal Photographic Society – a singular honour and a culminating one, because thereafter he threw all his energies into developing the 'New Photography' heralded by Röntgen's discovery.[52]

For rest of biography, see pages 114 and 215.

'We telephoned the General and Queen's Hospitals and asked them to send any case suitable, and the next night a woman came from the Queen's Hospital with a needle in her hand. This we photographed successfully and made a bromide print which we told her to take to the hospital in the morning. This she gave to the Casualty Surgeon, who was Mr. J. Hazelwood Clayton, and from the information it gave him he removed the needle. This was the first operation in the world done by x-rays ...'[50]

Clayton recorded details of this woman patient, Mrs Batry, in his note-books, which after his death were presented to the library of the Birmingham Medical School with other papers. Mrs Batry told him that some days before she had been busy sewing when she had accidentally run a needle into her hand. Clayton, on examining her at Queen's Hospital found the hand painful but could not find the position of the needle. However, Hall-Edwards' and Ratcliffe's 'shadowgraph' showed the needle clearly and enabled Clayton to remove it. The case of Mrs Batry was reported in the national and local press on 15 February, and Clayton described the details in a letter to the *British Medical Journal*.[53]

On 4 March 1896 Hall-Edwards addressed a meeting of the Midlands Medical Society on 'The New Shadow Photography'. He described the apparatus which he and Ratcliffe had used and discussed the clinical applications.[54] However, when he gave technical details of his work he chose to publish them in *The Photographic Review*,[55] a journal read by professional and amateur photographers, thus emphasising the initially uncertain status of x-rays in scientific circles. The overriding clinical application of Röntgen's discovery had yet to be established – thanks largely to the work of pioneers such as Hall-Edwards himself.

Hall-Edwards soon photographed patients with fractures of the limb bones, and before long he was invited to speak before the Birmingham Medical Institute. The audience was interested but critical, and one surgeon, Bennett-May, openly expressed his doubts. Always, he said, he should trust his fingers to detect a fracture rather than depend on radiographs. There was still no apparatus at the General Hospital or the Queen's Hospital, and Professor Poynting and his staff at Mason's College helped Hall-Edwards to meet the demand for x-rays from general practitioners. On 25 February they photographed the hand of a 16-year-old, a patient of Mr. Marsh, a surgeon at Queen's Hospital. It showed a needle, which Marsh successfully removed.[56]

In 1899 Hall-Edwards was invited to join the staff of the General and Royal Orthopaedic Hospitals as Surgeon Radiographer, as well as the Birmingham and Midland Eye Hospital and the Birmingham Dental Hospital. He installed an x-ray outfit in the General Hospital, which by that time had a tube with a platinum target and a Wehnelt interrupter, devices which shortened exposure times. When the South African War broke out later in 1899, Hall-Edwards volunteered his services because his experience with x-ray apparatus was almost unique. He went to South Africa in the following year, and spent 14 months making radiographs on the *veld*, see Chapter 10. Dr. Ratcliffe being, in his own words,[50] 'the only one who understood the set (at the General Hospital)', was appointed *locum tenens* and he carried on until Hall-Edwards returned.

Two other doctors in Scotland apart from John Macintyre are known to have produced radiographs in 1896. In Edinburgh the pioneer was Dawson Turner. On 5 February he demonstrated x-rays to members of the Medico-Chirurgical Society of Edinburgh and exhibited photographs of coins, a purse, and human extremities including a wrist.[57] Later in the year he injected the blood vessels of cadaveric specimens of human kidney and heart and made radiographs, which David Walsh reproduced in his textbook – one of the first anatomical applications of the new science.

DAWSON   FYERS   DUCKWORTH   TURNER, M.D., F.R.C.P.(Edinburgh), F.R.S.(Edinburgh) (1857–1928) was born in Liverpool to the wife of the Reverend Turner, headmaster of the Royal Institution School, he was educated at Shrewsbury School and went up to Oxford in 1877 as a non-collegiate student. He graduated in arts from Dalhousie University, Canada, and then M.B., C.M. with honours from Edinburgh, proceeding to M.D. in 1890.[58]

After postgraduate study in Vienna and Paris, Dawson Turner returned to Edinburgh as the lecturer in biological physics at Surgeon's Hall, and early recognised the importance of x-rays in medicine. He was appointed 'Assistant Medical Electrician' to the Edinburgh Royal Infirmary in November 1896, and remained associated with the x-ray service of the Hospital until he retired in 1925. He was a strong advocate and a pioneer in Britain of radium as a method of treatment. It is said that he started this work in Edinburgh by purchasing a small amount of the substance himself, and then placing it at the disposal of the Infirmary. When the new x-ray department was opened in 1926, a plaque was erected in the entrance to his memory, reading – 'Pioneer and Founder of Roentgen Ray and Radium Work in the Royal Infirmary, Edinburgh, 1895–1925'.[59]

For rest of biography, see page 125.

The other Scottish pioneer who merits a mention is the surgeon who verified the benefit of the great discovery personally by visiting Röntgen in Würzburg in June 1896.[60] This was the Aberdeen ophthalmic surgeon, James MacKenzie Davidson, whose interest in x-rays may have been stimulated by the Glasgow experimenters and whose visit to Germany may have been prompted by Macintyre's correspondence with Röntgen.

SIR JAMES MACKENZIE DAVIDSON, M.B., C.M.(Aberdeen) (1857–1919) was the first leader of the radiological profession and the first man to receive a knighthood for services to radiology.

Before he abandoned his ophthalmic practice for a career in radiology in London, he introduced radiography in Aberdeen.

Born in Buenos Aires of Scottish parents who later returned home for their son's education, MacKenzie Davidson graduated in medicine from Aberdeen University in 1882. His interest in physics stimulated him to study ophthalmology, and in 1886 he was elected the Honorary Ophthalmic Surgeon to the Aberdeen Royal Infirmary. He remained there for 10 years, until Röntgen's discovery convinced him that his future lay in the new science of radiology.[61]

For rest of biography, see pages 98 and 181.

MacKenzie Davidson's scientific curiosity manifested itself in Aberdeen where he combined radiography with his ophthalmic surgical practice. Using his own Crookes tube and an induction coil with a 10-inch spark,[62] he succeeded as early as February 1896 in making a radiograph of a broken needle in the foot of a patient.[63] He also x-rayed a fractured femoral neck and the foot of a girl with six toes. Illustrations of these cases were printed in the first number of the pioneer journal, *Archives of Clinical Skiagraphy*, which appeared a few months later. The science of x-rays was to prove the medium in which his inventive genius would flourish in London.[64]

No account of the early experimenters would be complete without referring to the numerous enthusiastic amateurs unattached to large hospitals who built their own apparatus and took x-rays. Often the beginning was no more than a sophisticated variation of the schoolboy steam engine or crystal set built at home. Primitive apparatus which generated x-rays could be constructed without much difficulty, even in the depths of the country, from spare parts which were readily available; only a scientific curiosity and aptitude were required. At first only enthusiasts built sets, but soon many doctors acquired apparatus to use in their practices.

This step was easier and the financial outlay was far less in those early days, compared with our own time. According to Dr. David Walsh who in 1897 published one of the world's first x-ray textbooks, *The Röntgen Ray in Medical Work*, 'with a good Röntgen apparatus and a trained mechanic somewhere within reach in case of breakdown, any medical man may teach himself to use the fluorescent screen and to expose the scientific plate'.

Notable members of this rural army of x-ray pioneers were:

LIEUTENANT-COLONEL JAMES WILLIAM GIFFORD (1856–1930), who gave one of the earliest public demonstrations of x-rays in London to the Royal Photographic Society at 12 Hanover Square on 21 January 1896. Gifford, a well-to-do lace maker of Chard, Somerset, had his laboratory in his home, where he and his wife produced 'electrographs', and where the reporter of *The Windsor Magazine* photographed him early in February 1896, surrounded by gas tubes, coils and other simple apparatus for generating x-rays. A cat's paw, a fish and a human extremity x-rayed by Gifford illustrated an article entitled 'Marvels of the New Light', written by Snowden Ward in the April issue.[65]

Gifford remained an experimenter, writing articles on x-rays for *Nature* and contributing to discussions on apparatus at meetings of the Röntgen Society, of which he was elected a member in 1897. In 1910 he presented his personal hoard of radium – 40 mg, then worth about £600 – to the Cancer Research Laboratories of the Middlesex Hospital.

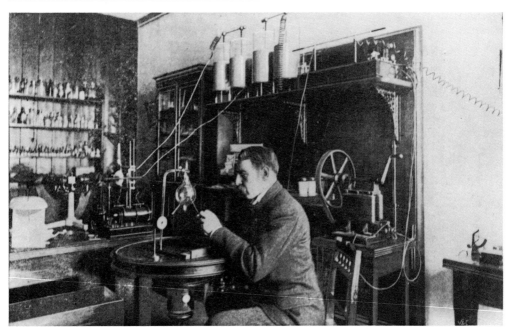

18. Colonel Gifford experimenting with a vacuum tube in his workshop at Chard, Somerset early in February 1896

DR. CHARLES SAVORY, surgeon at Haverfordwest in west Wales, who in March 1896 reported using x-rays to locate a needle in a patient's hand.[66]

DR. STANLEY GREEN, M.B., B.S., of Lincoln, a country doctor who during the first decade remained at the forefront of applying radiography to the diagnosis of chest diseases. By 1906 he had published more than ten papers. One of these, entitled 'The Position of the Radiographer in the Early Diagnosis of Pulmonary Tuberculosis', was one of the first radiological articles to contain references.[67] A quarter of a century later, Dr. Green was still in active practice in Lincoln.

PROFESSOR GEORGE WILLIAM WATSON, M.D., F.R.C.P. (1877–1956), who between 1919 and 1938 was Consultant Physician to the Leeds General Infirmary and St. James's Hospital and Professor of Medicine in the University of Leeds, was a 19-year-old youth at Keighley Grammar School in 1896. On 5 November of that year, *Nature* printed the following report:[68] 'We have pleasure in noting that 'a Yorkshire lad' G. W. Watson of Keighley obtained some wonderfully good Röntgen photographs by using an old home-made Wimshurst machine to illuminate a Crookes tube. The machine gave a spark about 1¾ inches in length and was without condensers. With this equipment, good radiographs of the bones of the hand were obtained in twenty minutes. One of these pictures, and also a radiograph of an abnormally developed elbow, have been submitted to us. . . .'

THE REVEREND FREDERICK WALTER, a Congregational minister in Norfolk and a friend of Harry W. Cox, the pioneer equipment maker, took his first x-ray photograph of a lesion in 1896 using an Apps 3-inch coil and a Dean tube – exposure time: 30 minutes. Ten years later, Mr. Walter x-rayed the same lesion using a Cox 10-inch coil and a Record tube

– exposure time: 5 *seconds*!.[69] At the time of Mr. Walter's death in 1955 aged 90 years – he was then the oldest member of the British Institute of Radiology, having joined the Röntgen Society in 1902 – his son remembered as a small boy in 1896 being bribed to lie still on a couch for half-an-hour, while his father took an x-ray photograph of his arm with a Crookes tube.[70]

Russell Reynolds towards the end of his long life named eight doctors and six scientists whom he considered to be the true pioneers of British radiology.[21] The doctors were MacKenzie Davidson, Robert Jones, Hall-Edwards, John Macintyre, Thurstan Holland, Sydney Rowland, W. S. Hedley, and George Batten. To this list should be added the name of Reynolds himself. The scientists were Lodge, Silvanus Thompson, Crookes, Campbell Swinton, Jackson, and Ernest Payne. The dominating role of the scientists as early x-ray experimenters is reflected in the number of scientific papers published by British workers during 1896. Of over 1,000 titles collected by Glasser from the world literature more than one hundred came from the British Isles:[60] Campbell Swinton – 20; Lodge – 20; Macintyre – 17; Rowland – 16; J. J. Thomson – 10; Lord Kelvin – 7; Silvanus Thompson – 7; MacKenzie Davidson – 5; Gifford – 4; Schuster – 3; Phillips – 2; and Hall-Edwards – 2.

Most of the doctors mentioned in this chapter went on to create hospital departments of radiology. Some of the non-medical pioneers became hospital physicists. We shall meet them in the next chapters.

Chapter 4

EARLY APPARATUS AND THE MAKERS

'An x-ray tube is a glass bulb surrounded by profanity'

Cuthbert Andrews[1]

'I really must take exception to the statement by Mr. W. E. Schall, that "before 1914 the x-ray industry in this country hardly existed" '

R. S. Wright (1928)[2]

The remarkable fact about the discovery that Röntgen made in November 1895 was this, that no new apparatus had to be invented before he could carry out his experiments. He used the standard equipment to be found in any physics laboratory round the world; indeed, Röntgen was simply repeating tests that had been performed on countless occasions for nearly 20 years by physicists and amateur scientists. He succeeded, where others such as Crookes, Jackson and Lenard had failed, because he recognised that the part of the glass tube which phosphoresced was emitting a penetrating new radiation that was fundamentally different from the cathode stream.

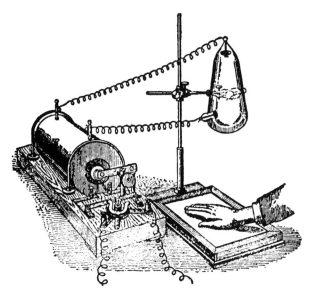

19. The experimental apparatus used by Professor Röntgen in 1895. A simple mechanical interrupter is mounted on the same block as the induction coil, connected by electrical cables to the battery (not shown)

PROFESSOR RÖNTGEN'S APPARATUS

Visitors to Würzburg in 1896 were shown the apparatus used for the Great Discovery by Professor Röntgen himself. It consisted of an ordinary Rühmkorff coil with a 4–6-inch spark gap charged by a current of 20 amperes; a mercury interrupter; wet (rechargeable) batteries; and a Hittorf vacuum tube, which was clamped in a wooden vice (*see* 19). Thin copper wires linked the batteries, coil and tube. Almost everything fitted on the same table.[3]

From this bench beginning – the bare essentials for the laboratory experiment – grew all the sophisticated x-ray apparatus of modern times.

HIGH-TENSION GENERATORS AND TRANSFORMERS

In 1896 a young engineer called Hermann Lemp, who was an employee of the General Electric Company in America, was given the task of finding a suitable exciting source for x-rays. In reviewing the state of the art in that year, he concluded that it offered the following options:[4]

1. *Induction coil* (Rühmkorff) with mechanical interrupter. This device, the apparatus used by Röntgen, gave unidirectional current but of a frequency on the low side for fluoroscopic work.
2. *Influence machine* (Holtz, Wimshurst). This device gave a steady unidirectional current of high frequency and potentials as great as 100,000 volts, but of low output. It was easily disabled by adverse weather and its great bulk rendered it impractical as a usual source for x-rays.
3. *X-ray high-tension transformer* (prototype built by Thomson and Lemp in 1896, the first commercial transformer patented by Snook in 1907). In order to convert the alternating current discharges of this apparatus, Lemp built a mechanical synchronous rectifier which yielded high-frequency unidirectional currents of such power that they rapidly damaged the gas tubes, by either melting the target or exhausting the vacuum.
4. *Dynamo with condensers*. This device gave unidirectional currents of high frequency but, like the influence machine, it had to be very bulky to be of practical use.

In Britain nearly all the early experimenters used the induction coil to generate their x-rays. The most notable exceptions were Lord Blythswood who built a Wimshurst machine on his estate in Renfrewshire which could produce 100,000 volts, and Dr. Lewis Jones who installed an American version, the Holtz influence machine, in the Electrical Department of St. Bartholomew's Hospital. James Wimshurst, F.R.S. (1831–1902), the inventor, who was an early recruit to the Röntgen Society, demonstrated this device to his fellow members at a meeting held in the Hospital on 7 June 1900 and compared it with his own machine.[5]

Induction coils of the Rühmkorff type were activated by the passage of an electrical current through the primary coil, which excited a current of high potential and high frequency in the secondary part. A coil with an interrupter produced a peak-shaped high-tension current, its positive phase being much higher than the negative; this implied theoretically – but not in practice – that rectification was not necessary. The tension delivered to the tube was measured in a primitive way by means of a variable spark gap mounted above the induction coil. With the primary current closed, the copper connecting wires produced the crackling noise associated with discharge phenomena; sparks could be seen in the dark. This 'corona effect' ionised the surrounding air, and electrically-charged dust particles were precipitated on the walls. The distinctive smell of ozone and dirty walls were hallmarks of the early departments. Excitation of the secondary coil depended on the frequency of interruption of the current – the 'make and break' of the primary, which was effected by rapidly vibrating the break or circuit interrupter, a noisy device with a notoriety of its own. The forerunner of several varieties was the platinum hammer break invented in 1898 and ousted only when coils became larger: a more efficient device was required for coils with spark gaps over 8 inches. One of the first and most successful of these consisted of a motor-driven piston alternating in and out of a pot of mercury. It was built by Harry W. Cox Limited to the design of Dr. MacKenzie Davidson and marketed in 1898 for £6 16s 6d; the advertisement claimed that it was 'easy to take to pieces and clean; light; will run hanging from a hook in the wall'.[6] A modification made by competitors in 1910 was claimed to deliver 10,000 interruptions a minute.[7]

Improvements to the mercury break included a rotary arm and a pneumatic buffer. It was noisy and smelly to use, and was gradually replaced by the Wehnelt break, an American machine operating on the electrolytic principle, which was less unpleasant.[8] Advertisers claimed that the Wehnelt with a molten state anode was the only reliable break, 'as it has caused a revolution in the construction of the x-ray tube and induction coil'.[9] Soon another variation stole the radiologists' fancy, the Wappler interrupter, because it gave the heaviest discharge of all.[10]

Four British-made induction coils were displayed for sale at the *conversazione* of the Röntgen Society in November 1898.[11] Harry W. Cox and Alfred Apps, who was the pioneer designer of Newton and Company, both demonstrated 18-inch heavy linkage coils. Their competitors, A. E. Dean and Company and Watson and Sons, also offered a range of coils, which were all bettered during the next ten years.[12] Progress towards greater output and shorter exposures was achieved by larger induction coils, faster interrupters and a condenser placed across the terminals of the primary circuit. Within ten years electrical insulating wire had improved sufficiently for very large coils to be constructed with spark gaps of 20 inches. Newton and Company in 1908 marketed a coil for instantaneous radiography, called the Instantia, which reduced exposures for chest radiographs to a few seconds. A four-fold increase in output was achieved by doubling the number of turns in the coil.[13] By 1907 the induction coil with interrupter had been perfected as a generator for x-rays from a vacuum tube to the point where further progress seemed to be unlikely.

In that year an American engineer, Homer Snook, perfected a new device which heralded the end of bench-top radiography. Snook set himself the task in 1903, when a graduate student in physics at the University of Pennsylvania, of finding ways of improving the discharge from an induction coil. He made an oscillographic study of the spark and was impressed by the amount of inverse discharge that he found. He then developed a synchronous series spark gap and built a synchronous reversing high-tension switch for the secondary circuit of the coil, in order to put both the direct and the inverse discharges through the tube. He obtained his discharges from a coil with a mercury interrupter, and further oscillographic studies revealed much time waste between the waves as well as poor wave form. Thereupon he built a motor-driven, close-core transformer for alternating current to which a high-tension rotary switch was linked in the secondary circuit (*see* 20). Snook, by applying Lemp's idea of synchronising the activities of the primary and secondary circuits of the coil mechanically, solved the problem of achieving more output for x-ray work. Even the earliest Snook models delivered 100 kilovolts at over 100 milliamperes – an output which was greater than the existing gas tubes could stand, as will be described later.

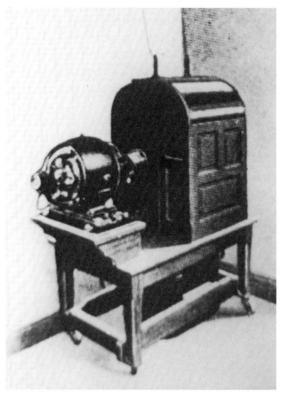

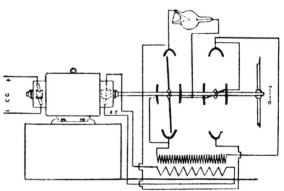

20. Snook's rectifier. Left *The first model ever built, which was installed in the Jefferson Hospital, Philadelphia in 1907 and continued operating until 1946.* Above *Wiring circuit*

Snook's mechanical rectifier earned the name of the 'interrupterless transformer' from American radiologists who, it is said,[14] were relieved at being rescued from the inequities of that noisy, smelly and unreliable instrument, the interrupter. The first Snook unit was installed in the Jefferson Hospital, Philadelphia in 1907 (it was still working in 1946). In 1908 Snook exhibited his invention in Europe, at the First International Congress of Electrology and Radiology in Amsterdam.[15] In the following year Newton and Company became the sole British agents. By July 1909 Russell Wright had built a British version which he demonstrated to fellow members of the Röntgen Society.[16] Some months later in Belfast at the annual meeting of the British Medical Association, Siemens Brothers unveiled a rotary high-tension rectifier – their company's version of the Snook apparatus.[17]

Advertisements of the Snook Manufacturing Company in 1907 claimed, 'The day of the induction coil is passing'. This line proved to be prophetic, because Snook's ingenious invention was one of the three developments that heralded the so-called Golden Age of Radiology. (The other two inventions were also American-inspired – Coolidge's hot-cathode tube and the Potter–Bucky intensifying grid). The enhanced tube output had one immediate benefit, namely instantaneous radiography, because exposure times were reduced to seconds. However, the price paid for this advance was high in terms of the damage to glass tubes. Snook's discovery showed up the Crookes tube for what it was, namely a valuable and fragile object best suited to bench experiments, and it hastened the development of a more robust alternative vacuum tube, see next section.

The hot-cathode rectifying valve (Kenotron) which replaced the Snook transformer in the 1930s was invented by another American, Saul Dushman in 1914. It differed from the conventional x-ray tube in that with a low anode tension a large current could pass in one direction and not the reverse. Dushman's high-vacuum valves eventually ousted the noisy mechanical rectifiers, but only in 1925, and until that time interrupterless transformers of the Snook type remained the best generator of x-rays available.

THE X-RAY TUBE

Technical milestones in radiology from Röntgen's discovery to the present time have been most closely related to the following developments in tube construction, each one introduced roughly ten years after the prevous, since 1900:[18]

1. *Gas-filled tubes* with induction coil generators.
2. *High-vacuum (Coolidge) tubes* and valves with Snook transformer generators.
3. *Self-protected tubes* (Metalix, Bouwers).
4. High-tension protected tubes and generators.
5. Image intensification and cinéfluorography.
6. X-ray television.

Only the first three developments come within the scope of this book.

1. *Gas Tubes*. Partially evacuated gas tubes became part of the experimental physicist's bench equipment after 1874, when William Crookes perfected the tube that subsequently bore his name. Professor Röntgen used a Crookes-type tube for his experiments in 1895, and thereafter for a further 20 years until superseded by the Coolidge tube, the gas vacuum tube was synonymous with the production of x-rays.

Röntgen's tube was pear-shaped, and had a flat circular cathode at its narrow end and an anode protruding in a small side tube. When activated, the cathode rays flew off at right angles to the surface of the flat cathode and struck against the glass wall of the bulbous end, producing a vivid phosphorescence, as well as heat and x-rays. 'The life of these tubes' – an early observer recorded[19] – 'was very brief: a few exposures at most, and the tube was either pierced by a spark or cracked on account of the heat generated by the bombardment of electrons.' Equally disappointing was the poor quality of the x-ray beam, because the cathode stream struck the glass wall of the tube and x-rays came off in all directions from it.

The first improvement was an attempt to focus the cathode stream, and thus to concentrate the beam of x-rays. A. A. Campbell Swinton modified a Crookes tube by fashioning the anode from a sheet of platinum and inserting it in the tube so that some of the cathode rays were received upon it and did not strike the glass wall of the tube. It was this tube which he used to produce the radiograph of the bones of his hand – the first made of a living person in England – in January 1896. The events surrounding this experiment are described in Chapter 3, and Swinton's radiograph is shown on page 26. Professor Herbert Jackson had designed his focus tube in 1894, albeit for purposes not connected with the generation of x-rays; and he probably knew of Crookes' original tube with a concave electrode. He replaced the flat disc of the cathode with a hollowed-out or dished disc and mounted the platinum anode at an angle of 45 degrees within the tube. These modifications brought the cathode stream to a focus on the platinum plate, which was either an independent pole (target, anti-cathode) or the anode itself. The source of the x-ray beam was thus concentrated to one spot, and the resulting x-ray photographs at once showed a wonderful sharpness and detail. Jackson's focus tube, 'the greatest advance since Röntgen's discovery',[19] launched clinical radiography.[20]

Soon the experimenters with focus tubes encountered the problems of their own success. By building larger and more robust gas tubes and heavier induction coils, the currents that could be passed through the tube were increased from 1–2 to 5–6 milliamperes. This level of output was more than the early sheet platinum anti-cathode target could stand, and it was melted by the heat. The search commenced for a target material which possessed a high firing point and a high atomic weight, as well as for devices to avoid overheating of its surface. Platinum because of high cost and 'softness' to the cathode stream, was soon discarded in favour of other metals. Iridium embedded in a copper block was also tried and rejected,[21] then MacKenzie Davidson and A. C. Cossor built a tube with an anti-cathode made from osmium.[22] In 1907 Siemens Brothers introduced the tantalum anti-cathode, after perfecting the production of this metal in ingots of sheets and wire for the filaments of electrical light bulbs. Two types of device were tried for dissipating heat from the target: a heavy copper backing of the anode extending to the exterior and serving as a metallic radiator,[23] and later a piped system of water-cooling, which was incorporated in the heavy-duty Gundelach and Macalister Wiggins tubes. By these means, currents of 50 milliamperes were eventually achieved with gas tubes.

None of these improvements removed the great defect of the gas tube, namely that the current could not be varied independently of the voltage applied. Moreover, as the tube's vacuum increased during use, the high-tension current passed only with difficulty due to gradually increasing electrical resistance; in radiographers' language, the tube 'hardened'. This erratic behaviour begged solutions at several levels. The practising radiographer had a rack of gas tubes for daily use, with which he was completely familiar.[20] In 1904 Ernest Harnack of the London Hospital produced a *vade mecum* for A. E. Dean and Company entitled 'Hints on the Choice of a Tube', in which he described his collection of tubes 'for the complete outfit':[24] '*No. 1 "Soft" variety*, which will ultimately pass into the condition of nos. 2 and 3, should be used for the following – tendons, limbs in children, the epiphyses in very young subjects and less dense structures. *No. 2 "Medium"*, where the bones grow lighter and there is much "fire" in the fluorescent screen. The thorax may also be examined, and should show the ribs of heart black. It is used for permanent records of the thorax, examination for renal calculi in thin subjects, limbs in adults and all the deeper structures a No. 1 tube fails to penetrate. *No. 3 "Medium-Hard"*, where the bones of the limb appear illuminated on the screen, and when examining the thorax the heart and ribs appear lighter but more distinct in character. It is used for screen work and in the detection of renal calculi in stout adults. (With this latter type of tube I have successfully radiographed the vertebrae and upper part of the pelvis in a patient weighing nearly 19 stone.)'

Scientific efforts were also made to overcome the gradual increase in hardness of the gas tube. The increased electrical resistance could be reduced by heating the tube with a spirit lamp or bunsen burner – but only temporarily; and many tubes were fractured by such treatment. Soon devices came into use by which a small volume of gas could be introduced into the tube. Crookes in 1874 had first done so, by heating a small amount of caustic potash secreted in a side arm of the tube, the gas when liberated immediately lowering the vacuum. Another ingenious plan, patented by Harrison Glew, involved placing small pieces of iron coated with sealing wax in a side arm: one of these was isolated by means of a magnet and then heated with a flame to liberate sufficient gas to lower the vacuum. Finally this technique, the acclusion method, was made to work automatically, sparks passing to the side arm as the resistance of the tube increased and liberating sufficient gas to lower it.

Dr. John Macintyre while serving as President of the Röntgen Society in 1900–1 offered a gold medal 'to the maker of the best practical x-ray tube for both photographic and screen work'. A committee of experts was formed to act as judges, and 28 tubes were submitted by manufacturers, both domestic and foreign. By a series of preliminary tests, the number of tubes was reduced to six, and the final test was made photographically. Under identical conditions of electrification, exposure, distance and development, the density and sharpness of the radiographic images produced by the six tubes were studied and shown to vary greatly. The two best were selected, further tests were made upon these two, and the cheaper one was awarded the gold medal. Afterwards, the committee discovered that both these tubes came from the same maker – C. H. F. Müller of Hamburg. The winning tube was presented to the Röntgen Society for its collection.

The Röntgen Society at the suggestion of the first treasurer, J. J. Vezey, at an early stage decided to make a collection of historical tubes and other x-ray apparatus. The original collection comprised 62 tubes which had been used to generate x-rays before 1908, and four screens. The donors included pioneer experimenters, radiographers and instrument makers in Britain: A. C. Cossor, Sir William Crookes, Dr. J. MacKenzie Davidson, E. Harrison Glew, A. W. Isenthal, Professor Herbert Jackson, Sir Oliver Lodge, Ernest Payne, J. Russell Reynolds, A. A. Campbell Swinton; and the German manufacturers E. Gundelach, C. H. F. Müller and Siemens Brothers.[25]

During the presidency of Professor C. V. Boys in 1906–7 arrangements were made with the trustees of the Science Museum, South Kensington for the safe custody on loan and the exhibition of the collection. Before it was handed over in 1909, Dr. George Rodman, an enthusiastic photographer, made 43 lantern slides of the tubes.[27] Rodman's slides were lodged in the Society's house, and today 37 of them remain, numbered in a different order, in the archives of the British Institute of Radiology. Although only a few gas tubes are on display at South Kensington, this priceless collection of radiological muniments remains in the Museum's custody.[26]

This historic collection is as symbolic of the passing of the gas tube as gravestones in a churchyard; Rodman's lantern slides and their captions are the inscriptions (see Table). The earliest items, donated by Sir William Crookes, were a fluorescent screen and three experimental tubes with concave electrodes and vacuum regulators which

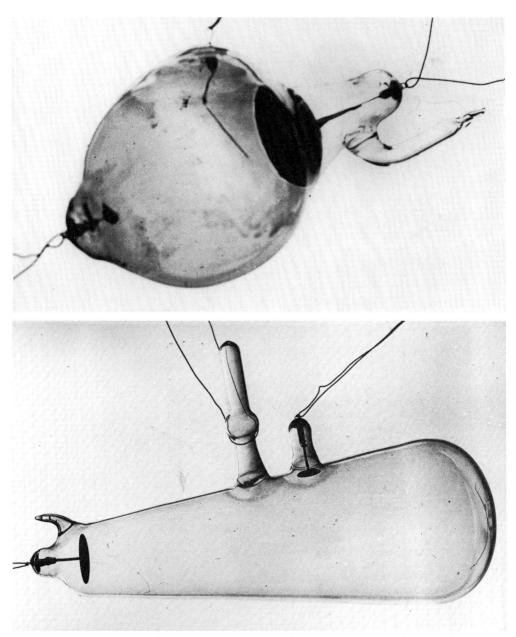

21. Early vacuum tubes in the Science Museum, London. Top *The original tube with a concave electrode, built and used by Sir William Crookes for conduction experiments in 1879.* Above *Pear-shaped tube used by Professor Röntgen*

Classification of illustrations (slides and photographs) of the collection of 62 x-ray tubes loaned to the Victoria and Albert Museum in 1909.

	Captions to list of 43 slides, January 1911	Plate number reference in the Gardiner paper of May 1909
1	Original Tube with concave electrode, used by Sir W. Crookes in 1879.	V, 3
2	Sir W. Crookes' original vacuum regulating Tube. Exhibited, 1879.	VI, 1
3	Radiant matter Tube. Used by Sir W. Crookes in 1879.	VIII, 1
4	Large Pear shaped Tube. Form originally used by Prof. Röntgen.	VIII, 3
5	Tube with Ring Anode, in 1896. By A. A. Campbell Swinton.	V, 1
6	Pear-shaped X-ray Tube.	none
7	X-ray Tube. Early Cylindrical pattern.	VIII, 4
8	X-ray Tube. Early Cylindrical pattern.	none
9	Prof. Herbert Jackson's First Focus Tube, 1896.	VIII, 5
10	Vacuum Regulating Tube. By F. H. Glew, 1896.	VI, 2
11	Tube with Auxiliary Anode, 1896.	none
12	Focus Tube for Alternating Current. By A. A. Campbell Swinton, 1896.	VIII, 6
13	'Penetrator' Tube, 1896.	VIII, 7
14	Tube with Platinum Anti-kathode. By A. A. Campbell Swinton, 1896.	none
15	Cylindrical Tube, with Vacuum Regulator.	VIII, 8
16	Black Glass Tube.	VIII, 9
17	Tube with Adjustable Anode. By J. C. M. Stanton and H. L. Tyson Wolfe. Feb. 1897.	none
18	Tube with sliding kathode.	VIII, 10
19	X-ray Tube with Osmium Anode. By J. Mackenzie Davidson, 1898.	VI, 4
20	Tube with side tube coated with Red Phosphorus. By Siemens, Berlin, 1899.	none
21	Tube with side tube for Charcoal.	none
22	Tube with Adjustable Anti-kathode. Designed by Dr. Russell T. Reynolds.	IX, 11
23	Tube with Automatic Vacuum Regulator. Made by Queen and Co., Philadelphia.	VI, 3
24	Actual Tube awarded the Gold Medal of the Röntgen Society in 1901. Made by C. H. F. Muller, Hamburg.	V, 4
25	"Ideal" Tube. By Dessauer of Aschaffenburg.	none
26	Small Bulb, non-sparking Tube.	IX, 12
27	Tube with Automatic Regulation, 1906.	IX, 13
28	Tube for medium Currents. By Max Levy of Berlin, 1907.	none
29	Tube with Porcelain covered Anti-kathode, 1907.	IX, 14
30	Modern X-ray Tube.	IX, 15
31	Tube with Water cooled Anti-kathode.	IX, 16
32	Gundelach Tube, 1908.	none
33	Very Heavy Current Tube, with Air-cooled Anti-kathode, 1908.	IX, 17
34	Tube for Special Therapeutic Purposes.	X, 18
35	Tube for Therapeutic Purposes, 1898.	X, 19
36	Tube for Special Therapeutic Purposes, 1902.	X, 20
37	Tube with Anti-kathode covered with materials of heavy Atomic-weight. Designed by Dr. Langer, 1896.	none
38	Tube with Hemispherical kathode. By A. A. Campbell Swinton, 1896.	none
39	Aluminium Tube. By Benjamin Davis, 1896.	X, 21
40	Aluminium Tube. By Benjamin Davis, 1896.	X, 22
41	Tube with Two kathodes and flat Anti-kathode for Alternating Current.	none
42	Platinum Funnel Tube. By E. Gundelach, Sept. 1896.	X, 23
43	Tube with Four kathodes, 1899.	X, 24
—	Sir W. Crookes' Grid, 1879.	VIII, 2
—	Radiograph of hand, 13.1.1896.	V, 2
—	Radiograph of foetal elephant skull.	none
—	View of Reid Knox Hall.	none

he built and used in the 1870s; one of them was described in the *Philosophical Transactions of the Royal Society* for 1874.[26] When assembled in 1908, the collection included examples of 'a modern x-ray tube', 'a very heavy current tube, with air-cooled anti-kathode' and a large Gundelach tube. But the majority of the tubes date from the turn of the century and were given by their makers, each of whom was an innovator in the young science. An example of Professor Röntgen's pear-shaped tube was included, as well as Müller's tube that took the Society's gold medal in 1901, and several from other German suppliers. Archibald Campbell Swinton and his assistant, J. C. M. Stanton contributed at least six items, including the celebrated photograph of his hand, and the tube that he had used to take it (*see* 21).

If Rodman inscribed the gravestones, then J. H. Gardiner, Crookes's assistant who was editor of *The Journal of the Röntgen Society*, wrote the eulogy. Gardiner's brilliant paper, 'The Origin, History and Development of the X-ray Tube' is one of the classic descriptions in the literature of radiology.[19] He used several of Rodman's photographs as full-page illustrations. In addition, the number of *The Journal* in which the paper appeared contained three more plates not referred to by Gardiner but obviously forming part of the historical collection. Gardiner's article was published in 1909, within a few years of Coolidge's innovation, and the gas tube was developed no further.

2. Coolidge Tubes. In 1913 an American discovery revolutionised x-ray equipment. A new tube was designed which enabled the current to be regulated independently of the tension across the electrodes, and the milliamperage and kilovoltage both to be increased considerably. This more controllable, higher-output tube was a scientific match for Snook's transformer, and it sealed the doom of the gas tube. The new discovery was the hot-cathode tube which William Coolidge invented in 1913 (*see* 22).

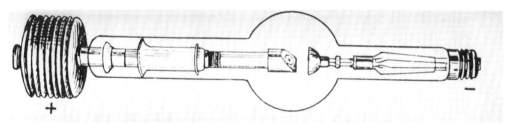

22. *The hot-cathode, high-vacuum tube perfected by William Coolidge in 1913, which enabled the tube current to be varied at will for the first time. The 1916 model shown in this illustration has its own radiator*

WILLIAM DAVID COOLIDGE, Ph.D. (1873–1975) was the other foreign national after W. C. Röntgen who through his scientific inventiveness exerted the greatest influence upon British radiology.

Born the son of a New England smallholder, Coolidge won a scholarship to the Massachusetts Institute of Technology to study electrical engineering and physical chemistry. After graduating in 1896, he carried out three years of research in Germany and gained his Ph.D. degree *summa cum laude* from Leipzig University. While in Leipzig, he is known to have met Röntgen, who visited the University as a candidate for a post in the department of physics. Coolidge returned to Boston and after teaching for five years joined the research laboratory of the General Electric Company of Schenectady, New York.[28] It was here that he was to make a series of discoveries in the course of the next 40 years, which altered the course of mankind. After retiring he worked on for another 30 years. When he died at the age of 102, he had patented a total of 83 designs and discoveries, and was loaded with scientific honours, including the Hughes Medal of the Royal Society, the Faraday Medal of the Institute of Electrical Engineers and Honorary Membership of the Röntgen Society (1918).

Coolidge attributed his idea for the hot-cathode tube to Edison's discovery of the electric light. Edison in the 1880s had demonstrated that, in the vacuum of the incandescent light bulb, current would flow from the hot filament to another electrode, and moreover that this emission could be controlled by varying the current which heated the filament. Then in 1913 the American Nobel Prizewinner Irving Langmuir showed that the electrical emission from a tungsten filament continued indefinitely within a vacuum. To all this, Coolidge added the one ingredient that gave the scientific facts a practical reality: in 1910 he produced a ductile form of tungsten, a substance previously regarded as an unworkable metal. By the time that Langmuir made known his work, Coolidge had described his new tube, 'A Powerful Röntgen Ray Tube with a Pulse Electric Discharge',[29] and in December 1913 General Electric installed the first model in the rooms of the New York radiologist, Lewis Gregory Cole.[14]

The hot cathode of Coolidge's tube consisted of a spiral of tungsten wire heated by a subsidiary electrical circuit. As Langmuir's work confirmed, the extent of electrical emission, i.e. the intensity of the current across the tube, could be controlled by adjusting the temperature of the anode. This was done simply by placing a variable resistor in the cathode circuit. The target of Coolidge's original tube was a solid block of tungsten, later it was made of platinoiridium embedded in copper.[21] The advantage of the tube over gas tubes was its enhanced performance – steady action with a tension as high as 150 kilovolts, and a current that could be varied at will.

Apart from the hot cathode, the other novel feature of the Coolidge tube that distinguished it from the gas tube was the high vacuum which ensured its reliability. The extraction of gases from glass tubes in order to create a very high vacuum was a problem that had been identified as early as 1896 by Sydney Rowland,[30] and several early experimenters including C. E. S. Phillips devised air pumps to overcome it.[31,32] Up to 1912 most laboratories used the carbon liquid-air method to produce high vacua, then new pumps appeared such as Gaede's molecular pump which Coolidge used, and which evacuated the residual gas more fully – in fact, so completely that no electrons could pass without heat being applied to the cathode. It was this absolute quality that gave Coolidge's tube its major advantage, namely the possibility of duplicating results with an accuracy never achieved with gas tubes.[14]

For British radiologists and x-ray manufacturers, the excitement over Coolidge's discovery was overshadowed by the outbreak of the First World War, which disrupted their lives and delayed its introduction.[33] In 1915 British firms manufacturing gas tubes had their stocks commandeered for military use, and, since their source of supply of soda glass in Germany and Belgium had been cut off, a critical shortage soon developed.[34] Cuthbert Andrews and others thereupon persuaded British glassmakers to produce soda glass and an independent gas tube industry was established before the end of the War.[35] As a result, the newer technological advances from America supplanted the conventional apparatus only slowly, and gas tubes remained in popular use in the early 1920s.[36]

3. *Self-Protected Tubes.* The decade of the 1920s produced x-ray tubes designed to conform with the requirements of protection. Bouwers, a Dutch scientist working in the research laboratory of Philips, in 1924 discovered a metal alloy which fused to glass, enabling x-ray tubes to be moulded cylindrically. He introduced a completely new hot-cathode x-ray tube, the Metalix, which was made of chrome-iron enclosed in a lead jacket. X-rays could be emitted only through a small window in the lead jacket, the beam being made just wide enough for practical purposes; and it could be further collimated. The smaller size and lighter weight of the Metalix, compared with gas tubes in their cumbersome protective boxes, prompted designers to adopt it for their x-ray couches and stands. At the Second International Congress of Radiology in Stockholm in 1928, most of the exhibitors showed tables and stands with Metalix tubes. In the next year Bouwers incorporated a rotating anode in his tube, later called the Rotalix.[18]

Self-protected x-ray tubes heralded the introduction of fully-protected generators and connecting cables which were electrically safe, i.e. shock-proof, as well as radiation-proof. Accidents, although rare, still occurred, and in January 1929, the *British Journal of Radiology* reported a death by electrocution in a large provincial hospital.[37] With these changes, for the first time the equipment of the x-ray room assumed an appearance that is recognisable to the present-day radiographer.

The Metalix portable unit, unveiled in Stockholm, consisted of a tube mounted in a metal shield and connected by flexible insulated cables to a portable high-tension transformer (*see* 23). The output of this unit was relatively high – sufficient for high-quality examinations of the chest and skull – and domiciliary radiography became a reality. More primitive mobile apparatus was used in November and December 1928 at Buckingham Palace to make chest radiographs of King George V during his severe illness. When pneumonia was complicated by empyema, the King's Physician, Lord Dawson summoned Dr. (later Sir) Harold Graham-Hodgson from King's College Hospital, and the radiographs were taken by Mr. Ferrier.[38,39]

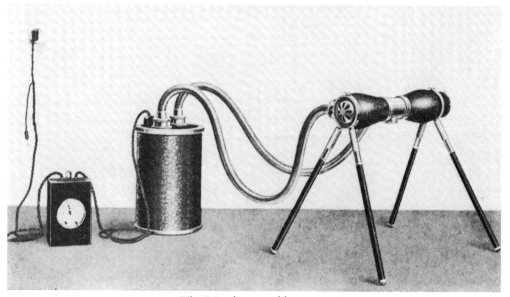

23. The Metalix portable x-ray unit

HENRY T. FERRIER, M.V.O. (4th Class), M.B.E., F.S.R., F.R.P.S. (1894–1967) was a distinguished pioneer radiographer who had charge of the St. John and Red Cross mobile x-ray unit in London. He received a diamond tiepin from the King, and later was elected a Member of the Royal Victorian Order.[40]

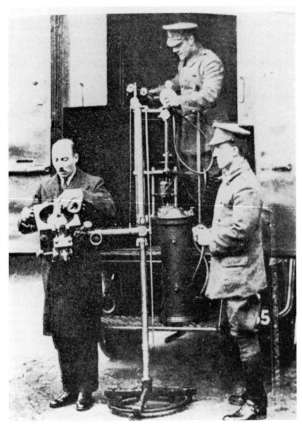

24. X-rays at Buckingham Palace. Mr. Henry Ferrier and his two assistants assemble the apparatus to make chest radiographs of King George V during his severe illness in 1928

COUCHES AND STANDS

Clinical enthusiasm for x-rays encouraged early users to build wooden stands and tables to simplify their task, which was mainly to examine the hands and feet of patients with fractures or foreign bodies. The transition from Röntgen's bench experiment to the first x-ray couch with a screen moving synchronously with the tube took less than six years to accomplish; so swift was the development of the British x-ray industry. The early couches and screening stands were built of wood, which was superseded by T-iron and later tubular metal.

One of the first purposely-built x-ray stands was the 'convenient foot and leg rest' illustrated in the *Archives of the Roentgen Ray* in 1898.[41] A simple wooden box enabled the operator to secure an x-ray plate in a vertical position beside the anatomical part to be examined (*see* 25). It was probably designed by Ernest Payne, a co-editor of *Archives*; other early non-medical radiographers who designed stands were Harrison Glew and J. H. Gardiner.

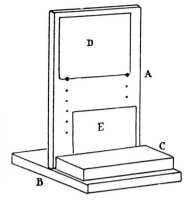

25. Radiography stand, 1898. A foot and leg rest consisting of an upright wooden board A fixed to a base B. A movable block C resting on the base was fixed a short distance from the upright, so that the plate E could be held in the gap between them

When doctors began screening and taking radiographs themselves, a new generation of apparatus designers was born. They could say what was needed and foretell future requirements, better than the apparatus maker working alone. Those doctors with inventive minds such as MacKenzie Davidson were great favourites of the makers. Davidson's radiographic couch, made before 1903 by Muirhead and Company, was the outcome of such fruitful collaboration (*see* 26).[42] The design was not ideal, because the upright pillars, while providing rigid support for the Crookes tube, impeded the patient's access to the couch; for the less mobile patient, getting on and off must have been a feat. Nevertheless, the couch was a milestone along the path of establishing radiography as a clinical discipline; and the design signalled the breaking point with the radiography of the laboratory where all the equipment stood on the same table.

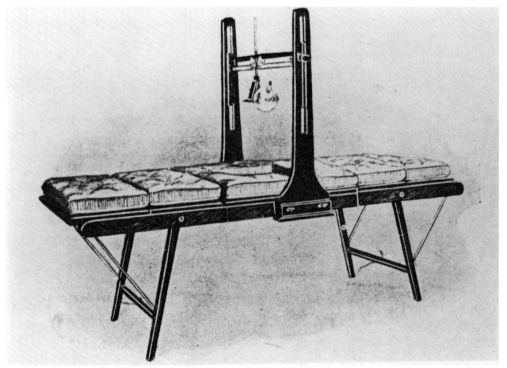

26. MacKenzie Davidson's x-ray couch, made in 1902 by Muirhead and Company

MacKenzie Davidson's couch spawned apparatus for x-ray fluoroscopy, of which
the begetter was probably Edward Shenton of Guy's Hospital, As will be described
in Chapter 5, Shenton by 1902 had introduced his 'System of Radiography', which
involved preliminary screening of each patient before radiographs were made. Essential
for this approach was appropriate apparatus, and this was the 'X-ray Localising Couch'
which Harry W. Cox installed in Guy's Hospital.[43] Cox made the original Shenton
X-ray Couch and continued to manufacture it for many years, soon copied by his rivals.
The Shenton–Dean Exploration Couch appeared in 1904,[44] and the Shenton–Sanitas
Couch in 1905.[45] Shenton's contribution was to fix the tube beneath the table and the
plate carrier (or fluoroscopic screen) above it; the carrier being arranged to move with
the tube and parallel to the table top. Cox's original model (*see* 27), a simple wooden
table with a canvas top, cost £14!

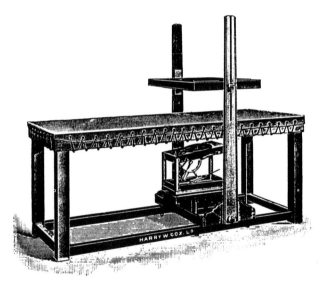

27. *Shenton's x-ray couch built by*
Harry W. Cox and installed in
Guy's Hospital in 1902. Cox's com-
petitors soon copied the design which
placed the tube beneath the table and
fixed the plate carrier (or fluoro-
scopic screen) above it

Shenton's couch underwent numerous modifications and refinements at the hands
of the five or six x-ray apparatus manufacturers that established factories in London
after 1900, as described later in this chapter. The table-top was made removable for
use as a stretcher, the foot switch for screening was coupled to operate with the room
lights, attachments for localisation were offered, and an overcouch tube was added by
A. E. Dean & Company in 1904 for stereoscopy (Harnack–Dean Precision Couch).[44]
Unquestionably, the most radical modification was that first made by Shenton himself
at Guy's Hospital. By attaching the two legs to the floor with hinges, the table could
be tipped on its end and used for upright screening. This innovation coincided with
the appointment to the Hospital in 1907 of Dr. Alfred Jordan as 'Medical Radiographer',
a title which reflected at that time the increasing importance of radiology in the diagnosis
of internal diseases. This primitive screening apparatus and its many copies – some of
them home-made contraptions such as A. E. Barclay's in Manchester (Chapter 7), proved
to be reliable and durable, remaining in use up to the 1920s.

Overcouch radiography owed its resurgence to Dr. (later Sir) Archibald Reid, who
conceived the novel idea of 'the fixed tube and the movable patient' (*see* 28).[46] In 1911

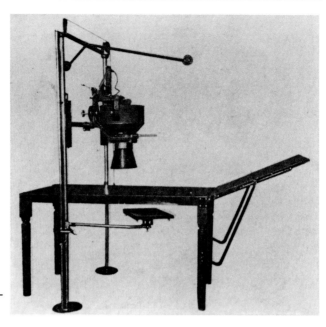

28. Dr. Archibald Reid's radio-graphy table, 1911

he introduced the prototype of his design to King's College Hospital. The tube (above table level) and the plate holder (beneath table level) were attached to the same floor-to-roof column, and the patient couch was free-standing. Thus, in addition to the tube being adjustable to the patient, the patient could be brought to the tube. Reid's design fathered the table for radiography, and supplemented the Shenton-type screening apparatus, of the modern x-ray department.

The last of the three American inventions to revolutionise the production of x-rays was the Potter–Bucky grid which reached Britain in the early 1920s. Gustav Bucky (died 1963), the co-inventor, whilst still in Berlin in 1914 had sent details of his remarkable anti-scatter grid for publication in the *Archives of the Roentgen Ray* in London,[47] but the outbreak of the First World War banished the prospect of introducing it. Only after Bucky emigrated to the United States and American x-ray manufacturers marketed the grid in 1921, did it appear in Britain.

The story of the changes that followed the introduction of these inventions in the 1920s belongs elsewhere because they lie beyond the scope of this book. As mentioned previously, the movement towards self-protected x-ray tubes of the Metalix type also brought shock-proof high-tension cables, oil-immersed generators and other sophisticated innovations. Gas tubes, induction coils and interrupters survived in wide use in the 1920s and beyond, because they were cheap. A gas tube cost six pounds, and private rooms could be completely equipped for less than £150![36]

SCREENS, GLASS PLATES AND FILMS

The third requirement for radiography after generators and tubes, which is mentioned in Chapter 1, is an emulsion sensitive to x-rays. When x-rays are produced the beam interacts with the emulsion to produce an image that may be viewed (fluoroscopy, screening) or permanently recorded by a chemical process (x-ray photography or radiography). Historically, fluoroscopy pre-dates radiography because Röntgen almost certainly screened his own hand before he took the x-ray photograph of his wife's.[48]

Röntgen himself started the quest for an improved emulsion immediately after making his astonishing discovery. He experimented with several chemical substances and then chose barium platinocyanide for his screen. At that time, the platinocyanides were well known as substances which fluoresced under gas-tube excitation, and he was performing experiments to find out why this phenomenon occurred, when he made the Great Discovery. First he disproved that the fluorescence was caused by the luminescence from the glass wall of the tube because he had covered his tube with a light-proof coat, thus showing that other invisible rays were responsible – a new kind of rays, which he called x-rays. Later on, others made experiments with emulsions which were known not to fluoresce, and confirmed that x-rays do directly affect the silver halide.[49]

The fluorescent property of the platinocyanides when activated by x-rays was turned to practical account a few weeks after Röntgen's discovery by Professor Salvioni of Perugia. He built an instrument which he called the cryptoscope.[50] The important component of this device was a sheet made of a substance opaque to light but capable of transmitting x-rays, such as cardboard, which was coated with the fluorescent emulsion – in Salvioni's case, barium platinocyanide. Much publicity was given to Salvioni's announcement in the press because it was believed that his invention allowed Röntgen's rays to be *seen*. Upon hearing the news in February 1896, several British experimenters immediately built their own cryptoscopes (*see* 29).

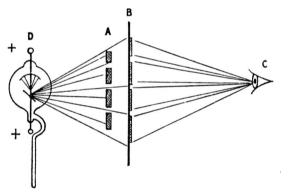

29. Diagram of Salvioni's cryptoscope in use. A, object or body casting image on a fluorescent screen B, which is seen by eye at C. D, focus tube

Professor Herbert Jackson at King's College, London, a chemist by profession, used the potassium instead of the barium salt of platinocyanide, which he applied in a gum arabic mixture to one side of a circular sheet of black cardboard. When placed in a beam of x-rays, the screen was found to light up with a vivid green colour.[51] When used with Jackson's focus tube (*see* 2,15), the quality of the screen image was at once superior to anything seen before, and adequate to demonstrate a needle in the tissues of a hand or foot. Jackson's cryptoscope was put into immediate clinical use by Dr. John Macintyre in Glasgow and by others, as described in Chapters 2 and 3. Soon it also became part of the impedimenta of fairground operators and other entrepreneurs who exploited the curiosity of the public to see their own bones.

Hurried experiments during the early months of 1896 gave the impression that all x-ray work could be satisfactorily carried out with the fluorescent screen. Thus the American inventor, Thomas Edison (who renamed Salvioni's device the fluoroscope), tested hundreds of chemical substances in his laboratory in a search for a cheaper and superior alternative to barium platinocyanide. In mid-March he sent Lord Kelvin a telegram which received worldwide publicity: 'Just found that calcium tungstate properly crystallized gives splendid fluorescence with Roentgen rays, far exceeding platinocyanide, rendering photography unnecessary'.[52] However, subsequent events proved the fallacy of Edison's enthusiastic verdict. While the instant image (and diagnosis) held great attraction for practical men such as Macintyre and Shenton, the fluoroscope failed to live up to its early theoretical promise. Radiation fog and the coarse grain of the screen obscured anatomical details. Most of the early experimenters continued their efforts to improve the photographic plate, particularly when its advantages were realised, namely: a permanent record, a better image, and – most important of all – the cumulative factor, which meant that a poor radiograph could be improved simply by prolonging the exposure time.

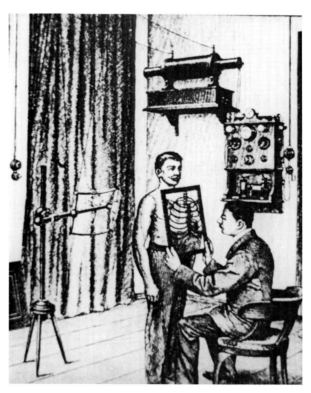

30. Chest fluoroscopy, 1898. A naive sketch of an early radiographer's consulting room showing an examination in progress. Fluoroscopy was popular after Edison discovered the calcium tungstate screen

A radiograph may be defined as a permanent shadow picture obtained through the action of x-rays upon a sensitive emulsion. Röntgen in the course of his crucial experiments to prove that this action was not caused by light rays, nonetheless used the instruments of the photographers. 'Of special interest' – he wrote[53] – 'is the fact that photographic dry plates are sensitive to the x-rays.' Accordingly, he and the early experimenters turned to the photographic industry to find the emulsion that best captured the x-ray image.

'What sensitive emulsion is best for x-ray work?' was a constant query in 1896.[54] The answers were usually quite contradictory, because each experimenter had his own preferences and no particular dry plate appeared to be superior. Two London photographers, H. Snowden Ward and E. A. Robins, in 1897 examined 17 varieties of plate used in x-ray work, and were able to draw one conclusion only, namely that thick emulsions were more desirable than those usually applied to plates. A German company, Schleussner, produced a revolutionary plate in 1896, with emulsion coating both surfaces of the glass, but it was too costly to find favour. The most popular plates for radiography were *Cadett Lightning and Professional, Paget Imperial*, Snowden Ward's '*S. W.*' *Roentgen*, and Wratten's *Drop-Shutter Plates*. The French *Lumière* plates were also used.

Wratten and Wainwright, one of the many photographic plate-making firms in London, was probably typical of the others. F. C. L. Wratten (1840–1926), when an assistant in a photographic shop in 1877, made a satisfactory gelatin dry plate which was about 15 times as sensitive as the collodion wet plate. He soon branched out on his own account, and a few years later marketed an improved version as *London Instantaneous Plates*. The plates were made in the Wrattens' home in Great Queen Street, Holborn. The emulsion was prepared by Mrs. Wratten in her kitchen, and it was poured onto the glass plates by hand from the spout of a teapot (a 'batch' of emulsion filled 20 teapots) and left to set on a chilled level surface. When dry, the plates were put in racks to set. Wratten later moved to a factory in Croydon and replaced his wife's teapot with a dry plate coating machine, and by 1896 had a thriving business.[55] In 1912 after the Company pioneered the introduction of colour photography, it was acquired by the American, George Eastman (1854–1932), the inventor of the box camera and founder of the Eastman–Kodak Company. Wratten and Wainwright's brilliant young scientist, Kenneth Mees, D.Sc., F.R.S. (1882–1960) then emigrated to America and established the Kodak research laboratories in Rochester, New York.

Many British plate-makers eventually found refuge under the blanket of Ilford Limited, and the early story of this company includes the names of those best known. At about the same time as J. C. L. Wratten, an Ilford man, Alfred Harman began to manufacture photographic dry plates in the basement of his home in Cranbrook Road. The plates were distributed by Marion and Company of Soho Square, London. Harman's venture succeeded and he soon established the Britannia Works Company with a factory on the outskirts of Ilford; in 1900 he changed his Company's name to Ilford Limited. The Company's scientific input came from F. F. Renwick (died 1943) who joined Harman in 1899 and served as director of research for three decades. Renwick was largely responsible for introducing the first British-made colour plates for photography in 1914 and for pioneering the manufacture of x-ray roll film at Brentwood in 1922. By the latter date, Ilford Limited had absorbed the following glass plate manufacturers:[14] Marion and Company of Soho Square, London (founded 1860); Imperial Dry Plate Company of Cricklewood, London (founded 1887); Thomas Illingworth and Company of Park Royal, London (founded 1890); Paget Prize Plate Company; Raja Limited; and General Dry Plate Company.

The manifest drawbacks of using glass plates for clinical radiography prompted several early workers to experiment with the bromide paper used by the photographic trade. This possibility was mentioned by Röntgen in his original report,[53] and enthusiastically advocated by George Eastman early in 1897. (*see* 31). However, Eastman failed to sell

AN IMPORTANT RADIOGRAPHIC DISCOVERY.

EASTMAN'S
...X=RAY PAPER

ENTIRELY SUPERSEDES DRY PLATES WITH THEIR ATTENDANT DRAWBACKS.

Of Unparalleled Advantage in Surgical Diagnosis by means of the Rontgen Rays.

MANUFACTURED SOLELY BY THE

EASTMAN Photographic Materials Co. Ltd.,
115=117 Oxford Street, London, W.
60 Cheapside, London, E.C.

PARIS: 4 Place Vendôme.
BERLIN: Eastman Kodak Gesellschaft, m.b. H., Markgrafen Strasse 91.

ROCHESTER, N.Y., U.S.A.
Eastman Kodak Co.

31. George Eastman's advertisement of February 1897. He was one of the first to claim that emulsion-coated paper was superior to glass plates for radiography

his paper, and several subsequent innovators also failed, because sensitised paper does not reveal anatomical detail and gradations of density as clearly as transmitted light.

The search for a permanent substitute for photographic plates became urgent when the First World War broke out, and supplies of Continental glass to Britain and the United States of America were halted. Attention then turned to the use of a celluloid base. As early as 1897 the Sandall Plate Company marketed a 'film' for radiography named Cristoid, in which the emulsion was first coated on glass and then stripped off; thus the 'film' was made of gelatin. A few years later, an American dentist devised a cellulose-base film suitable for examining teeth. Cellulose nitrate was a satisfactory base, but it was brittle and partly opaque, and – an alarming disadvantage – highly inflammable. Prior to 1914 Eastman–Kodak marketed a single-coated 14 × 17-inch film and in 1917 they introduced 'duplitized' (double-coated) film. Large stocks were shipped to England to replace glass plates, and soon they were used in the army hospitals. They were carried from Liverpool to London by road on Foden steam wagons because of the congestion of the railways.[56] Towards the end of the War, nitrate-based x-ray film was produced by Kodak at Harrow as a temporary measure. Eastman–Kodak's first 'safety film', with a cellulose acetate base, was placed on the American market in 1924, and production started at Harrow in 1928. Gevaert, the Belgian pioneers established in London since 1909, marketed x-ray films in 1929.

Soon all x-ray film was double-coated and this advance itself produced another considerable benefit. Such films could be used with intensification screens. These screens were thin cards coated with a fluorescent material such as calcium tungstate which enabled exposure times to be shortened considerably as a consequence of the x-ray enhancement by light from the screen.[20] Intensification screens, a *sine qua non* of modern radiography, owe their idea to the inventive mind of the pioneer, Archibald Campbell Swinton, who in 1896 recommended their use to reduce exposure times and improve image quality.[57]

APPARATUS MAKERS AND SUPPLERS BEFORE 1930

The British x-ray industry was founded by enthusiasts whose stimulus was fascination with the new science. Most of them were craftsmen producing scientific instruments and glassware, skilled trades that had flourished for a few hundred years in the alleys and courts off Fleet Street, London. It was work that called for manual dexterity and precision, as well as the ability to turn out a finished product: a superior pedigree for the founders of the new industry. The decision of the infant Röntgen Society to open its doors to them was a masterly gesture of encouragement which at once introduced the apparatus makers into the circle of the x-ray pioneers. The scientific exhibitors at the Society's first *conversazione* in November 1897 (Chapter 9) were the founders of the British x-ray industry. Britain was one of the first countries in the world to produce x-ray machines.[35]

Several firms entered the field early in 1896, and towards the end of the year their advertisements began to appear in the journals, offering manufactured items of equipment for sale. The leaders were Newton and Company, A. E. Dean and Company, Watson and Sons, and Harry W. Cox Limited. Within a few years these firms and others were marketing complete sets of apparatus. One of these offered a $2\frac{1}{2}$-inch coil, six bunsen-cell batteries, a focus tube with supports and a fluorescent screen for £7 10s. (*see* 32).

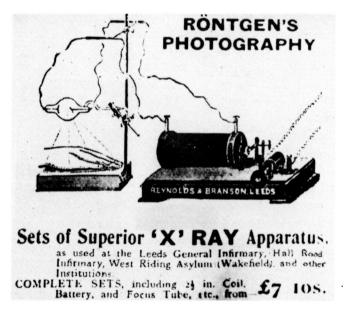

32. *Advertisement for a complete x-ray set, 1900*

NEWTON AND COMPANY, AFTER 1911 NEWTON AND WRIGHT LIMITED

Newton and Company were the oldest optical instrument makers in the world. The firm was founded about 1700 by the astronomer Isaac Newton (he was knighted by Queen Anne in 1705), and remained in the hands of his descendants. They held royal warrants from several monarchs as scientific instrument makers, and had supplied geographical globes to explorers, academics and the Prince Consort.

In 1896 the firm was controlled by Herbert Newton and his cousin Thomas Freshwater, but the impetus for entering the new x-ray field came from the brilliant young apprentice whom they had taken on some years before, Russell Wright. Other members of their successful team were the Clapham chemist, F. Harrison Glew and the electrical engineer, Alfred Apps. Glew and Wright claimed to have discovered the x-ray rectifier, having designed and built a prototype device for converting alternating to unidirectional current in 1900–1, thus anticipating Snook's ideas by several years.[58]

HERBERT C. NEWTON (1859–1940) was the senior partner of Newton and Company when x-rays were discovered, and he was among the first in Britain to confirm Röntgen's claims. He used a 2-inch induction coil, a bichromate battery and a 'Radiant Matter' tube of the type used by Crookes in 1879 (No. 3 of Table on page 52).

Newton was a Company man: he took the decision to enter the x-ray manufacturing field and presided over its subsequent success, becoming in 1912 chairman of the new x-ray company, Newton and Wright. Early commercial ventures, both highly successful, were the marketing of Professor Herbert Jackson's focus tube and manufacturing a range of fluorescent screens which, it is recorded,[59] Newton painted with his own hands. His interests were essentially photographic and in later life he became more involved in developing the photographic process, leaving electrical development to his colleagues. He was a founder member of the Röntgen Society.

RUSSELL STUART WRIGHT, M.I.E.E. (1876–1961) was the son of the well-known optical scientist Lewis Wright. He studied at King's College, London where he was befriended by Professor Herbert Jackson and witnessed Jackson's experiments with the original focus tube.

Russell Wright is one of the patrician figures of the British x-ray industry. Aged only 19 at the time of Röntgen's announcement and already an employee of Newton and Company, he served the firm for the rest of his life; after Herbert Newton's retirement, he controlled Newton and Wright. More than that, he identified with the first 60 years of British radiology. When he died in 1961 aged 85, he was the oldest member of the British Institute of Radiology and recalled being present at the original *conversazione* of the Röntgen Society in 1897 to hear Professor Silvanus Thompson deliver his presidential address.

Russell Wright was a great character, well known in North London where he lived. Keen on sport and physical fitness, he seldom used a car and was to be seen cycling between home and factory, head down and coat tails flying. He swam daily in the Highgate Ponds until over the age of 80.[35,60]

Newton and Company had premises at 3 Fleet Street and a factory occupying three floors of a building near Gray's Inn Road when they began to manufacture x-ray apparatus. Here Alfred Apps made his highly successful induction coils – they were always advertised with his name prefixed, as 'Apps-Newton' coils – and Wright and Glew designed and produced other items such as their rectifier, gas tubes (one of which remains reposited in the Science Museum, South Kensington) and a motorised mercury interrupter which was patented. Glew (died 1920), an enthusiastic contributor at scientific meetings and to the early literature, had an experimental laboratory behind his chemist shop in the Clapham Road. Later he was to become interested in the therapeutic uses of radium and his hands were severely damaged by contamination of his premises. In the 1950s his name was added to the British names on the Martyrs' Memorial in Hamburg with that of his son, E. Lowndes Glew, who also perished or radium-induced disease, see Chapter 11.[61]

Burgeoning demand for x-ray apparatus obliged Newton and Company to enlarge their factory, and in 1905 they moved to 471–3 Hornsey Road, Hornsey Rise, North London. Even though they secured the European manufacturing rights for the Snook rectifier and other American innovations such as the Coolidge tube,[50] they continued to produce gas tubes and induction coils until the 1920s. Two other pioneering engineers who worked for the firm were Evelyn Burnside who joined in 1905 and became a director of Newton and Wright; and H. W. Grover who joined after the First World War. Grover described the factory as he found it in 1918.[1]

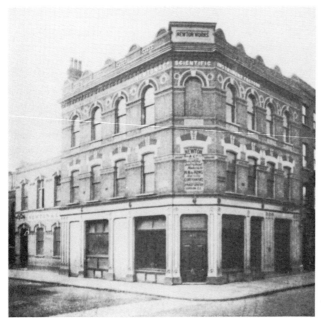

33. *Newton and Wright's premises, North London, 1918*

'Their works, typical of others in the industry, comprised a corner building with a basement and three floors in which all the manufacturing and other activities were undertaken. Factory personnel, in the main, were craftsmen, those of the machine shop possessing skills of turning, shaping and chasing threads with hand tools on simple lathes but producing components of the highest quality and finish; and here were made and assembled the tube stands, couches and screening stands equipped with supports of fibre and lead rubber to accommodate and protect the 8-inch gas tubes of the period.

'X-ray tubes were made on the top floor – some four or five glass blowers seated at a bench, their basic equipment being a variable gas flame, a pair of insulated tongs, and a good lung capacity. I well remember the skill and artistry which was required to balance and rotate with one hand the 7-inch or 8-inch glass bulb in the flame whilst simultaneously heating and rotating the anti-cathode assembly in the other, prior to making, at the critical moment, a union on the central axis. Even more complicated was the attachment of the regulator which was fitted at right angles to this axis. My sundry "off the record" attempts soon made me realize that tube making was not my *métier*.

'In the Winding Shop on the ground floor induction coils were still being manufactured in fairly large quantities. The plate was extremely simple, the sections of the

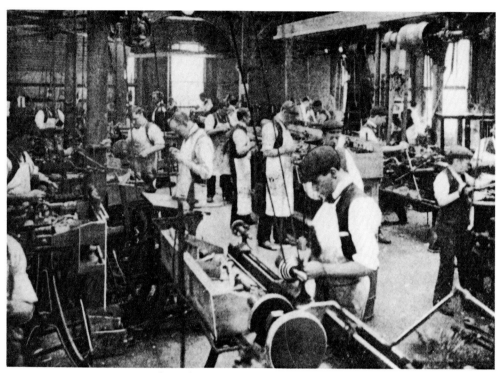

34. Machine shop, Newton and Wright Limited, 1918

induction coils being a series of pancake windings approximately 1/16-inch wide, wound between two metal discs. These pancakes were then immersed in wax and assembled on to a Micalite tube. If one of these pancake windings was inadvertently assembled in the reverse direction, failure of the coil on test was inevitable.

'It was the era of the mercury interrupter and the evil smell generated when cleaning out the base container and filtering the mercury through a muslin cloth would remain with one for days. . . .

'Adjoining the Winding Shop was the Woodworking Section in which were two unforgettable personalities. The cabinet maker, extremely short-sighted, with thick pebble lenses would work almost 12 inches from his material but could cut a perfect dovetail, and his cabinet and couch tops were a joy to behold. The polisher, who had been on the stage, would, in his lighter moments, tap dance around a couch, as he applied each consecutive coat to produce the gloss-like finish.

'Finally, the Packing and Despatch Department. London deliveries were made by horse-drawn van but in an emergency a lad would be taken from the shop floor to make a delivery of a gas tube by bus to the West End.'

In the 1920s Newton and Wright moved further out of London, to a site in Ballards Lane, Finchley, on which new premises were built. During the Second World War collaboration began with Metropolitan-Vickers of Manchester and in 1948, in one of the post-war mergers necessitated by the advent of the British National Health Service, Newton and Wright joined forces with the Victor X-Ray Company, the importing subsidiary in London of the General Electric Corporation of America. The new firm became a subsidiary of Metropolitan-Vickers.[14,62]

A. E. DEAN & COMPANY

Mr. Dean of Hatton Garden, the respected maker of scientific instruments and glassware was the principal competitor of Newton and Company. When his son, Alfred, realised in 1896 that Röntgen's discovery would create a demand for x-ray apparatus and proposed manufacturing it, he declined to be involved. The new x-rays had become the subject of newspaper cartoons and music-hall jokes, and he feared for his reputation.[12] At the end of the year young Dean, having failed to convince his father of the new direction, established his own company at 82 Hatton Garden.

ALFRED ERNEST DEAN (1866–1927) was a dedicated businessman who within eight years claimed to be the largest maker of x-ray apparatus in Britain. He had an eye for the market, and was soon the contractor to the War Office, India Office and Admiralty, as well as an exporter. Fluent in German and a frequent visitor abroad, he kept abreast of developments in apparatus design on the Continent. In the middle of 1897 he sold Surgeon-Major Beevor the prototype of his 'Portable or Field Service' apparatus for use in India, and later he supplied it to the British Army, see Chapter 10. Dean is also said to have marketed the first 'Ward Outfit', mobile x-ray apparatus for use by the bedside or in the operating theatre.[63]

Alfred Dean's greatest contribution to British radiological practice was the introduction of protective lead glass, the first being installed at the London Hospital in 1909, see Chapter 5.[35] This was an ironic feat, for Dean was himself a victim of radiation disease and subsequently had a finger amputated. He died of his injuries in 1927 and his name was added to the Martyrs' Memorial in Hamburg with other British names in the 1950s.[61]

GERALD PETER DEAN (1896–1976) joined his father in 1916. He worked in all departments – tubes, coil winding, assembly testing, final inspection, sales and service, and after 1927 as the managing director he proved himself to be a shrewd administrator. He was a life-long member of the Röntgen Society and British Institute of Radiology, serving as the vice-president in 1965. Gerald Dean retired in that year after completing a half century in the Company, and establishing a unique father-and-son partnership of 70 years in the manufacture of x-ray apparatus.[63]

The Deans gained a reputation for meticulous craftsmanship and reliability that earned their products praise as 'the Rolls Royces of x-ray apparatus'. Alfred Dean was the driving force in the early years. In 1898, after scarcely two years of manufacturing, he issued an illustrated 32-page prospectus of apparatus.[12] A 'complete installation' including six tubes cost £190, and a smaller complete unit £24! A wide range of vacuum tubes was produced, and Ernest Harnack, the radiographer of the London Hospital, contributed a section on their care.[24]

Alfred Dean's original tube-maker in 1896 was probably H. J. B. Aimer (1879–1951), the co-founder with his brother in 1904 of Aimer Brothers, later Aimer Products Limited, of Camden Road, London. Like Dean, Herbert Aimer was severely burned and eventually succumbed to his injuries, being commemorated after his death on the Martyrs' Memorial in Hamburg.[61]

As A. E. Dean and Company prospered, it outgrew the original Hatton Garden office and acquired other factory premises, first in High Holborn and then in 1939 at Waddon near Croydon. The remaining London office was destroyed by a German bomb in 1940: thereafter the Company made its headquarters at Croydon. After the Second World War, Gerald Dean invited the brilliant Australian engineer, John Caldwell (see below) to join the firm, and Caldwell succeeded him as managing director. In 1969 the Company was absorbed by the General Electric Company Limited and the name A. E. Dean and Company disappeared.

W. WATSON AND SONS, AFTER 1915 WATSON AND SONS (ELECTRO-MEDICAL)

The third company to start manufacturing x-ray apparatus in 1896 and which was to survive beyond the Second World War was Watson and Sons of High Holborn. Founded by William Watson in 1837, it made microscopes and other scientific apparatus, and by 1898 had won over 40 gold medals and other awards for excellence and achievement. The Company advertised as 'Opticians and Electricians to the British and Foreign Governments'. In the middle of 1896 Watson began to produce x-ray equipment, and within twelve months offered a wide range of items including a complete set. This set was 'Watson's Hospital Outfit', comprising a 10-inch spark coil, 12-volt accumulator, rheostat, three gas tubes and a fluorescent screen, complete in a strong case, for £53 2s 9d. The 'Penetrator', the top tube of the range, sold to the United States Army Medical Department at 35 shillings each ($8.75)! 'Mr. Campbell-Swinton's adjustable cathode tube' retailed at the same price. 'Dr. Hedley's Portable Localiser and Tube Holder' required no calculations and came with instructions for use, cost 30 shillings.

The apparatus was produced on the Company's premises at 313 High Holborn, where the x-ray department was lodged in a basement at the rear of the building. In 1903 when one of the young apprentices was Cuthbert Andrews (see below), Wimshurst machines were still being built, although the 10-inch spark induction coil was beginning to sell well. The demand from doctors for x-ray apparatus was then just beginning.[64]

Watson and Sons early established a name not only as a manufacturer of electromedical equipment but as an importer. For many years the firm represented the German manufacturers, Koch and Sterzel in Britain and imported Müller x-ray tubes, radiological contrast medium and other accessories. An early contract secured the company the franchise for radium from the Anglo-Belgian Mining Corporation in the Belgian Congo, and for several decades all radium applicators used in Britain and the Empire (except Canada) were produced by Watson and Sons.[35]

In 1915 a new company, Watson and Sons (Electro-Medical) Limited, was established under the dual directorship of C. H. Watson, who had successfully extended the traditional optical interests of the Company to enter the electromedical field, and Geoffrey Pearce.

GEOFFREY PEARCE, F.R.P.S. (died 1949) was an early convert to the new science. Cuthbert Andrews on Pearce's death recalled the apprenticeship they shared in the High Holborn factory in 1903. At that time, Andrews was still 'a microscope man', but Pearce was already energising Müller tubes with the Company's new induction coils.[65] By 1909 he was a director of Watson and Sons, and for the rest of his life the Company remained his sole interest. For many years all the radium used in the British Empire passed through his hands.

Geoffrey Pearce joined the Röntgen Society in 1905 and made several technical contributions at meetings on the reduction of exposure times.[66] He was elected an Honorary Member of the British Institute of Radiology in 1929 – the first (and one of the few) British apparatus makers to be so honoured.

In 1918 Watson and Sons was acquired by the General Electric Company of England – the first x-ray company to be swallowed up by a giant corporation. A large new factory was built in East Lane, North Wembley, and all manufacturing was concentrated there. The sales office remained in Sunic House, Kingsway, Holborn, retaining the original telegraphic address of 1896, 'Skiagram, London', and continuing to trade under the old name. By the 1930s the Company was the largest British manufacturer of x-ray equipment, a position maintained after the amalgamation with A. E. Dean and Company under the umbrella of the General Electric Company, when the name Watson and Sons (Electro-Medical) disappeared.

A great measure of the success of the Company after 1930 is ascribed to the brilliant Australian designer, John Caldwell (1903–70) – a man who, it is said,[63] altered the face of the British x-ray industry. Caldwell had charge of a small x-ray factory in Melbourne in 1936 when invited by the Chairman of the General Electric Company to join Watson and Sons. He modernised the administration, introducing innovations such as viable costing systems and a spare parts service, as well as radically improving design. Caldwell first motorised tilting tables for fluoroscopy and mobile units, and reshaped control desks. In 1948 he returned to Australia but, as mentioned above, he later took charge of A. E. Dean and Company. Geoffrey Pearce's mantle in the Company fell upon A. J. Minns (died 1974), a man like Pearce who joined as a young apprentice and stayed to serve all his life. In 1944 he was chief engineer, then for many years managing director, dying soon after his retirement.[67]

HARRY W. COX LIMITED

A 26-year-old London electrician Harry Cox, began manufacturing x-ray tubes and apparatus in 1896. Several years later he established his own company in Rosebery Avenue, later at 47 Gray's Inn Road, He regularly advertised his products in the radiological journals, using the line 'Actual Makers of X-Ray and Electro-Medical Apparatus'. A catalogue issued in 1905 showed a full range of items including couches and complete sets, and it confirmed his position as a leading supplier. He also imported German apparatus, and it was Cox's entry of the Müller gas tube which won the gold medal of the Röntgen Society in the competition for best design in 1901.[68]

Harry Cox and his works manager, F. R. Butt, were early radiation victims. They personally made the apparatus – without, it is said,[61] care or knowledge of protection. Until 1906 the gas tubes were tested for sharpness by holding a bare hand in front of the screen, and the focus was adjusted by holding up a lead pencil. Cox was invalided in 1908 and then ceased to manufacture apparatus. However, he continued to sell imported equipment until 1919 when he amalgamated his firm with the Cavendish Electrical Company, see below.

HAROLD WILLIAM COX was one of the first x-ray engineers to succumb to radiation damage, and his plight caused national concern.

For biography, see page 224.

FREDERICK R. BUTT AND COMPANY LIMITED

Established in 1908 at 147 Wardour Street, Frederick Butt within ten years built up a successful business. Until 1912 he was in partnership with Frank William Read (1880–1938), an x-ray engineer who died of aplastic anaemia after undergoing repeated skin transplants for radiation burns; his name is recorded on the Martyrs' Memorial.[61] In 1915 Butt's son, Freddy T. Butt, joined the Company. Manufacturing flourished, and in the following year the Butts issued a 148-page catalogue illustrating a wide range of apparatus, tubes and accessories.[69] Their military field sets sold well and after the War Butt's x-ray couches were popular.[70] They ceased to manufacture complete sets in 1948 but the Company continued to trade as a family business.

FREDERICK ROLAND BUTT (1877–1937), originally apprenticed to Harry W. Cox and his designer and planner, invented several pieces of apparatus, such as a device to prevent the passage of inverse current through the x-ray tube.[71]

In the early 1930s Butt's radiation injuries to his hands and chest began to cause pain; several fingers were amputated and eventually his left arm, and he finally died of disseminated cancer. In the 1950s his name was added to the British list on the Martyrs' Memorial.

A. C. Cossor

One of the earliest suppliers of gas tubes was A. C. Cossor who had his workshop at 54 Farrington Street, London (*see* 35). He was a founder member of the Röntgen Society and demonstrated a tube with an osmium anode at the *conversazione* in November 1897; and in the following year this tube was used by MacKenzie Davidson at Charing Cross Hospital to demonstrate kidney stones.[72] Cossor supplied gas tubes to many of the x-ray

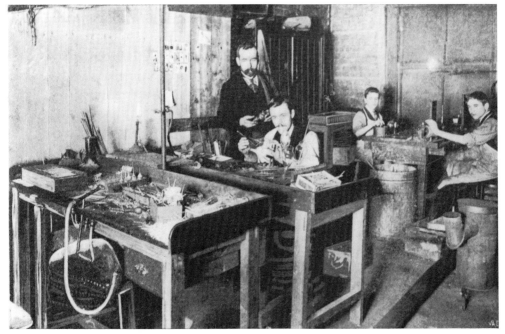

35. *Mr. Cossor's workshop in Farringdon Street, London in 1896, showing the glassblower at work. In the foreground A. C. Cossor stands beside his assistant, Mr. Hilliar, who was the first British radiation martyr*

pioneers, notably Sir William Crookes, Archibald Campbell Swinton and Colonel Gifford of Chard, and he made the three tubes which Surgeon-Major Beevor used during the Tirah Campaign in India in 1897–8, see Chapter 10. The photograph of Cossor's workshop which appeared in *The Windsor Magazine* in 1896 was taken during the early weeks of February of that year.[73] Next to Cossor in the picture is his chief assistant, Mr. Hilliar, who made the gas tubes. Hilliar is said to have been the first British victim of x-rays, dying of his injuries in 1902 or 1903 and being recorded among the British names on the Martyrs' Memorial.[61]

MILLER AND WOODS

Leslie Miller, A.M.I.E.E. was a frequent contributor of ideas of apparatus at meetings of the Röntgen Society, of which he was an early member.[64] His firm of manufacturing electricians in Gray's Inn Road made and supplied all the x-ray apparatus taken to Greece by Francis Abbott in 1897 as well as early kits for the larger London hospitals. In 1909 he wrote a book entitled '*Röntgen Ray Wrinkles*'.

A. W. ISENTHAL

A founder and loyal supporter of the Röntgen Society as well as a Council member in the early days, A. W. Isenthal, F.R.P.S. of 85 Mortimer Street, London was an early supplier of x-ray equipment. At the 1898 *conversazione* he exhibited 'a complete hospital outfit'. Isenthal spoke German (possibly he was an immigrant) and frequently visited the Continent. In May 1898 he was at Würzburg, returning with Professor Röntgen's fraternal greetings to the Society, and on other occasions he described developments in apparatus in Germany.[75,76] In 1898 he was the co-author of one of the earliest x-ray books, *Practical Radiography* with another enthusiast of the new photography, H. Snowden Ward. Half a century later in 1954 near the end of his very long life, A. W. Isenthal was elected an Honorary Member of the British Institute of Radiology.

SANITAS ELECTRICAL COMPANY

In 1902 two Germans, Willi Schwedler and Arthur Strich established a medical supplies company in Soho Square, London which sold x-ray apparatus. For ten years business grew and flourished, and an illustrated catalogue of 1910 advertised a range of equipment both locally made and imported from Germany. One local product, the Shenton–Sanitas Couch for screening and radiography was installed in hospitals in Glasgow and Edinburgh and at Guy's Hospital. In 1915 the Company was closed down under the Enemy Trading Act. The sales manager, Alfred Robert Winterson (1893–1922) then founded with E. H. Willis the Cavendish Electrical Company to build physical therapy equipment. In 1919 Cavendish amalgamated with Harry W. Cox to form the Cox–Cavendish Electrical Company Limited, with showrooms at 105 Great Portland Street and a factory at the Twyford Abbey Works, Harlesden. Winterson was only 36, and died three years later of radiation cancer after amputation of a hand and arm.[61] Cox–Cavendish ceased trading in 1922.

KARL SCHALL AND SCHALL AND SON, LATER SOLUS–SCHALL LIMITED

Karl Schall (died 1925) was a German instrument-maker who founded a company in Wigmore Street, London. He was one of three partners of a firm, Reiniger, Gebbert and Schall, in Erlangen, Germany, but decided to strike out on his own and settle in London in 1887. He employed as his works manager from 1893 to 1918 H. Rocky, the unusually gifted design engineer who later directed the firm, General Radiological Limited, see below. In 1913 Schall's son Willi joined him. Willi Schall, later a distinguished member of the British x-ray industry, formed his own company in 1925, Schall and Son Limited. He was an able engineer and his firm marketed high-quality products. He remained a leading supplier until 1931, and later the Second World War disrupted his markets. The company survived until 1946 when merged with the Solus Electrical Company as Solus–Schall Limited of 39 Welbeck Street.

WILLIAM E. SCHALL, Hon. F.S.R., B.Sc. (1888–1965) was a cultured, erudite and skilled man who was a familiar figure in x-ray circles in London for over 40 years; his spirited exchanges with Cuthbert Andrews at Institute meetings were long remembered. He was first elected to the Council of the Röntgen Society about 1914 and continued to serve almost continuously up to his death as the representative of the x-ray industry.[76]

Schall was active in many spheres connected with his Company. His book, *X-Rays, Their Origin, Dosage and Practical Application*, made him well known and he delivered several of the eponymous radiological lectures including the Silvanus Thompson Memorial Lecture in 1952. He was elected:

Member 1919, Treasurer 1956–65, Royal Institution
Founder Fellow, Institute of Physics, 1920
President, British Institute of Radiology, 1938–9
Honorary Fellow, Society of Radiographers, 1965.[77]

CUTHBERT ANDREWS

The Company started as a single-handed basement enterprise at 35 Hatton Garden in June 1910. Andrews was then aged 27, and had been allowed £100 credit by Müller to start his own business. He began to manufacture gas tubes, and this venture prospered until the First World War, when he was cut off from his Continental source of supply of soda glass. However, he persuaded the domestic glass-makers, Pilkingtons of Lancashire, to manufacture soda glass bulbs, and he was able to continue. For ten years after the war he was the only British maker of x-ray tubes. As the tubes grew larger, Andrews gave them appropriate names – the 'Mammoth' was followed in 1924 by 'Leviathan', the largest and last of the gas series. In 1928 he marketed his version of the Coolidge hot-cathode tube, and stopped producing gas tubes.

 Cuthbert Andrews moved his firm to Bushey Village, Hertfordshire in 1925, and his son, Richard, then joined the firm. For the next decade they manufactured a wide range of x-ray apparatus with great success, installing one complete set each week. Gradually this activity was given up, and in 1948 Andrews disposed of the tube manufacturing section of his company to General Radiological Limited. He once recalled that during the course of 38 years of manufacture, he had produced 30,000 tubes of 75 different types and ratings, ranging from early gas tubes to shock-free and line-focus tubes.

CUTHBERT ANDREWS, Hon. F.S.R. (1883–1972) owned one of the most successful and longest running small x-ray companies in Britain. He was a colourful personality, and when he died at the age of 90 years he was the *pater familias* of the British x-ray world.[35]

Born in Bloomsbury to the wife of a printer who died when he was young, he carried on the family business as a young man and became familiar with the technique of book production. His hobby and interest in botanical microscopy led him in 1904 to Watson and Sons, the leading microscope makers in High Holborn. The firm was then in the preliminary stages of their entry into the x-ray manufacturing business. Here he, Geoffrey Pearce, Arthur Gunstone and others in Watson's 'x-ray kindergarten' acquired the skill of radiography.[78]

The success of Cuthbert Andrews's business and his interest in x-ray affairs greatly benefitted the British Institute of Radiology, which he served as President in 1953–4 and of which he became an Honorary Member in 1956. He had joined the Röntgen Society in 1913 and was first elected to the Council in 1920, and thereafter he was continuously involved in its affairs. His counsel and advice in the 1950s led to the post-War modernisation of the Institute, starting with an alteration to the Memorandum and Rules which enabled income tax and rate rebates to be obtained and eventually the Royal Charter to be gained. He initiated the major reconstruction of the House in 1956–7 after negotiating a new 30-year lease until July 1984 at a modest rental, and he himself gifted the new seating in the Reid–Knox Hall. The 1962 edition of the Handbook, which embodied the Charter, was largely prepared by Andrews, his knowledge of printing and mastery of the English tongue contributing to its success.

Cuthbert Andrews had style. He covered his drive, hard work and determination with a good humour and ready wit which always brought a cheerful response. His passion for amateur theatricals and its rhetoric guided his life. Andrews was the brother of George Arliss, the famous actor, and modestly claimed himself as an effective contributor to the latter's success.[79]

After 1948 Cuthbert Andrews concentrated on establishing an efficient accessory business on mail-order lines, and the Company continued to flourish. Andrews's catalogues are collectors' pieces: Blue (1934), Orange (1939), Red (1952), Blue again (1955), Ivory (1958) and a 50-year anniversary Golden (1960) edition, called *Everything X-Ray*.

X-Rays Limited

This company in Gower Street, London was incorporated in 1919 with a capital of £75,000 derived, it is said,[35] from a potato merchant. Despite this large sum of money, financial problems beset its commercial operations, and it went into liquidation in 1932. However, two of its directors left constructive imprints on the industry. The first was Arthur Gunstone. The second Francis Owen-King, became a director of General Radiological Limited, see below.

ARTHUR CHARLES GUNSTONE (1889–1970) was a man of the x-ray industry rather than of one company. He was apprenticed to Watson and Sons of High Holborn in 1906 at the same time as Geoffrey Pearce and Cuthbert Andrews, and remained with the firm to design apparatus such as the 'Rectipulse' x-ray generator, a Snook-type rectifying device which he patented. From 1919 to 1925 he was associated with X-Rays Limited, and then left the company during one of the financial crises to establish with E. J. W. Watkinson a new company, the Solus Electrical Company of Judd Street (later Stanhope Street). Before Solus amalgamated with Schall in 1946, Gunstone moved to start his career with the Philips Electrical Company, which he served as technical adviser until he retired in 1959. He was a highly successful electrical design engineer despite his lack of higher technical education, and he personally knew Coolidge and Bouwers; 'a man of high integrity'.[80]

When he died aged 89, he was one of the three oldest members of the British Institute of radiology, having joined the Röntgen Society in 1913.

GENERAL RADIOLOGICAL AND SURGICAL APPARATUS COMPANY, LATER GR

This company was established in Great Portland Street, London in 1926 under unusual circumstances. Four years earlier, H. Rocky, the skilled instrument maker, obtained the franchise of Reiniger, Gebbert and Schall in Germany, who previously had marketed their products in England through a Swiss subsidiary. (Two of these names, Reiniger and Schall are familiar; the first in association with Siemens, and Schall is mentioned above.) Rocky became the first controlling director of General Radiological Limited, followed by Francis Owen-King, and later by Charles Rocky, his son.

H. ROCKY, A.I.M.E.E. (died 1943) was the unusually gifted and hard-working design engineer who for 25 years was Karl Schall's works manager. He is said to have been one of the first British engineers to appreciate the need for higher-quality construction of x-ray apparatus, and designed and built several of the earlier deep-therapy units. He was also one of the first to experiment with cascade high-tension transformers to produce high-voltage x-rays.[81]

The advent of the Second World War in 1939 saw General Radiological Limited pass into the hands of the Custodian of Enemy Property and into a state of near-suspended animation. This situation was partly relieved by the timely acquisition of drawings from Siemens by Rocky and his assistant, W. F. A. Kollibay, who had joined him from Germany in 1937 to help stimulate further expansion. After the War Kollibay launched Sierex Limited to carry the Siemens franchise and emerged as 'the only totally successful importer (of x-ray equipment) in the post-War years'.[35]

Chapter 5

EARLY X-RAY
DEPARTMENTS – I

THE MILLER, THE LONDON,
ST. BARTHOLOMEW'S, ST. THOMAS'S,
AND GUY'S HOSPITALS

Generally speaking, the first beginning of the x-ray department consisted of a cellar containing a small quantity of extremely elementary apparatus administered and controlled by some unqualified but clever men who had shown an aptitude for such work.

G. Allpress Simmons (1910)[1]

The first permanent x-ray units were acquired and installed in the more famous London hospitals between February and June of 1896 and immediately put into clinical use. A notable feature was the speed of this process, especially the prompt response with which doctors' requests were met by boards of management, hospital governors and other bodies responsible for paying for them. Some hospitals already possessed electro-therapeutic departments, and where they existed these departments were extended to incorporate the x-ray unit, and their staff were trained to operate it. Diagnostic and therapeutic x-rays at once became an additional clinical service of the electrical department.

Electrical treatment was itself the Cinderella of British medicine in 1895, in the days before hospitals had a mains supply. Electricity was utilised in the diagnosis of chronic injuries and to treat rheumatic and neurological disorders and a variety of skin lesions, notably lupus and rodent ulcer. Electric baths or hydrotherapy were popular as a mode of applying 'general electricization', a method prescribed in undiagnosed cases or for patients with debility or unexplained anaemia. Several leading hospitals in the 1890s, even before they were forced to meet the clinical demand for x-rays, appointed medical men to take charge of their electrical departments. All these doctors were of a similar type, combining scientific curiosity with a practical knowledge of electricity or photography. Usually the medical staff chose from among their colleagues the one most likely to be able to assess the value and validity of the various electrotherapeutic treatments then available. One of the first men to be styled 'Hospital Electrician' was Dr. W. E. Steavenson, who established the Electrical Department at St. Bartholomew's Hospital in 1882 and had charge of it until he died in 1891. His successor until his own retirement in 1912 was Dr. Lewis Jones, who expanded the Department early in 1896, to provide a diagnostic x-ray service in the Hospital; as we shall see later in this chapter.

THE MILLER HOSPITAL, GREENWICH

One of the earliest departments to open in a hospital in London – perhaps the first in Britain – was that in the Miller Hospital, Greenwich. Here Thomas Moore, senior surgeon to the Hospital, established an x-ray laboratory early in 1896 'soon after the publication of Röntgen's discovery'.[2]

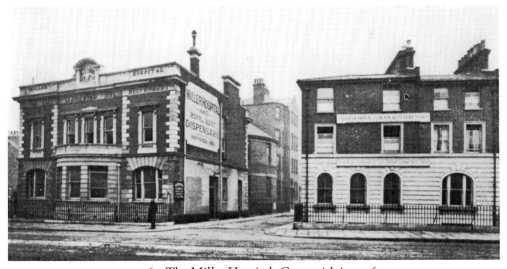

36. The Miller Hospital, Greenwich in 1906

Moore had his home in Lee Terrace, Blackheath, where a neighbour was the scientist William Webster, F.C.S. Like Sir William Crookes, Webster had experimented with vacuum tubes for over 20 years when the news of the discovery of x-rays reached England. In March 1896 he and Moore successfully made a radiograph of the fractured ribs of a child being treated in the Miller Hospital.[3] Other surgical x-rays followed and Moore, realising their clinical potential, persuaded the committee of the Hospital to install an apparatus. The partnership between Webster and Moore continued, more radiographs were made, and in October 1896 Webster developed a 'sunburn' of the skin of his right hand – one of the first instances of radiation dermatitis to be documented in Britain.[4] Webster was a founder member of the Röntgen Society.

THOMAS MOORE, F.R.C.S. (1838–1900) was an enthusiast for the new science. In addition to his pioneering work in the Miller Hospital, he served as the first Treasurer of the Röntgen

Society and for the three years up to his death as one of the early editors of the journal, *Archives of the Roentgen Ray*.

Thomas Moore was born at Halesowen, Worcestershire and trained at St. Bartholomew's Hospital, qualifying L.R.C.P. in 1865 and F.R.C.S. in 1867. For some years he practised at Petersfield, Hampshire, where he founded the Cottage Hospital. In 1880 he moved to Blackheath and joined the staff at the Miller Hospital as the surgeon. He was also consulting surgeon to the Brighton Children's Hospital.[5]

When he died, a memorial tablet was fixed to a wall in the Miller Hospital, which read: 'The X-ray Department in this hospital was founded in 1896 by Mr. Thomas Moore, F.R.C.S., Senior Surgeon. It was enlarged and refitted in 1901, the necessary funds being contributed by his friends as a tribute to his memory'.[6]

Moore's energy and pioneering zeal for radiology is reflected in the pages of the early volumes of the journal which he helped to edit. In 1897 he described and illustrated various cases, including a patient with a fracture of the olecranon process and another with obstruction of the oesophagus, which he had seen at the Hospital.[7] After the start of the South African War in 1899, Moore x-rayed war casualties on their return. Of one of these, an officer with a limb fracture, he produced a plate which showed excellent callus some months after the fracture had first been x-rayed at Wynberg Military Hospital, near Cape Town.[8]

In 1898 Moore invited another early pioneer to assist him at the Hospital, and this man expanded and continued the x-ray department after his death. He was John Jewell Vezey who, like Moore, was one of the first officers of the Röntgen Society and at one critical stage of its life, its mainstay, see Chapter 9. Vezey was a City businessman turned philanthropist-*cum*-amateur scientist. As the Hospital radiographer he was responsible for preparing the high-quality plates of Moore's patients which adorn the pages of the *Archives of the Roentgen Ray*.

On Moore's death Vezey and others contributed to the memorial fund which enabled the Miller Hospital to enlarge the x-ray department and equip it with more up-to-date apparatus. The apparatus, supplied by A. W. Isenthal and Company, consisted of a 12-inch coil with mercury interrupter, a couch for radiographic and screening work, 2 sets of 16-volt accumulators and a high-frequency apparatus. There were two sets of accumulators used for making mobile x-rays in the wards. Finally, the dark room was enlarged.[9] The local newspaper, in describing the newly-equipped x-ray department in October 1901, announced that Vezey was prepared to demonstrate the apparatus to visitors. He remained the 'honorary superintendent' for over five years, attending the Hospital each day to carry out his unpaid duties, until in 1906 he collapsed and died in the Department while examining a patient.[10]

Another personality was John Poland, F.R.C.S., orthopaedic surgeon and historian of the Hospital, and the author in 1898 of a book entitled *Traumatic Separation of the Epiphyses*.[11] This book was one of the first medical texts in which radiographs were used to illustrate the subject. It contained 45 plates, many of which were made at the Miller Hospital and most of which were demonstrated at the first *conversazione* of the Röntgen Society held in London in the Autumn of 1897.[12]

THE LONDON HOSPITAL

X-rays were introduced to the Hospital early in 1896 by W. S. Hedley, a retired Army medical officer who already had charge of the Electrotherapeutic Department. In that year Ernest Harnack was appointed as his non-medical assistant, and together they built up and began to provide an x-ray service to the outpatient department and clinicians of the Hospital. It was one of the first in the country.

WILLIAM SNOWDON HEDLEY, M.D.Edinburgh, M.R.C.S. (1841–1930) devoted a decade of his retirement to publicising and implementing Röntgen's discovery, and thereby ensured his place as one of the small band of true pioneers of British radiology.[13]

Educated at Edinburgh University, Hedley entered the Army upon qualifying in 1863. He served as an Army surgeon for nearly 30 years, in 1885 in the Sudan and then in the Nile Expedition, having charge of a field hospital. Thereafter he went to the London Hospital, where his presence as Head of the Electrical Department during the formative years of radiology enabled him to assist decisively in its gestation.

In April 1896 he contributed x-ray cases to the first issue of the new journal *Archives of Clinical Skiagraphy*, and in July 1897 after the name of the journal altered to *Archives of the Roentgen Ray*, he joined Sydney Rowland as co-editor. In 1900 when British electrotherapeutists started their own publication, *The Journal of Physical Therapeutics*, Hedley became its first editor, see Chapter 8.[14] He was the author of several books on the medical applications of electricity, and his frequent contributions of case material during 1897–1900 reflect the activity and high quality of the early x-ray work at the London Hospital. On the page-sized radiographs illustrating pathological conditions, Hedley always credited his 'Assistant', Ernest Harnack.

When in June 1903 the new outpatient wing which included a much-expanded Electrotherapeutic Department was opened and Reginald Morton was given charge of the Department, Hedley retired. When he died a quarter of a century later aged 89 years, an obituary notice in the *British Medical Journal* recalled at some length his army experience, but failed to mention his association with the London Hospital or his seminal contribution to introducing x-rays into clinical use in Britain![15]

Hedley and Harnack were practical men with military ability to organise, and their efforts after 1896 to establish an x-ray service in the Hospital recruited powerful allies among the clinical staff. A surgeon of the Hospital, C. W. Mansell-Moullin, was a particularly enthusiastic supporter of the new photography. He was one of the established leaders of the medical profession in London at that time, and his may have been the decisive influence behind its introduction at the London Hospital. Mansell-Moullin succeeded Silvanus Thompson as President of the Röntgen Society and later helped to edit the *Archives of the Roentgen Ray*, see Chapter 8.

Hedley collaborated with MacKenzie Davidson to devise his cross-thread device for localising foreign bodies which, although acclaimed,[16] was found by Barclay 'in a well-dusted and polished mahogany box . . . I doubt if it had ever been used or that any who worked in the department knew how to use it'.[17] Hedley also designed an obscure device of those early days, a reflecting stereoscope, which was praised when demonstrated to the Royal Society in May 1898.[18] On a more practical level, he and Harnack equipped the Department and probably helped to build the original apparatus. Harnack designed one of the first tables, the Harnack–Dean Couch, with tubes placed above and beneath it, for examining patients.[19] An early photograph of Ernest Harnack

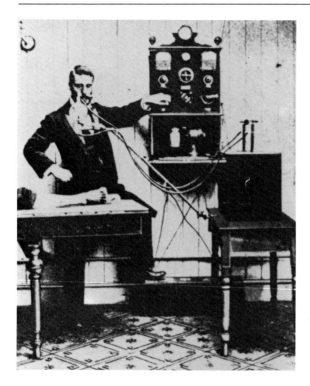

37. Ernest Harnack radiographing a patient's ankle at the London Hospital. He is using the portable military x-ray kit marketed by A. E. Dean in 1898, see 66

x-raying the ankle of a patient shows the equipment initially used – a Rühmkorff coil standing on a table with the vacuum tube held in a clamp, the controls and interrupter on a wall panel behind. Unshielded wires make the circuit: Harnack wears no protective gloves or clothing and stands close to the tube.[20] Working practice of the Department remained unchanged for a long time, the operator first testing the output of the x-ray tube by screening his own hands, before positioning the patient for radiography. This practice ceased only in 1908 as a result of the radiographers' injuries.

A corner of the curtain covering these early days and the activity of Hedley and Harnack was lifted by one of the Hospital's medical students in 1900, who later himself illuminated British radiology – A. E. Barclay. 'For a clinical student' – he reminisced[17] – 'there was no contact with the rooms in which x-ray apparatus was installed. I doubt if we even knew where the apparatus was housed that sometimes provided one's chief with the glass plates that were so easily broken and on which were to be seen blurred and vague shadows of bones. Few of the surgeons yet fully trusted x-ray plates and I remember a very heated argument between two of the honoraries, one of whom was an enthusiast for their use, the other maintaining that his clinical examination was more reliable. . . . Sometimes, hopefully rather than expectantly, x-ray plates were asked for of the chest, kidneys, bladder, or even the spine. . . . For practical purposes, however, the x-ray diagnostic service was confined to fractures and the detection of metallic foreign bodies, particularly the many cases of needles in the hand that came from the tailoring trade of Whitechapel. . . .'

'It was in the attempts to remove these under x-ray guidance that, as an Accident Room Officer, I became familiar with the x-ray department (on the top floor of the Out Patient Department). Nobody suggested that there might be danger in these operations either to ourselves or to our patients. The x-ray tube was operated at full capacity all the time. Fortunately for us, that capacity was small, in the region of 0.5 mA for screening, but even so the strain on the tube was severe for it often gave out and had to be replaced or coaxed back to a suitable hardness. For this reason, these operations were not popular for it was a serious matter if one of the two or three tubes fit for service was put out of action. It might well mean that it would not be possible even to attempt the next chest case that might be sent up. Not infrequently the department went out of action because there was not a single one of the dozen tubes that could be coaxed from that blue fluorescence, indicating that the tube had gone soft, to that sharply defined and welcome green that denoted a tube that was emitting x-rays of the type we needed. . . . At the time I did not appreciate the anxiety of Mr. Harnack for the welfare of his beloved tubes. . . . Mr. Harnack was in charge of the Department and Mr. Suggars was his assistant. They both already suffered from severe dermatitis of the hands, while the hands of Mr. Wilson (another assistant) were so bad that he had been taken off all x-ray work and had been made clinical photographer to the Hospital.'

Ernest Harnack and his three assistants, Reginald Blackall, Ernest Wilson and Harold Suggars, were the pioneer British radiographers. They were the first to be appointed 'x-ray operators', the first to receive radiation injuries, and the first to die of x-ray cancer. By 1903 all four men suffered from severe dermatitis of the hands and several had undergone amputations. Wilson before that date had been withdrawn to serve as the Hospital's first clinical photographer. A few years later, Harnack too was invalided due to his severe radiation injuries. When 'Cappy' Barnard joined the staff in 1907, Harnack had retired and Suggars was chief of the diagnostic section.[20] Wilson's death in 1911 caused an uproar, see Chapter 11. Suggars and Blackall were less severely affected and continued to work for a decade or more; both were active in establishing the Society of Radiographers in the 1920s.

The plight of the four radiographers and particularly their frightful mutilation was a cautionary lesson to their colleagues and it remained impressed on the minds of the next generation of British radiologists,[21] hastening the statutory introduction of protective regulations in the 1920s. A memorial plaque was placed in a corridor of the London Hospital to commemorate them, and their names are recorded on the Martyrs' Memorial in Hamburg.[22]

By 1903 radiography had been integrated into the clinical life of the Hospital and the work of the Department had outgrown the original provisions.[19] In that year a new outpatient wing was opened by the King and Queen and a large part of the second floor of the building was newly equipped as an electrical department. About 4,000 x-ray exposures were made, but nearly 20,000 patients were seen. The majority of these patients attended for electrical treatment of skin lesions, and in 1903 the Department was divided into two parts.

Dr. James Sequeira, skin physician at the Hospital, was given charge of the first part, called 'Departments for the Treatment of Diseases of the Skin by Light and X-Rays'. Here Finsen lamps were used for treating cases of lupus – in the previous three years over 750 had been treated, mostly by Harold Suggars. X-rays were used for skin lesions such as rodent ulcers and ringworm. This treatment was applied by means of apparatus installed by A. E. Dean, a conventional vacuum tube powered by a 15-inch spark coil

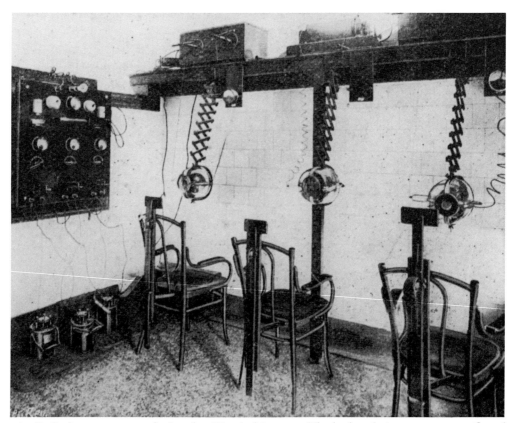

38. *Radiotherapy room at the London Hospital in 1905. The barber chair arrangement reflected
the main therapeutic use of x-rays at that time – ringworm of the scalp*

and a motor-driven dipper interrupter with an automatic cut-out serving as a primitive
dose regulator.[23]

The second part comprised the rest of the original Electrotherapeutic Department,
which was now concerned with utilising x-rays for medical diagnosis and treatment
other than skin lesions. The doctor appointed to take charge of this early department
of radiology remained, in the parlance of the day, an electrotherapeutist, but he was
to become one of the fathers of British radiotherapy – E. Reginald Morton.

EDWARD REGINALD MORTON, M.D., C.M.(Toronto), F.R.C.S.(Edinburgh) (ca 1865–
1944) succeeded Dr. Hedley as medical officer in charge of the Electrical Department when the
new department opened in 1903. He held the post for five years.

Born in Barrie, Ontario, and qualifying at the University of Toronto, Morton came to Britain
in 1891 to obtain the Scottish Triple Qualification and then took the Edinburgh F.R.C.S. After
helping in his father's practice in Canada for a while he returned to England and entered general
practice in Taunton. Here he pursued his hobby of electricity and – after Röntgen's discovery
became known – used x-rays in clinical work, until appointed to the London Hospital.[24]

Morton applied his great enthusiasm to all aspects of the department's work, but his main
interest was the treatment of patients. Consequently A. E. Barclay when his clinical assistant
in 1902–4, found himself responsible for all diagnostic work.[17] Morton – in common with col-

leagues such as Lewis Jones at St. Bartholomew's Hospital – correctly saw his duty as the Hospital's electrotherapist; the role of the diagnostic radiologist had yet to emerge.

He wrote two books, *Essentials of Medical Electricity* (1905) and *A Textbook of Radiology* (1915). For rest of biography, see page 109.

This pragmatic subdivision of the original Electrical Department was the first attempt in Britain to divorce the science of radiology from the world of water-baths, treatments with high-frequency and constant sinusoidal currents, and other mysteries. The treatment of inoperable malignancies with x-rays now commenced in the Hospital, a special room being set aside and details recorded in a case book.

The new diagnostic room, still presided over by Mr. Harnack (now called 'Chief Radiographer'), had a couch and Müller tubes energised by a 16-inch spark coil supplied by A. E. Dean. Mains electricity had reached the Hospital and current at 60 volts was delivered to it from a transformer mounted on the roof. A high-speed jet-brake could be put into circuit for screening by means of a two-way switch. Adjoining was a dark room suitable for processing x-ray plates and film, where the ailing radiographer, Edward Wilson practised his clinical photography.

Protective measures were slow to appear, despite the ever-present evidence of the hazards of radiation which Harnack and Wilson and their colleagues bore. But by 1908 some steps had been taken.[20] The radiographers no longer screened their hands before x-raying a patient, and a measuring device, a Bauer Qualimeter, was used to test the dose. The tube was encased in a lead-lined box, later in a lead-glass bowl with a protruding window of soda glass through which the x-ray beam could pass. Lead-lined cubicles with lead-glass windows were installed for x-ray therapy in 1909 – the first attempt in any hospital to protect the operator during treatment, see Chapter 11.

Until 1909 a ward patient requiring radiography faced a long journey down to the basement of the Hospital, through a tunnel under the road, and then up to the second floor of the outpatient department. It is true that a 'portable' set was available for emergencies on the wards – a battery of accumulators and a Müller tube mounted on a hospital trolley – but this primitive unit became increasingly unpopular with the radiographers because the tube had no protection at all. The only safety measure which they could adopt was to distance themselves from the tubing during the lengthy exposures.

These makeshift arrangements could not be endured indefinitely, and in 1909 a new department was established within the Hospital. Upon Dr. Morton's departure, Dr. Gilbert Scott was elected to take charge.

SEBASTIAN GILBERT SCOTT, M.R.C.S., L.R.C.P., D.M.R.E., F.F.R. (1879–1941) served the London Hospital for 21 years until 1930.

Scott was born into a family of architects – his grandfather and uncle were architects, his uncle being the celebrated Victorian, Sir Giles Gilbert Scott. He studied medicine at King's College Hospital, qualifying in 1904, and commenced his x-ray and electrotherapeutic work there as a clinical assistant to Dr. Archibald Reid.[25]

At the London Hospital, Scott became known for his enthusiasm for teaching diagnostic radiology to students preparing for the Cambridge Diploma, and for his unusual knowledge of skeletal lesions. In 1920–1 he served as President of the Electro-Therapeutical Section of the Royal Society of Medicine. He wrote two books, in 1931 *Radiology in Relation to Medical Jurispru-*

dence, and subsequently his Fellowship thesis *Radiological Atlas of Chronic Rheumatic Arthritis – The Hand* was published.

Dr. Scott was the first 'dedicated' radiologist of the Hospital – in the sense that he eschewed electrotherapeutics and confined his medical practice to x-ray work. Although his major interest was diagnostic radiology, he continued to treat patients with x-rays. Only on his retirement in 1930 was the first specialist radiotherapist appointed to the Hospital.

ST. BARTHOLOMEW'S HOSPITAL

X-rays were produced in the Hospital for diagnostic purposes within months of the announcement of Röntgen's discovery, and they were used to treat skin diseases before the end of 1896. As at the London Hospital, the new photography was made the responsibility of the Electrical Department, and the x-ray service was introduced as an appendage of Electrotherapeutics, sharing its space, staff and budget.

The Electrical Department was established in 1882 by Dr. W. E. Steavenson; it is said to have been the first in London to be fully equipped.[26] Dr. Steavenson's department was housed in the grounds of the Hospital in a disused lecture theatre which was divided internally by wooden partitions into rooms or compartments and lighted by a large central skylight. In 1905 there were six rooms in use – a waiting room, an examination room, an electrical bathroom, two rooms for electrical treatment, and an x-ray room. The basement had been converted for the treatment of lupus by light rays, for use as a workshop and a photographic dark room, and for housing the generator which supplied the Department with direct current.

Electric light mains carrying alternating current reached the Hospital in 1894, and the whole department was wired with sockets in each room, through which different voltages could be supplied by means of a transformer. The arrival of mains electricity in the Electrical Department, momentous as this event must have been, was soon overshadowed by a far more important development in electrotherapy – the discovery of x-rays.

The Hospital possesses Volume XXV of a register of 213 patients who were x-rayed between 1 June 1896 and 12 June 1897.[27] On page 1 there is inscribed: 'A few x-ray cases are entered in Volume XX at or near the end of the Volume. The apparatus set up for the Hospital's use commences with this book and at this date June 1 '96.' Unfortunately, the previous volume, recording the earlier radiography at the Hospital, is missing.

The position in 1896 was vividly recalled a decade later by the then head of the department, Dr. Lewis Jones, who succeeded Dr. Steavenson on the latter's death in 1891. '(The discovery of x-rays) at once opened up an unlimited amount of fresh work, and systematic x-ray work for the Hospital was definitely commenced in the electrical department in 1896. Those who were working with x-rays in those early days will not only remember the great interest which was excited among medical men by the discovery of x-rays, but will also recollect the great difficulties experienced at that time in meeting the ever-increasing demands of the surgeons for x-ray pictures of their cases. No sooner were these pioneers able to produce pictures of needles in the hands and feet than they were confronted with requests for photographs of knees, hip-joints, and renal calculi. While they wrestled with 20-minute exposures, and plates which on development often revealed nothing but gradations of misty fog, their efforts received but little thanks or appreciation. . . .'[26]

H. LEWIS JONES, M.A., M.D., F.R.C.P. (1857–1915) is the father of British electro-therapeutics. He introduced x-rays to St. Bartholomew's Hospital in the early months of 1896 and actively encouraged his assistant Hugh Walsham and others to establish a diagnostic and therapeutic service in the early years.

Born at Sheerness to the wife of a Naval chaplain, Lewis Jones won a scholarship from Shrewsbury to Cambridge and then to St. Bartholomew's Hospital. He qualified in 1881, and held several posts in the Hospital – demonstrator in physiology and casualty physician – before being chosen as medical officer in charge of the Electrical Department in 1891.

As soon as Lewis Jones went to Bart's, it was written in his obituary,[28] electrotherapy took an upward trend. Thanks chiefly to the introduction of x-rays, the Electrical Department assumed a greater importance in the Hospital, and his high professional reputation made him the leader of his specialty in the country. He was one of the founders and first President of the British Electrotherapeutic Society – the forerunner of the Electro-Therapeutical Section of the Royal Society of Medicine and he was the founder chairman of the Electrotherapeutic Section of the British Medical Association in 1904.

Lewis Jones's book, *Medical Electricity*, was a standard text of which six editions were printed. He joined the Röntgen Society in 1898 and took a lead in publicising the new science. In March 1900 he described his work at the Hospital in an important address to the Institute of Electrical Engineers:[29] he told them that x-rays were in daily surgical use including MacKenzie Davidson's stereoscopic foreign-body localiser, and that their use enabled physicians to diagnose lung tuberculosis at an earlier stage than with the stethoscope. Three months later the Röntgen Society met at St. Bartholomew's Hospital at Lewis Jones's invitation, to examine the Holtz type of influence machine recently installed in his Department.

Thereafter until ill-health obliged him to retire prematurely in 1912, Lewis Jones remained in the forefront of his specialty. Although not by inclination a radiologist, he contributed a number of cases to the early numbers of the *Archives of the Roentgen Ray*, and he is credited with first describing the association between cervical rib and atrophy of the intrinsic muscles of the hand.[29]

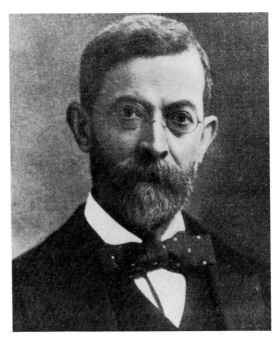

39. H. Lewis Jones

The demand for x-rays in the Hospital increased by leaps and bounds. From a total of 213 patients in the first year of operation (1896–7), it rose to over 1200 in six years. 'The Department is probably destined in a very few years to become the largest of all the special departments in the Hospital', Dr. Jones predicted in 1906.[26] Soon afterwards he re-organised the Department to meet the fresh demand, establishing a separate department for skin diseases and re-equipping the electrical department. A South American visitor to the Hospital in 1909 found Lewis Jones completely occupied with hydrotherapy, ionic treatment, electrodiagnosis and muscle testing, and the x-ray department under the care of Dr. Hugh Walsham.[30] There were two sets for diagnosis, Miller coils with Drault gas-breaks that could be operated at a distance of 2 metres, and two sets for radiotherapy.

HUGH WALSHAM, M.A., M.D., F.R.C.P., F.R. Astronomical S. (1856–1924) was the pioneer radiologist at St. Bartholomew's Hospital. Appointed for this purpose in 1896, he remained the departmental assistant for 16 years. When Lewis Jones retired, the x-ray division was separated from the Electrical Department, and Walsham was elected the first Radiologist of the Hospital, a post he held for five years before being forced to retire through ill-health. It is said that as early as 1901 the skin of his hands had broken down, and later fingers were amputated; eventually he abandoned all x-ray work. Walsham is one of the original 14 British martyrs whose names are recorded in Hamburg.

Born in Wisbech, Cambridgeshire as the younger brother of W. F. Walsham, who became a Surgeon to St. Bartholomew's Hospital, Hugh Walsham was educated at Caius College, Cambridge and St. Bartholomew's Hospital, qualifying in 1887. In 1894 he was elected to the staff of the City Hospital for the Diseases of the Chest, Victoria Park, first as the pathologist and two years later as the physician of the outpatient department. Simultaneously he became Lewis Jones's assistant at St. Bartholomew's Hospital. Thus he commenced a practice of two decades as the first chest radiologist in the world.[31]

Walsham in the early days of experimentation, when most pioneers were occupied with x-raying extremities and foreign bodies, was one of the first to realise the potential of the new rays in the diagnosis of diseases of the chest and great vessels. 'The amount of time and the energy which (he) put into his early work is legendary – seeing outpatients at Victoria Park and screening them himself, then spending the afternoon in an ill-ventilated little wooden hut in the electrical department using x-rays to treat and diagnose patients. . . .'[32] In 1899 he showed that pulmonary tuberculosis could be detected earlier with radiographs than by conventional physical examination, and its prognosis more accurately given. The publication of a succession of cases – cavitation, pneumonia, oesophageal cancer, aneurysm of the aorta – established Walsham as a chest specialist.[33] In recognition he was elected a Fellow and awarded a prize by the Royal College of Physicians a few years later. In 1906 he wrote with G. Harrison Orton, *The Röntgen Rays in the Diagnosis of Diseases of the Chest*, which is said to have been the first book to be published on the subject.

Walsham was a retiring man, a reluctant communicator who eschewed medical meetings, and when he died he was almost unknown to the younger generation of radiologists.

ST. THOMAS'S HOSPITAL

Stanley Kent's lecture before the Medical and Physical Society at St. Thomas's Hospital on 13 February 1896 is believed to have been the first practical demonstration of the new photography in a London hospital. He gave a brief description of the mode of production of x-rays and of the various vacuum tubes, and then made several x-ray exposures. One of the volunteer 'patients' was a medical student with a healed fracture of the head of the fifth metacarpal bone. Nearly a half-century later the student, then a middle-aged country practitioner, returned the faded print of his fractured hand for safe-keeping, as the first x-ray ever made in the Hospital.[34]

This early date may be taken as the day on which the clinical x-ray service commenced in the Hospital, because over the next three months Stanley Kent turned his success into a practical reality. 'Since the demonstration (in February)' – it was reported in the May number of the Hospital's *Gazette*[35] – 'Mr. Stanley Kent has been able by means of improved apparatus, greatly to simplify the process and to obtain photographs of deeply-seated organs of the body, the spine, showing details of vertebrae, the pelvic bones, etc. These advances have been chiefly due to the introduction of a new kind of Crookes tube (known as the "focus" tube) designed by Mr. Jackson of King's College, and manufactured by Mr. Müller. So greatly superior to the old form is this tube, that cases which it was formerly impossible to photograph in half-an-hour, are now easily accomplished in 5 minutes. . . .'

Later in 1896 provision was made for x-raying patients in the Hospital, in that part of the basement which was immediately underneath the existing Electrical Room. The original registers indicate that the Department opened and the first patient was examined on 16 October. However, by that date many radiographs had been made, and the greater significance of the opening is the fact that this Department may have been the first Hospital x-ray department. 'As far as one has been able to ascertain' – claimed the reporter in the Hospital's *Gazette* in 1897[36] – 'this special department was the first to be established in a hospital and was fitted up for the sole object of utilising the x-rays in the examination of cases.'

This early x-ray department consisted of three rooms and the basement corridor outside. Patients waited in the corridor. They were prepared in the first room which was lighted by an incandescent gas lamp which also served for making bromide prints. The second room, the x-ray laboratory, was described in the *Gazette*. 'The examination room is very conveniently fitted and everything has been done to make the greatest use of the space available. Shelves around the room at the level of the top of the doors give good accommodation for drying the photographic plates and storing the negatives. The window can easily be closed with a shutter, so that it is possible to work with the fluorescent screen in comfort and without crushing, many being able to see the shadow at the same time. There are electric wall plugs and gas connections for Bunsen burners so placed as to be available in any part of the room. A large table occupies the space in front of the window, the height being arranged so as to allow the couch (which can be raised at either end and is provided with rollers which move at the slightest touch) to be placed beneath it out of the way. This table also allows for the beds from the wards on which the patients are brought down in the lift, to be run directly into the room and immediately beneath the vacuum tube which is attached to a movable arm fixed to the edge of the table, so that the patient is not disturbed from the time when he leaves the ward until he returns.

'The apparatus consists of 2 large coils giving a 6 to 8 inch and 10 to 12 inch spark in air respectively; the larger one is fixed to the table, and the smaller one is on a movable stand, arranged to hold all the apparatus necessary, so that if it is essential 2 patients can be examined at the same time, or both coils can be used on the same case at the same time, the whole stand and apparatus moving with the greatest ease on large casters. These coils are worked by 3 large accumulators which are charged in turn.

'The Tesla coil is worked from the mains and is also situated on the shelf in front of the window. Tubes in various degrees of exhaustion are kept always ready, so as to have some in the proper condition for meeting every requirement for the examination of the different tissues.'

The third room was fitted out for developing the plates, a photographic dark room, complete with lead-covered draining surfaces, glazed sinks, a hypobath – 'What more could the heart of man desire?' the anonymous reporter asked. Then he answered the question himself, perhaps unwittingly, by describing the fuel gas stove in the corner of the room – an essential item of equipment in those early days, for heating the vacuum tubes to soften them!

The anonymous correspondent of the *Gazette* can be identified by his enthusiasm and his distinctive turn of phrase as Barry Blacker, a pioneer radiologist who was also the first British medical casualty of the new rays.

ARTHUR BARRY BLACKER, M.D., B.S., L.R.C.P., M.R.C.S. (died 1902) established the x-ray department in St. Thomas's Hospital and had charge of it up to his death from radiation cancer.

Blacker studied at St. Thomas's Hospital and graduated M.B. from the University of Durham in 1885 and M.D. in 1890. In the opening months of 1896 he was an assistant to Dr. Hedley at St. Bartholomew's Hospital, during the period when x-rays were introduced in the Electrical Department,[26] and he accepted the post of 'Superintendent of the X-ray Department' at St. Thomas's Hospital when the Department opened later that year. He also attended the Brompton Hospital for Consumption in the same capacity. He was an early member of the Röntgen Society, and served on its Council, attending and contributing frequently at meetings.[37]

In 1897 Blacker selected and personally tested the x-ray apparatus for the British Red Cross medical team serving with the Greeks in the Graeco-Turkish War. When the South African War started two years later, one of his technical assistants, Henry Catlin, volunteered for service and in 1900 he forwarded a report from Catlin to the Editor of the *Archives of the Roentgen Ray* for publication, see Chapter 10.[38]

Barry Blacker by the mode of his death came to be even more widely known to the new young profession that he had been in life. Severe x-ray dermatitis had early befallen him, and in 1902 he perished of an axillary cancer. Twenty-five years later the way of his dying had still not been forgotten.[21] His name is recorded incorrectly on the Martyrs' Memorial in Hamburg as 'Blacken'.[39]

The young Department seems to have found immediate acceptance as an established clinical service. In 1897, the first full working year, 416 patients were x-rayed, of whom 114 were inpatients. The following extracts from the original register illustrate the type of work done and the long exposure times then required to obtain satisfactory results:

Case No. 1. 16.10.96. Fracture of right leg – bicycle accident. Result: fracture shown; four-inch spark gap, 15 minute exposure.

Case No. 2. 16.10.96. Examination to show a bullet wound from an air gun in the head. No details are given but apparently the bullet was successfully shown on two glass plates.

Case No. 18. 26.11.96. Mention is made of the first screening examination of the heart, but no comments are made in the register.

Case No. 19. 27.11.96. Thimble in abdomen. Seen on a glass plate after an exposure of 35 minutes.

Case No. 41. 11.12.96. Left elbow. Bullet wound received at Krugersdorf (*sic*).

Case No. 48. 8.1.97. Patient was screened for the presence of a pin in the throat. The pin was seen on screening but the plate, with half-hour exposure, did not show it.

Case No. 91. 26.3.97. Tumour of radius. Reported as a possible ossifying sarcoma.

After Blacker's death Dr. Arthur H. Greg, F.R.C.S., was appointed, and he had charge of the X-ray Department until 1911 when he resigned. Another arrival in the Department at this time who, however, remained there for the rest of his working life was Cyrus Luther Winch (1881–1958). He was appointed as Dr. Blacker's technical assistant in 1901, and remained radiographer of the Hospital until he retired in 1933. He was a founder member of the Society of Radiographers, and President of the Society shortly before his death.[40] The later years of Dr. Greg's term as radiologist saw the original basement department overwhelmed by a steep rise in the demand for diagnostic x-rays:

1897 – 416	1912 – 6475
1908 – 797	1913 – 6501
1901 – 1253	

The Department moved to a new site in 1909. When Dr. (later Sir) Archibald Reid succeeded Dr. Greg at the beginning of 1912, he wrote:[41] 'The Department possessed in the way of apparatus two Miller induction coils, one 12-inch for radiography and the other 10-inch for treatment, a simple tube stand (which at first offered no protection to the operator, but afterwards a lead glass bowl was used to enclose the tube), and a small hand screen. The coil was used from a 65-volt direct current motor generator, the latter being derived from the alternating current mains, and the greatest output it was capable of was about $1\frac{1}{2}$ mA through a medium vacuum tube. Practically no radiographical examinations of the chest and abdomen were done during that period. There was very little x-ray treatment and even that was of a very rough-and-ready description.'

SIR ARCHIBALD DOUGLAS REID, K.B.E., C.M.G., M.R.C.S., L.R.C.P., D.M.R.E. (1871–1924), the eminent British radiologist, moved from King's College Hospital to become Radiologist of St. Thomas's Hospital at the age of 41 years, and he remained there up to his death 12 years later. His first year there saw a 12-fold increase in the number of patients examined, compared with the number seen in 1897, and the pattern of the modern department was soon established.

For rest of biography, see pages 95 and 186.

The X-ray Department of St. Thomas's Hospital in 1912 was one of the most complete and advanced in Britain. Reid re-organised it when he went there, and he described his changes to his colleagues when the Electro-Therapeutical Section of the Royal Society of Medicine visited it in January 1914: 'The original large room set apart for radiography has been divided into two, the largest half being equipped with a modern 16-inch coil worked from the direct-current mains at 220 volts by means of an elaborate switchboard. The tube is now enclosed by an ample protection shield capable of taking compressor diaphragms of various sizes and fitted with a stereoscopic and self-centring plate-board capable of being used underneath a special X-ray couch when necessary. The whole of this apparatus has been designed so that ward patients can be sent down to the Department in their beds, and the bed being wheeled under the compressor, negatives can be taken of most parts of the body with the minimum of discomfort and inconvenience to the patient. The smaller room has been made light-tight, and contains an elaborate screening apparatus fitted with a rotating turntable, by means of which the patient, either seated or standing up, can be examined in any position with the least possible trouble. In addition, by means of special cassettes and a tube shift, both worked by electro-magneto, it is possible to obtain stereoscopic radiograms of the chest and abdomen in about two seconds. This apparatus, as well as a large negative examining box and a stereoscope was erected during the middle part of 1912, and the first radiograms under the new regime were taken on September 1. At the present time working in the Department are three qualified clinical assistants, two other assistants, and one developer. The nursing staff consists of a sister and two nurses.'

Unlike the situation at some other teaching hospitals at that time, therapy and skin patients did not preponderate at St. Thomas's Hospital, where the majority of x-ray examinations was made for diagnostic purposes. Most of the 6501 cases seen in 1913 were examined to exclude fractures or to localise foreign bodies, usually in the extremities. However, the following were included: 'Number of chest examinations, 378; number of abdominal examinations, 196. Seven cases of undoubted enlargement of the sella turcica; one case of a safety-pin embedded at the bifurcation of the trachea; one case of a bullet lodged in the dorsal spine, the bullet being located in the spinal canal by x-rays and abstracted by the surgeon (? murder or suicide); a case of retropharyngeal abscess before and after treatment; one case of enlarged thymus; a fracture of every carpal bone of the wrist except trapezium and trapezoid; dislocation of semilunar bone of the wrist *per se*; several cases of bilocular stomach, none of which have been diagnosed clinically; one case of undoubted obstruction of the caecum; four cases of fracture of the spine; one case of an extraordinary abnormality of the lower cervical and upper one or two dorsal vertebrae believed to be a spina bifida. . . .'[42]

GUY'S HOSPITAL

Less than a fortnight after Silvanus Thompson gave his lecture to the Clinical Society of London on 30 March 1896, the *Guy's Hospital Gazette* printed a news item from America which described Thomas Edison's discovery of the calcium tungstate screen beneath the title: 'X-ray spectacles which will avoid the unnecessary cutting'.[43] However, a year elapsed before an x-ray apparatus was installed and the first 'skiagrams' were made. In April 1897 a man was admitted with a suspected bullet after a shooting incident, and radiographs were hurriedly attempted. The results were unsatisfactory and the report in the *Gazette* inferred that the newly-acquired apparatus was still incomplete or the dark room was unready. 'It seems likely' – the *Gazette* continued[44] – 'that as at St. Thomas's Hospital the skiagraphic work will become part of the work of the electrical department. . . .'

Later in that month the following notice was printed'[45]

Skiagraphy in the Hospital.

PREPARATIONS for installing the new skiagraphic apparatus go on apace, and at present comprise a 10-inch spark coil of English make, by Messrs. Millar & Woods of Gray's Inn Road; and two special double pole vacuum tubes, one of high resistance for skiagraphing the thicker portions of the body, and the other of low resistance for obtaining clear and rapid impressions of the hand and foot.

There are also 50 ampère-hour accumulators by Messrs. Watson Bros. of Cockspur Street, Charing Cross, and a 12in. by 9in. double coated platinum platino cyanide screen from Berlin, for instantaneous work.

The bedroom belonging to the Sister in Accident ward has been given up for the purpose, and when completed will contain the apparatus, which is at present in the electric department, and a special universal jointed bar bracket for placing the tubes in position to take any portion of the body. The place itself will be lighted by electricity.

It is intended that the room when ready shall for the present be available for skiagraphy, and the electrician be in attendance from 12 till 12.30, and 2.30 till 3 o'clock every week-day except Saturday, when the time will be from 12 till 1 p.m.; rules no doubt being issued to this effect.

The autumn of 1897 saw the start of this early x-ray service based on the Accident Ward. Late in October the *Gazette* printed an article 'How to Take a Skiagraph' – a naively-phrased essay presumably directed at the medical students – which reported local technical experience. 'At Guy's a hand generally takes from 8 to 10 minutes and other thicker parts proportionally more time. This is a pity, for it wastes not only time but electricity. I think it is due to the tubes. . . .'[46]

The author of this article, 'J.T.D.', has not been identified, but the early protagonists of radiology were two medical students, A. H. B. Kirkman and E. W. H. Shenton, both of whom were appointed 'radiographers' to the Hospital in 1899.[47] Kirkman qualified in that year and joined the army for the South African War, but Edward Shenton remained to create the Radiology Department of Guy's Hospital, He did not graduate until 1901, therefore – like the young Sydney Rowland at St. Bartholomew's Hospital – he qualified as a radiologist before he was a doctor.

In October 1899 Kirkman and Shenton read a paper entitled 'The Röntgen Rays as a Means of Diagnosis' before the Pupils' Physical Society in the Hospital.[48] They showed 20 lantern slides made from radiographs of pathological conditions and demonstrated how the rays are generated. The majority were of accident cases, peripheral fractures or dislocations, but several were more interesting. Their final slide was a chest radiograph 'taken while the patient held her breath: *the exposure was one minute*'. It showed the pulmonary vessels clearly because the patient had remained still for the whole time. This was not usually so, and a surgeon writing in *The Lancet* had recently questioned the reliability of the x-rays to reveal foreign bodies such as bullets in the chest. Kirkman and Shenton were able to stress the importance of exerting quality control by reducing exposure times.

EDWARD WARREN HINE SHENTON, M.R.C.S., L.R.C.P. (1872–1955) was the medical student who created the x-ray service in Guy's Hospital and remained 'Surgical Radiographer' to the Hospital for 20 years.

His claim to be honoured by posterity is the Department of Radiology that he established which, visitors claimed, was one of the most modern in London. Shenton combined the practicality of the pioneer with an inventive flair and a loyalty to Guy's Hospital which fitted him for his role as the begetter of the new science.

All Shenton's publications reflect his commitment to his department and its equipment. His 13-page contribution to the Hospital's *Reports* in 1901, 'Notes on the Setting Up and Working of an X-Ray Installation' is a model of clarity and good sense.[49] Figure 53 of this paper illustrated 'Shenton's X-ray Couch', the table made to his design by Harry W. Cox, and later by A. E. Dean[50] and the Sanitas Electrical Company (page 58).

Even before that date, his other interests were clear – the radiological diagnosis of urinary calculi, and a simplified method of localising foreign bodies in the soft tissues. He described his first case of urinary calculus in 1899, perhaps one of the first three to be recorded,[47] and in 1903 he reviewed his technique and case material in an important article. By 1906 he had collected 1,600 cases.[51] His interest in skeletal and joint lesions prompted many papers – 'Shenton's line' in the diagnosis of congenital dislocation of the hip was described in 1902,[52] and his book *Disease in Bone, its Detection by the X-Rays* appeared in 1911. Shenton was an early recruit to the Röntgen Society and served on the Council for several years after 1901. As the Society's librarian he indulged yet another interest, the study of the normal. 'There is an anatomy for surgery, an anatomy for medicine and there is a special anatomy for radiography', he wrote on the occasion of presenting the Society with a set of normal radiographs.[47] Later he threw his weight behind the British Electrotherapeutic Society and contributed material to its journal.

Shenton resigned from Guy's Hospital in 1919 after serving it for two decades. From 1933 until he retired in 1950, he was honorary radiologist to Saint Bartholomew's Hospital, Rochester, Kent.[53]

Shenton stamped his mark on the early department. Soon he established an examination route for each patient which consisted of preliminary screening (radioscopy) with the patient lying supine, followed by exposure of a single print, either plate or print (radiography). This 'system of radiography' had diagnostic advantages in those early days, as he illustrated to the Röntgen Society in February 1901.[54] Radiographs of the body cavities were invariably spoilt by movement blur since the exposure times were as long as one minute; foreign bodies such as bullets could easily be missed. 'Anyone can be taught to place a plate beneath an injured limb, to adjust a tube above it and with a small knowledge of photography to produce a radiogram. If such work as this is to be accepted as a scientific use of the Roentgen rays in medicine, there is no such thing as radiographic diagnosis . . . Careful screening is the basis of radiographic examination.' Shenton's system appears to have been the first attempt to lay down procedures for x-ray examinations in Britain.

Since the radiography of foreign bodies accounted for much of the work done in the department, Shenton devised his own simple fluoroscopic method of localisation, which he explained as follows:[55] Suppose there is a needle in the hand. Place the hand in contact with the screen and adjust the tube so that the anode is parallel to the surface of the screen. When the needle is clearly visible, the screen and hand are swayed from side to side. The bones and the needle will be seen to be moving across the screen, and the relative rate at which they move is the key to the depth of the needle. If the needle is quite superficial, that is, close to the screen surface, its image moves a shorter distance than the images of the bones. A rough and ready method, Shenton admitted, but it was effective and time-saving. 'Dr. MacKenzie Davidson's method is a very scientific and exact mode of localisation, but the time, patience and material required render it suitable for the occasional case only. It would be impossible to x-ray all the cases of foreign body at Guy's by MacKenzie Davidson's method, and have time to do anything else . . .'[48]

In 1904 three separate electrical and allied departments were established in the Hospital and doctors took charge of each:

Electrotherapeutics (Dr. Arthur F. Hertz)
Actinotherapeutics, Light and X-Ray Treatment (Dr. Iredell)
Radiography (Dr. Shenton, Dr. P. J. Morton, and Dr. Alfred Jordan)

Not only did this arrangement complete the divorce of radiology from conventional electrotherapeutics, but a further innovative subdivision was itself soon created within the Radiography Department in 1907. Shenton was styled 'Surgical Radiographer' and Alfred Jordan was appointed 'Medical Radiographer'.[56]

ALFRED CHARLES JORDAN, C.B.E., M.D. Cantab., M.R.C.P. (born 1877) pioneered the diagnostic use of x-rays in internal medicine. He described himself as 'an x-ray specialist interested in the diagnosis of thoracic and gastro-intestinal diseases'.[57]

Born in Cheshire and educated at Sidney Sussex College, Cambridge and St. Bartholomew's Hospital, he qualified in 1898, and proceeded to M.D. in 1902 and was elected M.R.C.P. in 1911. Following an early interest in x-rays, he took medical charge of the X-ray and Electrical Departments of the Metropolitan Hospital and the Queen's Hospital for Children in 1906. In the following year he was elected Medical Radiographer at Guy's Hospital, an appointment which he combined with that of Honorary Radiologist to the National Hospital for Diseases of the Chest.

After the First World War, Dr. Jordan retired to private consultant practice in Wimpole Street.

Jordan's appointment tacitly acknowledged the new importance of the radiologist in clinical diagnosis. Hitherto most radiologists found their time occupied by examining limb injuries and acute surgical cases. Systemic study of the thorax and abdomen required a more planned approach and more sophisticated apparatus. This heralded the tilting table suitable for screening the patient in the erect position, which was built for the Hospital by Harry W. Cox. The unit was, in effect, Shenton's couch standing on an end, with its x-ray tube mobile in upward and downward directions (*see* 40). In front of the table was parked a lead-fronted frame surmounted by the fluoroscopic screen. A bicycle saddle served as a seat for the patient during screening. The modern radiologist will see, in the photographs of this primitive contraption which appeared in the *Archives of the Roentgen Ray* in 1909,[58] the humble predecessor of the fluoroscopic juggernauts of the present day. Even the blue bulb for lighting the x-ray room was linked to the primary current and could be switched on and off by the screening foot pedal.

Foreign visitors found Guy's Hospital the best-equipped department after the London Hospital. 'The whole installation' – wrote a South American professor in 1909[30] – 'is

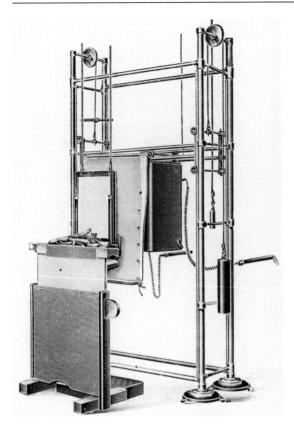

40. *Screening apparatus at Guy's Hospital, 1909*

most modern and complete, the vertical support, the chair, and all the other accessories being of the most recent model as used by Albers-Schönberg in the St. George Hospital at Hamburg.' The reviewer of Shenton's book for the *Archives of the Roentgen Ray* in 1911 probably expressed a generally agreed sentiment when he wrote: 'We congratulate Guy's Hospital on its school of Roentgenography. Drs. Hertz, Shenton, Morton and Jordan have all done good work for English Radiography.'[59]

Chapter 6

EARLY X-RAY
DEPARTMENTS – II

OTHER LONDON HOSPITALS

If one pays a visit to one of the great London hospitals, one is struck with the enormous progress which has been made of late in the provision of adequate space for the x-ray departments. . . . The qualified radiographer is watching the evolution of most interesting and rapidly growing branches of medical science. . . . Where will you get a picture of moving bones and joints, of heart, of stomach and intestines, better than from the fluorescent screen of the x-ray department?

Archives of the Roentgen Ray (1911)[1]

KING'S COLLEGE HOSPITAL

The Electro-therapeutic and Radiographic Department of King's College Hospital was a well-established entity soon after the turn of the century. Colleagues from abroad considered it to be one of the five hospitals worth visiting in London, the others being the London, St. Bartholomew's, Guy's, and Charing Cross.[2]

Archibald Reid, later the radiologist of St. Thomas's Hospital, was a King's man. After qualifying in 1901, he remained at the Hospital and, encouraged by its famous surgeon Sir Watson Cheyne, developed an interest in electricity. Soon he was appointed 'Electrical Medical Officer' to King's College and 'Radiographer' to the Evelina Hospital.

SIR ARCHIBALD DOUGLAS REID (see page 89) in the early part of his career introduced x-rays to King's College Hospital. Before he moved to St. Thomas's Hospital, he made significant contributions, not only to medical organisation in London, but also to radiological knowledge. In the year 1905 alone, papers appeared in *Medical Electrology and Radiology* under his authorship in which were described a case of achrondoplasia, the technique of examining the stomach with bismuth subnitrate, and the diagnosis of urinary-tract calculi.[3]

For rest of biography, see pages 186 and 187.

Reid was born a leader, and even in the first part of his radiological career at King's College Hospital, his talent for solving problems was manifest. The x-ray equipment in his department was up-to-date and he kept it so. In 1911 he heralded a revolution in radiographic technique by introducing the overhead tube. Hitherto most operators had utilised the Shenton table with an undercouch tube for taking x-ray plates, but Reid in that year devised an entirely new apparatus (*see* 28). This was the floor-standing column on which the tube was mounted above the level of the table and the film holder below it. This simple apparatus, the descendant of which can be seen in any modern x-ray department, was soon widely adopted. Reid's illustrated paper, 'The Technique of Skiagraphy', is a landmark in radiographic history.[4]

When Reid left for St. Thomas's Hospital in 1912, he was succeeded as head of the Department – the post designated as 'Radiographer to the Hospital' – by Robert Knox. Like Reid, Knox also was destined to be a luminary of British radiology, their names often linked.

ROBERT KNOX, M.D.(Edinburgh), M.R.C.S., L.R.C.P. (1867–1928) served King's College Hospital for 15 years. At the time of his death he was described as the leading British radiologist, the one most widely known at home and abroad.

For rest of biography, see pages 187–188.

SIR HAROLD KINGSTON GRAHAM-HODGSON, K.C.V.O., M.B., F.R.C.P., F.F.R., D.M.R.E. (1890–1960) was appointed honorary radiologist to King's College Hospital in 1924, a post he held for 9 years.

Graham-Hodgson, the son of a doctor at Eastbourne, was educated at Clare College, Cambridge and qualified at the University of Durham in 1916. He interrupted his undergraduate studies to serve as a despatch rider in France, and after qualifying returned there as a regimental medical officer. His interest in radiology was aroused in 1918 when posted to the Second Northern General Hospital at Leeds, but after the War he practised as a family doctor in Chislehurst for some years before turning to radiology. On obtaining the Cambridge Diploma in 1923 he was appointed honorary radiologist to the Central London Throat, Nose and Ear Hospital in Golden Square and the following year to King's College Hospital.

The Golden Square appointment enabled him to study the radiological features of the paranasal sinuses and ears, and he became the acknowledged expert in this field. In 1930 he described the radiological technique which he evolved for examining the sinuses, and it remains the standard technique.[5] His private practice in Upper Grosvenor Street was reputed to be the largest in London, and he caught the eye of Lord Dawson, who in 1928 selected him to carry out his radiological examination of King George V during his illness. He was created C.V.O. in the following year, and in 1950 was advanced to K.C.V.O. for his continued services to the Royal Family.[6]

In 1934 Graham-Hodgson left King's College Hospital to plan and start a separate department of diagnostic radiology at the Middlesex Hospital.

For rest of biography, see page 98.

THE MIDDLESEX HOSPITAL

Soon after Röntgen's discovery became known, the Middlesex Hospital purchased a small coil and vacuum tube for £14 – the minimum apparatus then regarded as necessary to keep up to date.[7] This x-ray kit was housed in a room above the Out-Patient Department and used in cases with suspected fracture or foreign body of the extremities. An administrative official, C. H. March, took charge and made the x-ray photographs when required.

Medical demand soon outgrew this primitive arrangement, and in 1902 an Electrical Department was established for diagnosis and treatment. No space could be found in the building at that time, and a temporary structure was erected in the forecourt of the Hospital close to the East Wing. Until the extensions on the west side provided the space required for a new department, this building, popularly known as the 'Tin House', met the x-ray and electrical requirements of the Hospital.

Three pioneers, all of whom were radiation martyrs, staffed the Tin House. They were Sister Ellen Clark, Mr. Reginald Mann and Dr. Lyster. R. F. Mann (1881–1916) as a youth became Mr. March's assistant in 1899 and served Dr. Lyster until 1916, taking diagnostic radiographs and carrying out x-ray treatments up to a few months of his death. In 1906 when only 25, radiation changes appeared in his hands, which countless operations over the next ten years failed to arrest; and he died of disseminated cancer. Lyster's other assistant, Sister Clark (died 1941) joined Mann in 1907 and spent 14 years treating the scalps of children with ringworm. 'Clarky' retired to live in the Hospital's convalescent home at Clacton-on-Sea and survived to old age, displaying radiation burns on her arms and hands to the students who visited her.[8]

CECIL R. CHAWORTH LYSTER, M.R.C.S. (1860–1920) was an enthusiastic innovator of the new photography who introduced x-rays into clinical use in the Middlesex Hospital. He was a pioneer of radiotherapy, publishing in 1903 promising results of treating cases of lupus, breast cancer and other neoplasms. He also described a novel radiographic method of foreign body localisation.[9]

Before taking charge of the Electrical Department of the Hospital in middle age, Lyster was attached to the Charing Cross Hospital, and also served as superintendent of the Bolingbroke Hospital. But he dedicated the last 17 years of his life to the Middlesex, eventually creating with his loyal assistants a fully integrated department.

Apart from his hospital work, Lyster made two significant contributions to the infant profession. In 1917 he attended the meeting at MacKenzie Davidson's house at which the British Association of Radiology and Physiotherapy was formed and the decision was taken to persuade the University of Cambridge to establish a Diploma course, see Chapter 9. According to Lister's obituarist,[10] he initiated these discussions. In 1918–9 he served as President of the Electro-Therapeutical Section of the Royal Society of Medicine.

Lyster contributed most significantly in the field of radiation protection. With the distinguished physicist, Professor Sidney Russ, who was his colleague, Lyster established the first radiation monitoring service at the Middlesex Hospital in 1918.[11] At the time of his death, Lyster served on the British X-Ray and Radium Protection Committee, see Chapter 11. He suffered patiently from his radiation injuries for the last decade of his life, losing several fingers of his right hand. His is one of the original 14 British names on the Martyrs' Memorial in Hamburg. The names of his assistants, Sister Clark and Reggie Mann were added in the 1950s.

In 1933 a benefactor, W. H. Collins, donated £35,000 to build and equip a diagnostic x-ray department, and subsequently when the Hospital had been re-built, he gave more money to endow the new department. This gift enabled the final separation of the diagnostic department to be made from the therapeutic side, which Dr. J. H. Douglas Webster already directed.[12] The challenge of designing, equipping and directing the new diagnostic x-ray department fell to the radiologist at King's College Hospital, Dr. Harold Graham-Hodgson.

DR. HAROLD GRAHAM-HODGSON (see page 96) joined the staff of the Middlesex Hospital in 1933 and remained Director of the Department of X-ray Diagnosis until his retirement in 1956.

The Department which he planned had revolutionary features at the time, but was later accepted as a model by many other hospitals. It quickly built up and maintained a reputation for teaching and became one of the foremost centres for postgraduate radiological instruction in Britain. One of Graham-Hodgson's young team was Dr. T. V. L. Critchlow, a familiar and loved figure in London, and another was a radiographer whom he took with him from King's College Hospital to be his superintendent, Joseph Kenny (1902–55).[13] Graham-Hodgson was a big man with an adventurous spirit who was popular and respected by his colleagues and associates. Apart from his knighthood, he received many hours:

> Founder Fellow of the Faculty of Radiologists, later a Member of Council
> President of the Section of Radiology of the Royal Society of Medicine
> Honorary Fellow of the American College of Radiologists
> Treasurer, International Congress of Radiology, London, 1950.[6]

CHARING CROSS HOSPITAL

Foreign radiologists visiting London in the early 1900s were directed first to Charing Cross Hospital where the various electrical departments were combined under the charge of a doctor.[2] The only satellite unit was that of Dr. McLeod, the skin physician who applied x-ray and light treatment to patients with skin complaints in his own department.

The first radiologist at Charing Cross Hospital was the ophthalmic surgeon from Aberdeen, Dr. (later Sir) James MacKenzie Davidson, who settled in London in 1897 after visiting Röntgen in Germany. Davidson while in Aberdeen developed a system of localising foreign bodies of the eye with x-rays which brought him national recognition after he demonstrated it to ophthalmologists in 1898. The method is based on using three co-ordinates of a point, and if all three can be obtained, the position of any fourth point (such as a foreign body) can be determined. From this time forward, the history of localisation for surgical purposes of foreign bodies not only in the eye but in other parts of the human is largely the history of the development of Davidson's method.[14]

SIR JAMES MACKENZIE DAVIDSON (see page 41) was about 40 years old when elected to the staff of the Charing Cross Hospital, and he remained the 'Consulting Surgeon to the X-ray Department' for two decades until he died. Charing Cross possessed a link with Aberdeen through its physician, Dr. Bruce who had been a contemporary of Davidson's at Aberdeen, and whose nephew, Ironside Bruce, later was Davidson's assistant.

The summer of 1897 found Davidson already working in the Hospital which remained the testing ground for his scientific curiosity for the rest of his life. In July of that year he published a radiograph of a bladder stone in the *Archives of the Roentgen Ray*, drawing attention to the importance of the x-ray diagnosis of urinary calculi.[15] The first device that he invented, the cross-thread localiser, was developed with W. S. Hedley as already noted; and they described their invention in *The Lancet* in October 1897.[16] The localiser used the principle of triangulation and, although not practical enough for the liking of many radiologists, was to remain popular with ophthalmologists. Davidson's localiser was adapted by the Army and used in South Africa and during the First World War. The other subject to which his grasp of physics allowed him to contribute was stereoscopic viewing of the x-ray picture. He built an attachment which enabled a stereoscopic effect to be obtained on the fluoroscopic screen: in 1900 it was described as 'one of the most interesting pieces of equipment ever devised'.[17] This subject remained a lifelong interest of Davidson's, and his last lecture, published posthumously,[18] was entitled 'Stereoscopic Radiography'.

Other products of Davidson's inventive mind were a motor-driven paddle mercury interrupter which was made by Harry W. Cox and widely used after 1900. In the last year of his life he devised a new table for x-ray localisation.[19]

Davidson's obsession with the physics of radiology was the basis of his professional life. But he owed his success in the field of medical politics to the other components of his personality – his outstanding ability to communicate and his qualities of leadership, which singled him out as the leader of the new profession.

For rest of biography, see pages 181–182.

In 1908 (just before Archibald Reid introduced his overcouch tube) a visitor to the x-ray department of the Charing Cross Hospital wrote:[2] 'In London one never sees a focus-tube above the table, since the English radiographer desires above all to obtain a previous examination with the screen, using it as a photographer uses his ground-glass focussing-screen. In this way he is able to adjust the focus-tube, rectify the position of the patient, or alter the field at will. Then by simply replacing the screen by a photographic plate, he is able to take his skiagram. The patient does not move since he is lying down. . . . Dr. Ironside Bruce's table has above it a frame, which carries a plumb-line indicating the position and direction of the normal ray. He uses a Bauer tube and a gas break, similar to Drault's gas interrupter, a form very common in England. With a spark-gap of 4 inches, he obtains a current of $1\frac{1}{2}$ milliamperes through the tube. With this installation an exposure of 15–20 seconds is sufficient for the thorax, and two minutes for the kidney . . .'.

Dr. Ironside Bruce, who became MacKenzie Davidson's assistant after the South African War, was a talented young Scot whose death from a radiation-induced aplastic anaemia in 1921 at the age of 42 shocked the British radiological world. It produced an outcry which led directly to the creation of a national protection committee.

WILLIAM IRONSIDE BRUCE, M.D. Aberdeen, D.M.R.E. (1879–1921) was the son of a doctor at Dingwall and the nephew of a physician at Charing Cross Hospital. He qualified at Aberdeen University in 1900 and went immediately to South Africa as a civil surgeon to the South African Field Force. There he witnessed the early use of x-rays in the diagnosis of war wounds, and this experience may have influenced him in his future career.[20]

Bruce was in post by 1905 at Charing Cross and also at the Hospital for Sick Children, Great Ormond Street. He was then 26, and he retained both appointments up to his death. He soon made his presence felt in London, lecturing regularly and finding a place on the City's radiological committees. A steady flow of papers came from his pen on radiological subjects, such as the diagnosis of urinary calculi, sinusitis, dilated bowel and chronic arthritis. He helped to establish his reputation by publishing a book in 1907, *A System of Radiography; with an Atlas of the Normal*, which was highly favoured by the reviewers, one of whom claimed that it was the first British book to reach the high standard of German texts.[21]

Bruce's interest in the x-ray diagnosis of blood and other malignant diseases may have contributed to his early death. His is one of the original 14 British names on the Martyrs' Memorial in Hamburg.

Cochrane Shanks was a postgraduate student at Charing Cross in the early 1920s. 'The Department was a modern one of its day, for its director was an intelligent, forceful

Scot who was one of the foremost figures in a rapidly developing speciality . . . (It) was up-to-date in that it was on the top floor of the Hospital instead of the more usual basement, and consisted of one large room and a cupboard that served as a dark room. The staff consisted of Dr. Bruce, a radiographer (both of whom attended on 3 afternoons a week) and a sister in charge. On average 5 cases were x-rayed on each of these 3 afternoons, consisting of fractures, chests and urinary tracts, with an occasional barium meal. Glass x-ray plates were still in use, the largest being 12 × 10 inches and the intensifying screen was still something of a novelty. The equipment consisted of a 16-inch coil, gas tubes, a canvas topped couch and a primitive screening stand. The screen was held in the observer's hand against the patient's chest or abdomen . . .'.[22]

Dr. Russell Reynolds, who as the London schoolboy had built an x-ray set when Röntgen's discovery was announced, succeeded Bruce in 1921.

THE ROYAL FREE HOSPITAL

Sydney Rowland in the summer of 1896 described patients in the *British Medical Journal* who were x-rayed at the Royal Free Hospital,[23] but the doctor who introduced x-rays was a remarkable graduate of the Medical School. She was the country's first woman radiologist, Dr. Florence Stoney.

In 1901 Dr. Stoney brought back from America an x-ray tube – said to have been given to her by a colleague of Coolidge[24] – and she thereafter specialised in x-ray work. She established the first clinical x-ray service in the Royal Free Hospital and the Elizabeth Garrett Anderson Hospital. No separate room was available for x-ray work and the apparatus could only be used when the room in which it was installed was not required for other purposes. There was no assistant, and the plates were often taken home and developed in the bathroom at night. Casualty house officers used the apparatus out of hours for emergency cases, and it was frequently out of order. In those days the radiologist was not a member of the Staff and was not even a member of the committee discussing the organisation of the x-ray department.

FLORENCE CONSTANCE STONEY, O.B.E., M.D. London, D.M.R.E. Cambridge (died 1932), Britain's pioneer woman radiologist, was born into a talented Dublin family. Her father and her brother were Fellows of the Royal Society and her sister was a mathematical physicist. Florence, when denied entry to Dublin University which was not open to women, entered the London School of Medicine for Women and took the London University M.B., B.S. degrees with honours, and proceeded to the M.D. in 1898. Hoping to be an anatomist, she worked as a demonstrator at the School for several years, giving up only when she found that there was no prospect at that time of a woman being appointed to the lectureship.

In 1902 she specialised in x-rays and continued to practise at the Royal Free Hospital until the outbreak of the First World War. Immediately and against much opposition, she then led an all-women medical corps to Belgium and established a 135-bed surgical hospital for wounded soldiers. When bombed out the corps moved to France, where they re-established a Hospital in a chateau near Cherbourg. Conditions were primitive and Dr. Stoney and her helpers had first to adapt a waterwheel in the grounds to generate the electricity required to light the building and power x-rays. In 1915 she was the first woman doctor to be accepted for full-time work by the War Office, and was given charge of the radiological department of the 1,000-bed military

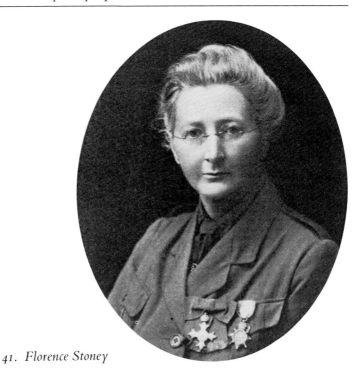

41. Florence Stoney

hospital at Fulham. For several years she was the only woman member of the large medical staff, and won surgeons' plaudits for her skilled x-ray localisation of bullets, a task which was aided by her training in anatomy. On being demobilised she was awarded the O.B.E.

After the War Dr. Stoney settled in Bournemouth, and combined a large radiological practice with appointments in local hospitals until she retired in 1928. She was the founder and President of the Wessex branch of the British Association for Radiology and Physiotherapy (now the British Institute of Radiology). When the University of Cambridge initiated the Diploma course, she was awarded the Diploma *honoris causa* in recognition of her distinguished pioneering and war work.

In 1907 the Royal Free Hospital elected Dr. Harrison Orton to take charge of a combined Department of Radiology and Electrotherapy. This appointment appears to have been made over the head of Dr. Stoney, who continued to work in the Department and who pioneered deep x-ray treatment in the Hospital. In 1912 she presented the results of x-ray treatment of exophthalmic goitre at the Annual Meeting of the British Medical Association in Liverpool. Dr. Stoney's association with the Hospital ceased when the War broke out. Dr. Orton resigned his appointment in 1913.

UNIVERSITY COLLEGE HOSPITAL

In 1907 two departments existed. The Electrotherapeutic Department ('open five days a week') was under the charge of Dr. E. S. Worrall, and the Radiographic and Photographic Department ('open daily in the afternoon from 1:30 to 4') under Dr. Higham

Cooper.[25] Cooper, who was also radiographer to the Hospital at Tottenham, was Worrall's assistant. Worrall wrote a paper about patients with lupus and rodent ulcer whom he treated in the Hospital in 1906 and he also lectured to members of the Röntgen Society on the diagnostic value of x-rays.[26]

WESTMINSTER HOSPITAL

In 1907 Dr. M. D. Sale-Barker had charge of the Department of Electrotherapy and Radiography in the Hospital.[25]

ST. MARY'S HOSPITAL

Clinical x-rays were made in the Hospital as early as 1896,[27] but no department was organised until Dr. G. Allpress Simmons joined the staff nearly a decade later. The radiographs were taken by the theatre instrument beadle with a primitive set kept in the basement, at times when he could be spared from his duties of looking after the surgical instruments. 'Considering his limitations' – commented Dr. Simmons[28] – 'his work was extremely good.'

By 1907 two departments had been established: one for electrotherapeutic work under Dr. Wilfred Harris; and one for radiography and x-ray treatment under a 'medical officer in charge of the x-ray department'.[29] When Dr. Simmons left shortly afterwards to open an x-ray department in St. George's Hospital, Dr. Harrison Orton was appointed to this post.

GEORGE HARRISON ORTON, M.A., M.D., D.M.R.E., F.F.R. (1873–1947) served St. Mary's Hospital as its Radiologist for 27 years. He was a junior colleague of Lewis Jones and Hugh Walsham at St. Bartholomew's Hospital in his young days, and his fingers were badly mutilated. When he died his obituarist described him as 'perhaps the last martyr pioneer of radiology'.[30]

Born to the wife of a London surgeon, Harrison Orton was educated at Trinity College, Cambridge and St. Bartholomew's Hospital. As early as 1905 he was a Clinical Assistant in the Electrical Department there and in the following year he collaborated with Hugh Walsham in a book *The Roentgen Rays in the Diagnosis of Diseases of the Chest*, which was hailed as an early authoritative work. In 1907 he was placed in charge of the X-ray and Electrical Department of the Royal Free Hospital and other appointments followed: Honorary Radiologist to the National Hospital for Diseases of the Chest, and Mount Vernon Hospital. The most important appointment came in April 1908 when Orton succeeded Simmons as Medical Officer in Charge of the X-ray Department of St. Mary's Hospital.

Dr. Orton identified with the young profession in London, and especially with the newly created Electro-Therapeutical Section of the Royal Society of Medicine in 1907, serving on the first Council and later as Secretary and President. In 1917 he attended the meeting in MacKenzie Davidson's house, held to form the British Association of Radiology and Physiotherapy and to persuade the University of Cambridge to initiate a Diploma course. Subsequently he was one of the four guarantors of the bank overdraft which acquired the lease of 32 Welbeck Street as a home for the British Institute of Radiology.

Dr. Orton was a British pioneer of deep x-ray therapy and one of the first users of high kilovoltages in London.[31] His interest in this field grew in the 1920s when he served as co-secretary with Professor Sidney Russ of the British X-ray and Radium Protection Committee. However, he remained a diagnostic radiologist by instinct all his life. In 1935, 23 years after writing an early monograph on the x-ray examination of renal and ureteral calculi,[32] he delivered the Mac-Kenzie Davidson Memorial Lecture on 'Calcium Changes and their Importance in Diagnostic Radiology'. Orton's name was added in the 1950s to the British names on the Martyrs' Memorial in Hamburg.

H. COURTNEY GAGE, M.R.C.S., L.R.C.P., O.I.P.(Francaise) (1885–1947) became Director of the Radiology Department of St. Mary's Hospital when Harrison Orton retired in 1935, and he held the post up to his death.

Gage when young worked for MacKenzie Davidson as his technician. During the First World War he served in France with the American Red Cross and was responsible for the radiography of war casualties and civilians, and at the end of the war his service was acknowledged by the French Government. Several techniques devised by him for investigating spinal injuries were published in the *Journal de Radiologie* in 1916.[33]

After the War Gage enrolled as a student in St. Mary's Hospital Medical School and qualified in 1924 when aged 39. In 1926 he was appointed Assistant Honorary Radiologist and succeeded to the Directorship of the Department nine years later. He was a man in Orton's mould with local loyalties strongest; always he put patients, colleagues and the Hospital first. He was Editor of the *British Journal of Radiology* during a difficult time, from 1940 to 1943, and for this service the British Institute of Radiology bestowed the rare honour of Honorary Membership on him. Over the same period he acted as medical adviser to the Norwegian Forces, and King Haakon created him a Knight of the Royal Order of St. Olaf, a unique honour for a person not born in Norway. Gage's name was added with that of Orton's in the 1950s to the Martyrs' Memorial in Hamburg.

ST. GEORGE'S HOSPITAL

St. George's Hospital was the last of the London teaching hospitals to establish an electrical department. X-ray and light treatment were provided by the dermatologist, Dr. Wilfred Fox, but in 1907 diagnostic x-rays were still made for the Hospital's clinicians by a non-medical operator, F. T. Addyman.[25] Frank Addyman was a science graduate of London University, a laboratory technician who had gained experience of radiography during the South African War. He was an early member of the Röntgen Society, and the author of one of the first radiographic manuals, *Practical X-Ray Work*.

The first medical officer in charge of the x-ray work was Dr. G. Allpress Simmons, who was appointed 'Senior Radiographer' of the Hospital in 1907. Previously he had held the same post at St. Mary's Hospital. The moving force behind his appointment was Dr. Fox, who persuaded the Hospital authorities to establish a properly equipped and staffed electrical and x-ray department.

Posterity has reason to be grateful to Simmons for publishing his lecture to the Section of Radiology of the Annual Meeting of the British Medical Association in 1910.[28] He described and illustrated the first x-ray department of the Hospital, which he established on a floor area measuring 50 feet × 25 feet that had previously been a 12-bed ward (*see* 42). At the one end were two light-tight diagnostic x-ray rooms equipped with apparatus for screening patients and taking x-rays – 'instantaneous skiagrams can be made in a

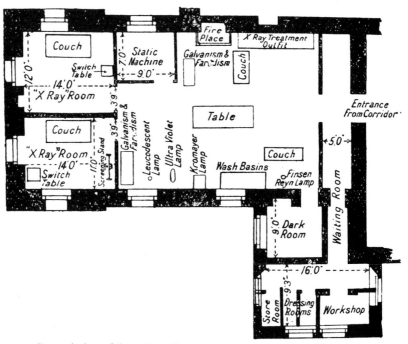

42. Ground plan of the x-Ray Department, St. George's Hospital, 1910

fraction of a second – a very useful possibility for children and for heart and lung cases'. When the one room was in use, the other doubled as a changing room. The rest of the old ward remained open, and stationed along the walls were the various lamps then fashionable for electrical therapy, which was given mostly for skin lesions. The Finsen-Reyn and Kromayer lamps were used successfully for lupus, the ultraviolet lamp for alopecia, and other apparatus provided treatment with galvanic, faradic or sinusoidal currents or electrocautery. Cases of non-skin cancer – still empiric and ill-defined diagnostic territory – were treated by a static machine and an 'x-ray treatment outfit'.

'There is hardly any known skin condition that is not treated electrically nowadays,' Simmons wrote, 'while a great many patients are also sent from all departments, in-patient and out-patient, medical and surgical, for all forms of treatment from rodent ulcer to hysteria'.

In keeping with the practice in most departments, written records were kept of each patient and plate. Each patient brought a requirement (request) form with him to the department, signed by a member of the medical staff. There was a sturdy record book called the x-ray register, into which an entry was made for each patient at the time of the examination, comprising date, name, age, name of physician or surgeon, ward, exactly what was required, and a brief clinical history, as well as technical notes (size of plates, position of patient, exposure time etc.). The plate was developed on the same day and a report made on it, and the plates and reports were sent out to the surgeon or physician on the next day.

'It may be of interest to describe a day's routine in the x-ray department. This is opened by the Sister in Charge and the mechanic at 9 am, and immediately treatment cases begin to arrive and an occasional screen case or two from the casualty department, any case other than a trivial one being kept for the radiographer. At about 1.15 the radiographer attends. . . . The outpatient physicians and surgeons arrive at one o'clock, and cases begin to come at once. The cases from the wards, for which requirements are generally sent in the morning, are now sent for, and everybody becomes very busy. . . . In the intervals, yesterday's plates are examined and reports of them entered in the book, and treatment cases seen and treatments prescribed. . . . After the departure of the radiographer there is more treatment work for Sister and nurse, and development for the mechanic to do, and there is also a good deal of bookwork to be done by the Sister . . .'. Finally Simmons identified what he believed to be the three main duties of the diagnostic radiologist – namely, to ensure that plates and reports go out promptly, to be selective and only send out plates which show the lesion clearly, and to keep careful and accurate records ('almost as important as doing good technical and expert work').

The eminent radiologist of St. George's Hospital between the two World Wars was Stanley Melville.

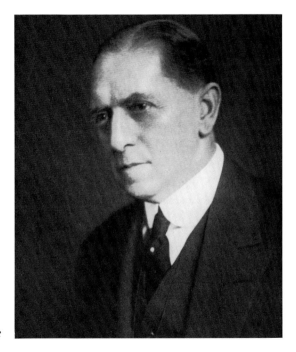

43. Stanley Melville

STANLEY MELVILLE, L.S.A., M.R.C.S., L.R.C.P., M.R.C.P., M.D.(Brussels) (1867–1934) was one of the architects of modern British radiology. His achievements rest on his skill as a planner and negotiator, which in turn were founded on the esteem in which his colleagues held him as a practising radiologist.

He was an unusual man.[34] A small Lancastrian with an eye-glass and meticulously correct in speech and dress in later years, he had left Liverpool as a young man and entered University College, London to read law. After being called to the Bar at Lincoln's Inn, he studied medicine and qualified in 1891. He had a flourishing general practice in Nevern Square five years later when Röntgen discovered x-rays, which with great courage and enthusiasm he gave up in 1898 to devote his time to the new science of radiology. He was an early recruit to the Röntgen Society and the Electro-Therapeutical Section of the Royal Society of Medicine but, unlike

Thurstan Holland and some of the pioneers, he published few of the innovations which he introduced into his own departments.

Melville's professional life was shared between the three hospitals of which he was the honorary radiologist – St. George's, the West London at Hammersmith, and the Brompton Hospital. He lived and practised at 9 Chandos Place and, thanks to his drive and the esteem in which his colleagues held him, this address became in the late 1920s the powerhouse of British radiology – as the home of MacKenzie Davidson had been in the previous generation.

His drive and charm took him to the top, and he served and led most of the radiological committees in the land:

Joint Secretary (with Russ), British X-Ray and Radium Protection Committee 1921–34
Secretary-General, 1st International Congress of Radiology, 1925
British representative, International Protection Committee, Stockholm, 1928
A founder and second President 1923–6, Society of Radiographers
President, Electro-Therapeutical Section of Royal Society of Medicine, 1924–5
President, British Institute of Radiology, 1934
Medical Editor, *British Journal of Radiology*, 1934.

Radiation injuries to Melville's hand marred his later years and produced great discomfort, but they did not shorten his life. Melville's is one of the original 14 British names inscribed on the Martyrs' Memorial in Hamburg.

THE BROMPTON HOSPITAL

It is known that Dr. Barry Blacker soon after establishing the x-ray department in St. Thomas's Hospital, attended the Brompton Hospital for Consumption to take radiographs for diagnostic purposes.[35] But the true begetter of chest radiology was Stanley Melville.

'When first I went (there)' – Melville reminisced in his Presidential Address to the British Institute of Radiology in 1933[36] – 'I found a small, 8-inch coil with Miller interrupter (the latter at that time a great advance), a small Cox Record tube on a wooden stand. There was no provision for taking a radiograph even were this possible, and there was a natural apathy among my medical colleagues who did not think much of this gross and rather foolish innovation. As showing the unimportance of radiography in chest disease in the early days, my contract with the Hospital was to attend two afternoons a week, when one might screen two, or even on a really busy afternoon, four or five patients, but I do not think it was of any medical assistance.'

The Brompton Hospital was the scene of Melville's major professional achievements. A primitive x-ray kit in the basement room with black-painted walls soon went, replaced by apparatus reflecting his advanced ideas – high performance transformer, rotating anode Coolidge tube, generator placed outside the x-ray room.[37] Melville introduced the 'standard chest' radiograph – taken at a distance of six feet from the tube and with the patient erect – which became the British practice, and he helped to establish 'The Brompton' as the Mecca for chest radiologists round the world.[38]

On Melville's death Dr. R. W. Rawlinson succeeded him as Director of Radiology at the Hospital.

THE CANCER HOSPITAL (FREE), FULHAM

The Cancer Hospital (now the Royal Marsden Hospital) was one of the first to recognise the therapeutic use of x-rays in the treatment of malignant disease. The first x-rays were produced there in 1903 when a 'very complete x-ray department' was established under the charge of Dr. J. D. Pollock.[39] Technical charge of the apparatus was in the hands of a remarkable early radiographer, George Westlake (died 1941). All x-ray work fell to him to carry out until Dr. Robert Knox was appointed in medical charge in 1911, and Westlake is credited with helping to lay the technical foundations of radiotherapy in Britain.[40] Originally the pharmacist of the Hospital, Westlake gave devoted service to the early x-ray department. As the first secretary of the Society, he was one of the founders of the Society of Radiographers.

In 1911 a Research Institute was established at the Hospital, and as part of the scheme new electrical laboratories were built. For this purpose, a two-storey building was erected at the rear of the Hospital in Fulham Road. When equipped, it was – according to the reporter of the *Archives of the Roentgen Ray*[39] – 'a model of what a Roentgen laboratory should be'. Dr. Knox co-operated with Siemens Brothers to create the most modern department of its day, utilising the experience of the first decade of practice to introduce new concepts in the design of the building and the choice of equipment. The illustrations of the *Archives* article take the reader into the building and provide

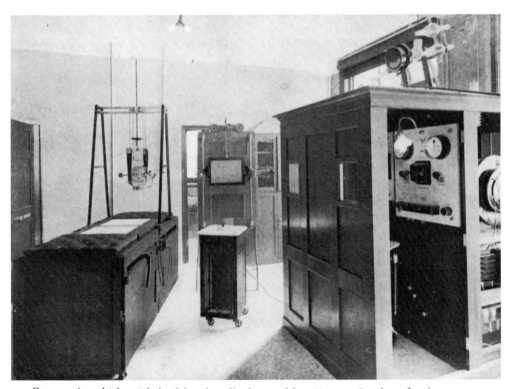

44. Operator's cubicle with lead-lined walls designed by Siemens Brothers for the x-ray room of the Cancer Hospital, Fulham in 1912

a unique view of an early x-ray department. Since the building had been erected purposely to house the Electrical Institute, the Cancer Hospital can claim to have possessed the first professionally designed x-ray department in Britain; one of the few not sited in a disused corridor or basement. Novel features of the building were hot-water central heating, comprehensive electrical wiring ('plugs and switches every few feet'), and piped cold air to cool the x-ray tubes. The ground floor consisted of the waiting room, doctor's office and diagnostic x-ray room. The first floor housed the electrotherapy department, including the radium area and three lead-lined cubicles. These cubicles were, in fact, insulated rooms and a logical improvement of the system pioneered at the London Hospital (*see* 44).

The diagnostic x-ray equipment on the ground floor was as novel as the building. The upright screening table working on the same principle as the contraption rigged up by Dr. Shenton at Guy's Hospital, was factory-built by Siemens Brothers to the design of Professor Rieder of Munich. The hanging screen was coupled to the tube and both were perfectly balanced, so that the operator could move them simultaneously with ease. The x-ray couch was designed by Dr. Knox along conventional lines, i.e. it had a sturdy mahogany frame and the tube was mounted underneath. However, the protective tube cover distinguished it as an advance on Shenton's original design.

The most interesting novelty was the control table, which was the first Siemens 'Single Impulse Outfit' to be installed in Britain. This apparatus had a large induction coil, capable of giving a 16-inch spark at heavy currents for instantaneous diagnostic work. The unusual feature was the new type of single impulse switch which could not only interrupt but reverse the secondary current. The outfit was mounted on the sides of a box-like structure about the size of a garden shed, which served also as the operator's cubicle.

The period 1911–27 saw the Electrical Department of the Cancer Hospital and Institute grow and flourish under the inspired leadership of Robert Knox. An important member of Knox's team, apart from George Westlake (who retired in 1927 when Knox died), was the pioneer x-ray physicist, C. E. S. Phillips.

WEST LONDON HOSPITAL, HAMMERSMITH

Radiographs were made before the turn of the century at the Hammersmith Hospital, which was an early British centre for the treatment of cancer by the combined surgical and radiotherapeutic approach. The pioneer was the cancer surgeon, Chisholm Williams, who held the titles of Electrotherapeutist and Radiographer to the Hospital, and Lecturer on these subjects at the West London Postgraduate College.

JOHN CHISHOLM WILLIAMS, L.S.A. (1891), F.R.C.S.(Edinburgh, 1898) (died 1928) was a medical student with scientific interests at St. Thomas's Hospital, who practised as an orthopaedic surgeon in London for the first 15 years of his career. However, his main interest was electrotherapeutics, and in 1903 he commenced his electrotherapeutic work at the Hammersmith Hospital. It is said that he verified Röntgen's discoveries within five weeks of the news of his discovery becoming known, with x-ray apparatus that he built himself.[8]

Chisholm Williams treated his first patient with x-rays in February 1900, a 61-year-old man with an epithelioma of the tongue. Five years later he recalled that, while the first 16 cases which he treated in this way all died, the seventeenth one survived – a patient with a recurrent tumour which cleared up after six treatments.[41]

Chisholm Williams was a luminary of the British Electrotherapeutic Society, serving as editor and vice-president prior to being the Society's last President before it became a section of the Royal Society of Medicine in 1907.

He suffered severe radiation burns of his arms and hands, and he is one of the original 14 British names recorded on the Martyrs' Memorial in Hamburg. Soon after the First World War he lost one hand and two fingers of the other hand, and was obliged through ill-health to abandon x-ray work. In 1927 on the occasion of the annual prize-giving ceremony at St. Thomas's Hospital, the Duke of Connaught presented Williams with the bronze medallion of the Carnegie Hero Fund for his services to mankind, and he was awarded a pension in the Civil List.

A colleague of Williams's at the West London Hospital was David Arthur, Lecturer of Pathology in the College, who also treated patients with x-rays and described a new vacuum tube for undercouch work in 1906.[42] He was the author with John Muir of an early textbook of radiology, *A Manual of Practical X-ray Work* (1909). The book was compiled from the notes of Arthur's lectures in a postgraduate course which he gave to army and navy surgeons. A reviewer claimed that the book contained 'the information necessary to enable the student to take and interpret a skiagram – exactly what is wanted in a practical textbook for x-ray work'.[43]

Williams's early radiotherapeutic work received a powerful impetus in 1909 when Reginald Morton resigned from the London Hospital and became the Radiographer of the Hospital.

EDWARD REGINALD MORTON (see page 82) was one of the men who introduced deep x-ray therapy into Britain soon after the end of the First World War. He visited Erlangen to study the work of Professor Schrumph and on his return introduced these techniques, and also the work of Wintz and Voltz in the measurement of dose. These fundamental advances helped to lay a scientific basis for radiotherapy and led, soon after Morton's retirement in 1926, to the separation of therapy from diagnosis and the appointment of the country's first radiotherapists.

During the First World War the Hospital was used by the military authorities, being called The Military Orthopaedic (later Special Surgical) Hospital, Hammersmith. War-injured soldiers were invalided back from France, some spending many months there in treatment and rehabilitation. One of these was a young soldier who later became a respected teacher of radiography, William Watson. He was a patient there for the last 30 months of the War, working as a helper in the X-ray Department, and this experience led him to qualify later as a radiographer. His recollections of the 1920s, recorded in 1961,[44] not only entertain but provide an immediate picture of an x-ray department at the end of the pioneering stage described in this chapter.

'The x-ray room consisted of two maternity rooms; the dark room had been a kitchen, the office a washroom. Other rooms were the doctor's office and the plate-storage rooms. The radiologist (a term not used then) was the radiographer or skiagraphist and was assisted by three V.A.D. nurses taking turns at the switchtable, the dark room, the office or marshalling the ever-growing queue of patients. There seemed to be days allocated to different parts of the body; femur days, kidney days, bone graft days, skull days and bismuth-meal days. Much original work was done in surgery especially in bone-

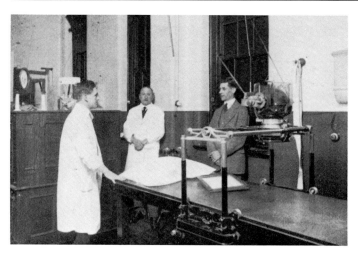

45. *X-ray Department of the West London Hospital, Hammersmith in 1918. Left to right are three pioneer radiographers, William Watson, T. Azeal and Charles Stockham*

grafting. Forearm bone grafts did not present much of a problem but lumbar spines and kidneys did. A sergeant-major's kidneys required not less than two minutes' exposure with a spark gap of 5 in. and 5 mA at a focus-plate distance of 24 in.; this could be reduced to 20 in. by a sort of shoehorn manoeuvre between the compressor (now called a cone), and the abdomen. Two minutes of hope versus anxiety often resulted in a packet of broken glass; otherwise, the result was a picture, passable (largely thanks to the compression technique), but clearly demonstrating the impossibility of seeing a small object inside a large one.

'The high-tension generator was a disc-rectified Snook, the second to be installed in this country, with a beautifully balanced motor, a 10 in. milliamperemeter, and a bare transformer mounted on bricks, all housed in a fine example of the cabinet-maker's art. There were three transformers really; one in use, one on the way to be repaired and one on the way back. Anything over 5 mA meant a call to 'panic-stations' and an inspection of the transformer's stalactites and stalagmites of melted wax. Control of input was by resistance only, plus a regenerative manipulation of the X-ray tube and spark-gap. Gas-tubes tended to get hard with use and required repeated softening by shunting the current through a small glass cylinder containing a 'rare' chemical which would release the requisite number of ions; the 'rare' chemical was common washing soda. Sparks there were galore which were very impressive, inducing a state of whole-hearted co-operation 'or else' in the mind of the patient. There was a clockwork time-switch. It required resetting every 20 seconds and a manual closing of an openwork switch connected directly to the mains. The nurse at the time-switch usually did some knitting while the patient was 'cooking' after the style set by Madame Defarge (but more sympathetically): it worked out something like half-a-row of a sock for an ankle and up to two rows for a lumbar spine.

'X-rays plates were of temperamental glass with a generous coating of emulsion on one side, each packed in a black envelope. They were developed in dishes, fixed in dishes, washed in a tank and dried over a hot radiator. Breakages were numerous. We became adept at passepartouting the irreplaceables. Of course, glass-plate radiographs could not be kept with the patients' case sheets, so they were all neatly stacked in racks – literally tons of them. Giving them out on inspection days was quite a business. They were sorted and marked and one staggered into the radiologist's office with a pile, having put the best ones on top. There were plenty of stereos of the thicker parts; the future for laterals of the 5th lumbar was very dim.

'Early in 1918 Capt. Stanley Melville took charge of the department and many innovations occurred for the better. By 1923 we had a Coolidge tube, a Potter-Bucky diaphragm, a Snook generator giving a real 100 mA, auto-transformer control, filament transformer, double-coated film and tungstate intensifying screens. We accepted the films with some diffidence, still ordering a few plates, and continued with dish development. Plates fought a losing battle and were definitely on the way out.

'Each innovation had a dramatic effect. A surgeon seeing for the first time a lumbar spine taken on film with a pair of screens through a Potter-Bucky diaphragm would be full of praise and delight. Double-coated film and tungstate screens had cut chest exposures down to 1/10 second at 6 ft. F.F.D., remarkable because with glass plates and no screens the exposure had been 2 to 12 seconds at 36 in. No doubt the quality obtained revolutionised chest radiology. A time-switch was not provided for brief exposures so an acquired dexterity was necessary for fractions of a second; a short, medium, or long 'flash' with a bare knife-switch was the usual variation.

'Potter-Bucky diaphragms were not built into the couch, so we became very muscular by lifting them on and off.

'Ward work there was in plenty in the 1920s. A single antero-posterior view of each of 15 femurs on one side of a ward constituted a morning's work. A similar dose on the other side of the ward completed the day. An exposure for a femur would be about a minute at 20 in. F.F.D., with 3 mA on plates without screens. The mobile sets (we had two) had a 12-inch induction coil, a mercury interrupter and a gas tube. The lot weighed over half a ton, the prime power being 24- or 48-volt accumulators. Compare these with the modern mobile set. The older ones had to be fed and watered every night if they were to remain trusty steeds whereas the modern set seems to thrive on neglect, and it does not kick the unwary. . . .'

When Dr. Melville died in 1934, Dr. Duncan White, a radiologist in Edinburgh, was appointed Director of the Diagnostic Radiology Department of the Hospital.

JOHN DUNCAN WHITE, O.B.E., M.B., Ch.B., D.M.R.E., Hon.F.S.R. (1896–1955) was Melville's *protégé*, at whose feet he trained as a radiologist.

White qualified in medicine at the University of Edinburgh in 1917, and after taking the Cambridge Diploma in 1921 spent several years in London as Melville's assistant before returning to Scotland. He worked in Aberdeen and then in 1932 was appointed to the Royal Infirmary, Edinburgh.

He remained Director of the Radiological Department of the Hammersmith Hospital for 21 years, until forced to retire prematurely by his x-ray injuries. These were attributed by one of his obituarists to the effects of his early work with radium, but Brailsford believed that they were the result of White's 'great enthusiasm for screening'. With G. H. Orton he was one of the last practising radiologists in Britain to die of radiation injuries.

Duncan White helped Melville to found the Society of Radiographers, he gave the first Stanley Melville Memorial Lecture of the Society, and he served as its President in 1942–4. He succeeded Melville in 1934 when aged only 38 as President of the British Institute of Radiology. During the Second World War he was placed in charge of the Army X-ray School at Millbank, and at the end of the War he supervised the chest radiography of 100,000 former prisoners of war.[45] White's was one of the British names added to the Martyrs' Memorial in Hamburg in the 1950s.

Chapter 7

EARLY X-RAY
DEPARTMENTS – III

HOSPITALS IN THE PROVINCES AND BEYOND

In the average county hospital, if you look for the darkest, steepest, and most awkward stair below ground, you will generally find that it takes you to the x-ray department . . .

A. E. Barclay (1923)[1]

THE QUEEN'S HOSPITAL AND THE GENERAL HOSPITAL, BIRMINGHAM

The early history of radiology in Birmingham is an account of the career and martyrdom of Dr. John Hall-Edwards. For the 25 years that followed upon Röntgen's discovery, Hall-Edwards remained the torch-bearer of the new science in his home city and achieved national recognition as a result of his injuries and his work. On his return from South Africa with experience of campaign radiography (see Chapter 10), he resumed the post that he had vacated at the beginning of the Boer War as 'Surgeon Radiographer' to the Birmingham hospitals. Later, as fashions changed, this title was altered to 'Medical Officer in Charge of the X-Ray and Light Departments' and then to 'Radiologist', and it was from this last office that he finally retired in the 1920s.

During this period the x-ray service grew to be an established feature of the clinical life of Birmingham. The scope and extent of the work done can be gauged by the contributions which Hall-Edwards made to contemporary medical literature. He was a prolific writer (and editor) and before 1910 the *Archives of the Roentgen Ray* and *Medical Electrology and Radiology* printed over 25 articles, case reports and lectures from his pen. They treat the following subjects:

X-ray diagnosis of urinary calculi;
The diagnosis of obscure fractures by x-ray;
Case reports of tuberculous osteitis of a metacarpal bone and syphilis of the radius;
A dermoid showing teeth;

A micturating cystogram in a child;

Ten years' experience in the localisation of foreign bodies by means of x-rays (1906);

Recent advances in diagnosis by x-rays (1907);

An instantaneous shutter for teleradiography.

Hall-Edwards's preoccupation with x-ray treatment is evident from his writings, which increasingly dealt with his efforts to treat patients with skin and glandular cancer. They also recorded his own mounting misfortunes. He wrote papers on the treatment of lupus, rodent ulcer, nasal epithelioma and lymphadenoma, and in an article in 1906 he speculated on ways of measuring the x-ray dose. Thereafter he concentrated his attention on the deleterious effects of x-rays on the tissues of the body, with reference to special case material – himself.

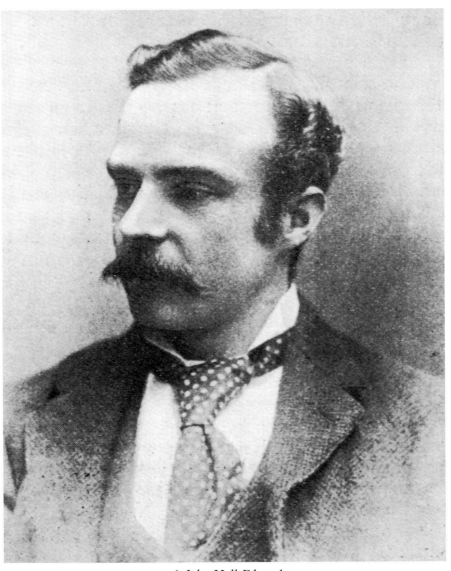

46. John Hall-Edwards

DR. JOHN HALL-EDWARDS (see page 39), at the time of his return from South Africa, already showed irreversible signs of radiation dermatitis. He suffered from its complications for the next 25 years, and he lost his life as a result of malignant transformation. Sir Gilbert Barling, his surgeon, gave a graphic description of Hall-Edwards's plight.[2] The state of the skin of his hands gradually became more precarious until in March 1908 some of the warts on the left hand were shown microscopically to be epitheliomatous; Barling amputated the left forearm. But the right hand was also affected, and soon all the fingers had to be removed, leaving only the thumb. When this news became known, there was a national outcry of concern: Sir Oliver Lodge chaired a public meeting in Birmingham to launch a fund to assist Hall-Edwards, and £800 was subscribed immediately. The *Archives of the Röentgen Ray* in an editorial commiserated with him and it described the welcome that he received from Reginald Morton, President of the Section of Electrotherapeutics when he arrived to attend the Annual Meeting of the British Medical Association in Sheffield in 1908.[3] Later, the *Archives* published Hall-Edwards's important observations on his own case, 'The Effects Upon Bone due to Prolonged Exposure to the X-Ray'. Post-amputation radiography revealed areas of destruction of the phalanges which corresponded to the site of the pain that he had experienced. 'In explaining the pain to my friends' – he wrote – 'I had been in the habit of saying that it felt as if bones were being gnawed away by rats. I was therefore not unprepared to see such changes in the deeper tissues'.[4]

Colleagues testified to the stoicism and fortitude with which Hall-Edwards bore his misfortunes. Indeed he put his experiences to good account by actively broadcasting, locally and nationally, the occupational hazards of radiation. His address to the Electro-Therapeutical Section of the Royal Society of Medicine on 20 November 1908, entitled 'On X-Ray Dermatitis and its Prevention', was one of the first authoritative descriptions of the problem by a radiologist, and it helped to hasten the introduction of the control measures outlined in Chapter 11.[5]

Hall-Edwards's is one of the original British names inscribed on the Martyrs' Memorial in Hamburg. His contribution to the application of x-rays to medicine and surgery was recognised in two other ways: in 1908 he was awarded a pension in the Civil List for services to the Nation, and in 1922 he received a Carnegie Hero Fund bronze medallion and pension, being the first civilian doctor to be so honoured.[6]

Beyond Birmingham Hall-Edwards served as:

Editor, *Archives of the Roentgen Ray*, 1904–5
President, British Electrotherapeutic Society, 1906
Vice-President, Röntgen Society, 1915.

In later years he became involved in local affairs in Birmingham, serving as a City Councillor, and he used his lecturing talents as a cancer publicist. He also took up painting, holding the brush between his remaining right thumb and an artificial finger, and some of his paintings were hung in medical exhibitions. He died, a victim of radiation, in 1926 in Edgbaston, only a few miles from his birthplace in the city of his life's work. He bequeathed a unique collection of early x-ray tubes to the University Department of Physics which are now lodged permanently in the University of Birmingham Medical School.

For rest of biography, see page 215.

Dr. James Brailsford reminisced on his appointment to the Queen's Hospital in the 1920s, on the state of the x-ray departments in the latter years of Hall-Edwards's career: 'The x-ray equipment was unchanged materially for over 20 years. It was maintained by the good man who did all the handywork, opening drains, mending pots and pans, etc. If any part showed defect, it was replaced. . . . Then a good combined couch and screening stand could be obtained for less than £200, and a Coolidge tube for £38. Apparatus was relatively simple, non-shock-proof, and the radiographs were still produced on glass plates. Radiography remained a surgically-oriented speciality – good for fractures, foreign-body localisation and the treatment of skin cancer.'[7] According to the annual report of the Birmingham General Hospital in 1912, 2,000 patients were radiographed, and 250 were screened. These included 922 cases of fracture or suspected fracture, 369 of foreign-body examinations (199 needles, 107 steel fragments, 51 bullets or pellets, 61 objects swallowed, etc.), and 1,709 patients received x-ray treatments.

Dr. Hall-Edwards had two partners, Drs. Black and Emrys-Jones, and the three radiologists attended each hospital for a day or so each week. Before 1914 Franklin Emrys-Jones was a fellow-contributor with Hall-Edwards of case material to radiological meetings and journals; he may have been trained by Thurstan Holland in Liverpool.

The First World War was the catalyst. For the first time chest radiographs were used routinely to detect tuberculosis in soldiers and this work, added to the casualty cases requiring examination, led to an enormous expansion of routine work. This expansion bred its own men, and a talented group of young technicians appeared on the scene in Birmingham to take charge of the x-ray departments of the military hospitals. They were the first generation of professional radiographers and two of them later served as presidents of the Society of Radiographers. George Lovell Stiles, M.B.E., J.P. (1891–1965), the veteran Derby superintendent radiographer, started work in the X-Ray Department of the Birmingham General Hospital under Dr. Hall-Edwards in July 1910 and had x-ray charge of a military hospital during the 1914–18 War.[8] The other President who launched his career under Hall-Edwards was W. H. J. (Harry) Coombs (born 1898), who worked as a youth in the X-Ray Department of the Queen's Hospital until he joined the Army in 1915 as a radiographer. He retired in Sheffield in 1962 after 50 years of hospital work.[9] Two radiographers in the military hospitals were to remain in Birmingham for their professional lives – James Brailsford and William Smith, who worked together for 44 years.

JAMES FREDERICK BRAILSFORD, M.D., Ph.D., F.R.C.P., F.F.R., Hon.F.S.R. (1888–1961) was a young Birmingham laboratory technician-radiographer who studied medicine after the First World War and became one of the world's leading authorities on skeletal diseases.

Born of humble parents, Jimmy Brailsford found work in local laboratories, first at the University and then in the city's public health service. His duties included the examination of specimens of sputum to diagnose tuberculosis, and later he personally recalled the scepticism of the early physicians in relying upon chest radiographs for this purpose. Young Brailsford's ability was recognised by the Medical Officer of Health, Sir John Robertson, and by 1914 he had been promoted sanitary inspector of the City. When the War broke out, Robertson arranged for him to take charge of the x-ray departments of the 1st and 2nd Birmingham War Hospitals sited in the Hollymoor and Rubery Mental Hospital. Brailsford joined the Army and with the rank of sergeant attended the Queen's Hospital to learn the essentials of radiography. Then for four years he produced glass plates with primitive non-shock-proof apparatus for Drs. Hall-Edwards and Black who each visited the Hospital twice a week. For much of the time Sergeant Brailsford was the radiologist.

The War over, Brailsford was discharged from the Army and immediately enrolled – then aged 30 – as a medical student in Birmingham, pursuing his studies with the zest and application that he brought to all tasks. He qualified with honours in 1923, and was immediately appointed assistant radiologist to the Queen's Hospital. Other appointments followed, the more important of which were to the Royal Cripples' Hospital and the Robert Jones and Agnes Hunt Orthopaedic Hospital at Oswestry. His reputation as a bone radiologist increased as his career went from strength to strength. He became known round the world in 1934 with the publication of his book *The Radiology of Bones and Joints*, which ran to several editions and brought him invitations to lecture in many countries.

Honours came from many sources, usually non-radiological ones, and particularly as recognition for work done. From surgeons he received the Robert Jones Medal of the British Orthopaedic Association in 1927 for a paper on deformities of the lumbosacral spine; and in 1935 he was a Hunterian professor of the Royal College of Surgeons of England – the first radiologist to be so honoured. From the University of Birmingham he received a Ph.D. degree in 1936, and the title of 'Honorary Director of Radiological Studies in Living Anatomy'. On his death the University established in his memory the James Brailsford Prize in Radiology. Perhaps the greatest compliment of all was paid to him by his own colleagues, who in 1934 elected him the first President of the British Association of Radiologists (now the Royal College of Radiologists).

James Brailsford was a man with strong convictions who never hesitated to speak his mind. In later years there was an aura of pugnacity about the great radiologist which sometimes hampered clinical communication. 'Bone biopsy is not necessary' – he declared when this diagnostic technique first came to the fore – 'the radiographs provide the diagnosis'. His friends knew that the dour attitude he adopted to some colleagues was the result of his fanatical devotion to his specialty, but it robbed him of some of his earlier high reputation and status. According to one obituarist,[10] Jimmy's colleagues in the Radiologists' Visiting Club saw his best side: he could relax among old friends, the pioneers of British radiology, beyond the reach of his detractors.

THE ROYAL INFIRMARY AND THE WESTERN INFIRMARY, GLASGOW

On 6 June 1896 the *British Medical Journal* carried the following report:[11] 'A Röntgen laboratory has been established in the Glasgow Royal Infirmary. The electrical apparatus in the Hospital is now very complete. . . . Photographs with the Röntgen apparatus have already been taken in the Hospital and it will now form a part of the ordinary work of the electrical department.'

This announcement heralded the start of the first hospital x-ray service in Glasgow. Dr. Macintyre conducted his preliminary experiments in his rooms at 179 Bath Street, but before the end of March – as Lord Kelvin revealed in a letter to the journal, *The Electrician*, 'Dr. Macintyre has converted an arrangement for use in the Royal Infirmary of Glasgow by which already in his own house he has examined bones of patients suffering from disease.'[12] Macintyre 11 years previously in 1885 had been elected 'Hospital Electrician' of the Infirmary and had created a department in a small room which he now expanded to include a pioneer Röntgen laboratory.[13]

This laboratory – claimed by some Scots to be the first department in any British hospital[12,14] – was generously equipped by its benefactors, a small group of well-to-do Glaswegians. It was housed in a room in the Lister Ward of the Infirmary. A photograph shows it to have been fitted out with a patient couch, an upright tube stand and a wall-mounted control panel. Several racks of x-ray tubes are visible on a wall. There were also induction coils, the latest mercury interrupter supplied by Baird and Tatlock, a mechanical interrupter, and several of the focus tubes then recently perfected by Professor Herbert Jackson in London. Using this apparatus, Macintyre continued the remarkable series of experiments already described in Chapter 3. He and his assistants in the Electrical Department also began to deal with large numbers of patients who were referred to them for x-ray examination. In 1901, in addition to frequent screening, over 1,400 radiographs were made of about 1,000 patients. These demands soon out-stripped the facilities available, and in 1901 Macintyre was obliged to ask the Hospital managers for a new department.

The new Electrical Pavilion of Glasgow Royal Infirmary was opened in 1902.[15] It was built alongside the corridor that linked the east and south blocks of the old Infirmary. As had happened in 1896, the entire cost of the building and equipment was borne by local benefactors. One of these was Lord Blythswood, who also donated a Wimshurst static machine built in his laboratory at Renfrew. The Pavilion consisted of four rooms, of which three housed the conventional apparatus of an electrical department, including an electromagnet for extracting metallic foreign bodies, a Finsen lamp and other apparatus for the treatment of skin lesions. The fourth room contained all the x-ray apparatus for diagnostic and therapeutic work, with dark-room accommodation.

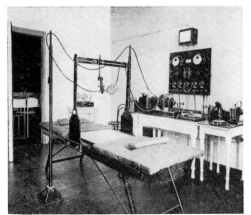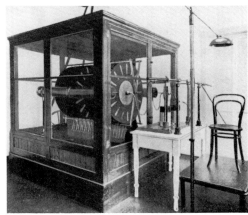

47. *Electrical Department, Glasgow Royal Infirmary in 1902.* Left *x-ray room equipped with a MacKenzie Davidson couch.* Right *Wimshurst machine built and donated by Lord Blythswood*

This room was one of the first purposely equipped x-ray departments in the world under the charge of a medical specialist. Macintyre himself described the apparatus and photographs in the following terms: 'Four large coils, capable of giving 14 to 12 inches spark respectively, have been added to the installation. All the well-known forms of interrupters have been fitted up, including the mercury, MacKenzie Davidson, and Wehnelt. A specially designed switchboard has been attached to the wall, with rheostats for motors, volt- and ampere-meters. There is also a special set of switches, so that any one of the interrupters with suitable condensers can instantly be employed as required for different purposes. Stands and vacuum tubes, Queen's, Dean's, and Cox's 'Record' designs have been provided as well as fluorescent screens, and all the most recent accessories for therapeutic as well as photographic purposes. Two couches have been provided for taking photographs from above or from below. There is also a localizer of the most recent design for detecting the situation of foreign bodies. All the apparatus necessary for the taking and demonstration of stereoscopic photographs have been added to the Department.'

The Electrical Pavilion served for 12 years as the X-Ray Department of the hospital, until the Infirmary was rebuilt. Electrical work in this period increased six-fold, due mainly to the greater demand for x-rays; the rest of the patients, a steadily declining proportion, were seen for electrical treatment or muscle testing:

    1901 – ? patients, 1400 x-rays
    1906 – 3140 patients, 2730 x-rays (87%)
    1914 – 6266 patients, 5725 x-rays (94%)

DR. JOHN MACINTYRE (see page 31) was not only the most distinguished British medical pioneer of x-rays but one of the first medical directors of a hospital x-ray department. Like Hedley and Lewis Jones in London, Macintyre was a medical electrician of some years' standing when Röntgen wrote to Lord Kelvin at the beginning of 1896. He remained in charge for two more decades, and was responsible for establishing the pattern of the x-ray service in Glasgow.

But Macintyre was never a practising radiologist in the modern sense of the description.[17] His inventive curiosity spanned all medical applications of electricity – as befitted the most senior consulting medical electrician in Glasgow – but he never lost sight of his original special interest, otolaryngology.

'Although I have been engaged in the general application of Röntgen's rays' – he wrote in 1896[12] – 'my main work will consist in its application to laryngeal surgery'. One of his earliest cases (in March 1896) was a boy who six months previously had swallowed a coin, which had impacted in his gullet. Macintyre was able to locate its level by means of the fluorescent screen prior to operative removal. This case was described by Lord Lister, then the Regius professor of surgery in Glasgow, when in his Presidential Address to the British Association in Liverpool in September 1896 he referred to 'the wonderful penetrating power' of x-rays. Macintyre never altered his view of his primary profession. In 1914 at the Aberdeen meeting of the British Medical Association when at the height of his radiological fame and he delivered a lecture on the comparative value of x-rays and radium in malignant disease, he styled himself simply 'Surgeon for Diseases of the Throat and Nose, Glasgow Royal Infirmary'. Less than half of his considerable output of scientific papers that he published – 45 out of 111 – dealt with radiological subjects.[18]

In the early days Macintyre was a giant in the new science, and soon he made his mark. Already in 1900 when chosen as the fourth President of the Röntgen Society, he was introduced as 'one of the chief pioneers of the practical application of Röntgen Rays to medicine and surgery'.[19] To the end of his life he never lost his interest in the department or the specialty which he helped to create. John Scott, the respected Glasgow radiographer, when a young member of the staff, was sent regularly to sit by the bedridden doctor to tell him the departmental news.[14]

Dr. Macintyre acquired his first assistant, John Gilchrist, in 1900, but Gilchrist soon moved to become the medical electrician of the Royal Hospital for Sick Children and to take charge of the ophthalmic department of the Infirmary. Penetrating wounds of the eyeball are a common occurrence in any industrial city, and the introduction of radiological localisation pioneered their successful treatment by a powerful electro-magnet. These advances prompted the professor of ophthalmology in Glasgow of that time, to observe that hitherto there was not 'as far as I am aware, a single instance on record of a foreign body having been removed from the vitreous chamber, and the sight at the same time being saved'.[16] When the Electrical Pavilion opened, another medical doctor, James Riddell, was appointed Medical Electrician to assist Dr. Macintyre. In 1903 they were joined by Samuel Capie and in 1906 by two more, styled Assistant Medical Electricians – Archibald Jubb and Catherine Chapman.

JAMES ROBERTSON RIDDELL, F.R.F.P.S. (1874–1935) was the first doctor in Glasgow to confine himself to the practice of diagnostic and therapeutic radiology – thus the city's first radiologist, as the title is now understood.[20]

Riddell was in family practice on the south side of the City in 1899 soon after qualifying, when his interest in the new photography encouraged him to become John Macintyre's assistant at the Infirmary. He abandoned his practice completely in 1902 when appointed Medical Electrician to work whole-time in the new Electrical Pavilion. He served the Glasgow hospitals for 30 years, for the first 18 at the Royal Infirmary, and thereafter at the Western Infirmary until he retired in 1932. James Riddell was the first doctor to be appointed by the University of Glasgow as 'Lecturer in Electrical Diagnosis and Therapeutics', a post which was created in 1916 at the Royal and then transferred in 1920 to the Western Infirmary.[12]

After Macintyre withdrew from active work, Riddell was the senior radiologist in Glasgow. He built up a large practice and was in great demand. In his private rooms at Newton Place he installed the radiotherapeutic apparatus developed by Professor Wintz of Erlangen. He advised many West of Scotland hospitals seeking to establish x-ray departments. Although no writer of articles for the medical press, he was the author of a textbook, *Radiology and Medical Electricity*, published in 1928.

Riddell's life was cut short by his radiation injuries – he underwent many small operations on his face and hands to remove small growths[21] – and his name is one of the original British names on the Martyrs' Memorial in Hamburg.

With the rebuilding of the Glasgow Royal Infirmary, the present x-ray department, then named the George V Electrical Institute, was opened in 1914. It came just in time to handle the huge increase in work occasioned by the War. 'Sixty or eighty photographs may be taken in an afternoon of soldiers and sailors suffering from injury,' it was reported soon after that date. In the first seven months of 1916, 7,000 radiographs were made. The staff had grown to four assistant medical electricians.[12]

At the Western Infirmary, Glasgow's other great hospital, Donald Macintosh, the medical superintendent, was an early x-ray pioneer. Using the simplest equipment and concentrating on those injuries in which x-rays could be of immediate clinical value, he accumulated an interesting collection of cases which he put to good use. In 1899 he published a comprehensive atlas of photographic plates, with brief notes on treatment by a surgeon, G. H. Edington. Macintosh's *Skiagraphic Atlas of Fractures and Dislocations* was one of the first radiological textbooks.[20]

Macintosh carried out photographic and electrical work as part of his general duties as medical superintendent of the Infirmary until 1907. In that year his position as Medical Electrician was confirmed by the hospital managers, and a properly organised department was established, being arranged on the lines of the department in the Royal Infirmary. Three assistants were then appointed – Joseph Goodwin-Tomkinson, later a dermatologist; Archibald Hay who resigned in 1920; and William Francis Somerville, the electrotherapeutist of later years. In 1920, the year in which James Riddell moved from the Royal Infirmary, over 6,000 x-rays were made in the Western Infirmary.

THE ROYAL SOUTHERN HOSPITAL AND THE ROYAL INFIRMARY, LIVERPOOL

The story of radiology in Liverpool started on 7 February 1896 with the case of a 12-year-old boy from Waterloo who had accidently shot himself in the wrist. On that day

Dr. Thurstan Holland, then a young general practitioner in the Princes Park part of the city, served as the boy's escort to the physics laboratory at the University College. Apart from Robert Jones and Professor Lodge, others present in the laboratory to witness the radiograph being made were E. E. Robinson, Lodge's assistant, and the surgeon, Mr. Houlgrave. Holland's name was not mentioned in the case report published by Jones and Lodge in *The Lancet*,[22] but his own account confirmed that he witnessed the 'various attempts and many exposures' made that afternoon which culminated in the historic success.[23] Holland, who admitted that he knew nothing of electricity or vacuum tubes at that time and had never seen an induction coil, was fascinated by the proceedings. Robert Jones had already grasped the potential significance of radiography in his own field and he remarked a few days later in Holland's presence that 'someone in Liverpool must be found to take it up seriously'. He then turned to Holland and asked, 'If I pay for an apparatus, will you undertake it?' Holland jumped at the offer, recalling nearly 40 years later, 'From that moment the whole course of my life was to be revolutionised, and a wonderful career was opened up for me.'

Within months Holland established an x-ray department for Robert Jones in the Royal Southern Hospital. On 29 May 1896 he made his first radiograph, his own hand (exposure time, two minutes). Immediately the surgeons of the hospital began to refer patients to him for radiographs; practically all of them had skeletal lesions. By October the experiment had proved itself and Holland was given an honorary post and found a room in the Hospital. This event inaugurated clinical radiology in Liverpool. No beginning could have been less auspicious from the standpoint of space, apparatus and financial reward. The 'department' was a ground-floor room containing a stone floor and a cold-water sink which was entered from the yard; it had no fireplace or heating apparatus – 'probably no more unsuitable room could have been chosen', Holland recalled,[23] but here he installed his apparatus and developed his plates.

This apparatus was one of the first 'x-ray kits' to be marketed by Newton and Company of London. It was largely untried and found to be unsuitable for clinical work – virtually still an experimental apparatus. The induction coil had a platinum flapper interrupter and gave a 3-inch spark, which proved inadequate and suitable only for extremity work. A panel of Groves batteries produced, when working, a current of 10 to 12 volts, and because of their inconvenience of use and unreliability had soon to be discarded. (Mains electricity had not yet reached the Royal Southern Hospital.) The tube also did not last: it was a pear-shaped vacuum tube without an anti-cathode, consequently when working it disgorged x-rays in all directions from its glass walls, it was soon replaced by one of Professor Jackson's focus tubes which made x-ray work a practical reality. The cost was £30! The difficulties were enormous and continuous, but Holland secured the future by his dogged and down-to-earth approach to problems. 'There was no one in Liverpool to turn to for help and assistance, as one felt one could not be running to a busy physicist like Lodge when every little difficulty arose. The result was that things had to be worked out, and one had to do the best one could for oneself . . .'[24]

Holland's note-book of the work done in 1896 is an x-ray record unique in the world. Before the year ended he had exposed 261 plates, and made the following list:

'A number of plates for testing purposes.
Several cases of exostoses.

Congenital deformities of various kinds – club hand, talipes, equino-varus, cases of
deformities of the bones and hands.

Fractures, old and recent, to show cause of non-union, follow-up cases.

Pieces of needle, mostly hands and feet.

Rheumatoid arthritis.

Osteitis.

Hypertrophic pulmonary osteo-arthropathy.

Strumous dactylitis.

Tuberculous disease of various joints.

Various dislocations, traumatic.

Congenital displacement of the patella.

Congenital dislocation of the hip.

Enchondromata.

Osteoma.

Foetuses.

Coins in the oesophagus.

Foreign bodies such as bullets, swallowed coins, swallowed tooth plate, foreign body
in the eye (an attempt to show), a swallowed trouser button (seen in the rectum
and afterwards passed).

A series of children's hands to show bone growth.

Rickets.

Metatarsalgia.

A piece of an iron fork in a bone and resulting bone changes.

Attempts to examine chests and even the abdomen.

To show the density of various stones.

To show the density of diamonds and paste.

To demonstrate a "mummy bird".

X-ray of a fish to show the bones.

Sprengel's deformity.

Osteomalacia, etc.'

Perhaps modesty prevented Holland from recording in this list the radiograph which
he made of the hand of Lord Lister, President of the British Association which met
in Liverpool in September 1896.

The foundations had been laid. Holland remained at the Royal Southern Hospital
for over seven years, and he admitted that this period was the testing time of his career.
Conditions gradually became better as the service proved its use to the surgeons, another
room adjoining the operating theatre was found, and in 1902 the original x-ray equipment was replaced. The new apparatus included a 10-inch Apps-Newton coil, a Mac-
Kenzie Davidson interrupter and a wall-mounted switchboard which connected the
apparatus through suitable resistances to the city supply of 230 volts. Holland reported:
'The apparatus is so arranged that no harm results if the break is stopped before the
current to the coil is turned off, and is altogether so simple in its arrangement that it
is quite easy for the house surgeons to use it for screening purposes. A large amount
of work is done, many medical cases chiefly of chest diseases, being examined in addition
to the ordinary surgical cases.'[25]

When Holland transferred his work to the Liverpool Royal Infirmary, he left David Morgan at the Royal Southern Hospital as 'Surgeon in Charge of the Electrical Department'.

DAVID MORGAN, M.B., C.M.(Edinburgh, 1884) was, after Holland, the earliest established radiologist in Liverpool. He practised at 46 Nelson Street. Between 1903 and 1908 he contributed a dozen or more papers to the *Archives of the Roentgen Ray*, and he served on the editorial committee of the journal in 1904. One of Morgan's papers was entitled 'Examination of the Urinary Bladder by X-Rays after Insufflation with Oxygen'.[26] Most of the others dealt with skeletal lesions, and he shared their authorship with Robert Jones.

In 1912 when the British Medical Association held its Annual Meeting in Liverpool, Morgan was Vice-President of the Section of Electrotherapeutics, Holland being the President. Morgan's name disappeared from the *Medical Directory* after 1913.

The Royal Infirmary, the principal hospital in Liverpool, was not far behind the Royal Southern Hospital in acquiring apparatus for radiography. The proximity to the physics laboratories of the University College was an advantage, and not long after Professor Lodge's historic experiment a small set borrowed from the University was installed under the main stairs of the Infirmary. The driving force appears to have been the pharmacist Prosper H. Marsden, F.C.S., who persuaded the University authorities to loan him the apparatus.[27] He was an early enthusiast of the new science, being elected to the Röntgen Society in March 1898. He acquired practical experience of radiography in the Infirmary, and was styled as 'Radiographer to the Royal Infirmary' as early as December 1897, when he delivered a lecture on his experiences.[28] Marsden contributed several cases with page-sized plates of excellent quality to the *Archives of the Roentgen Ray* between 1898 and 1904, including superb dental radiographs illustrating an article entitled 'On Radiography Applied to the Dental Surgeon'.[29] Another described the radiograph of a child with a stenotic lacrimal duct in which a probe had been placed.

Marsden's technician continued to work with Thurstan Holland and remained to become a radiation victim. He was C. R. L. Woods, who received severe radiation burns and lost both hands and forearms, dying of radiation-induced carcinoma of the nose and face. Charles Woods (died 1938) was the Liverpool martyr, and his name was added to the Hamburg Memorial in the 1950s. He was awarded the Röntgen Metal, and his disabilities in 1923 earned him the bronze plaque of the Carnegie Hero Fund, which was presented to him by the Duke of York (later King George VI) during a visit to Liverpool.

When Thurstan Holland was appointed to the staff of the Royal Infirmary in 1904, a new x-ray suite had already been equipped by public donations. It occupied the old operating theatre, and consisted of at least three rooms – x-ray room, waiting room, and dark room.[25] The new apparatus was similar to the modern set installed at the Royal Southern Hospital. A second apparatus was soon acquired for x-ray treatments. By 1900 several other Liverpool hospitals possessed equipment for radiography. At the Mill Road Infirmary, the medical superintendent was Nathan Raw, who was elected to the Röntgen Society with Marsden in 1898 – two months before Thurstan Holland. As early as December 1896, Raw showed a group of Manchester doctors radiographs of specimens of human kidney and other organs of which he had injected the arteries with plaster of paris. By 1900 Raw had installed x-ray apparatus in a room opposite

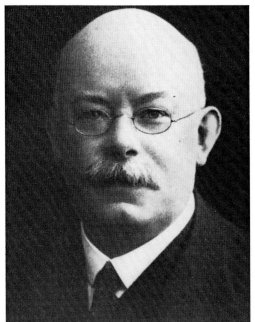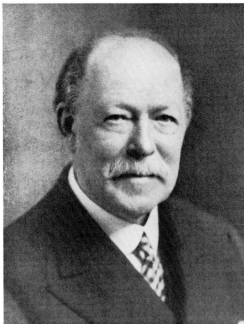

48. The Liverpool pioneers. Left *Prosper Marsden.* Right *Thurstan Holland in later life*

the operating theatre in order to examine patients immediately before and after opera-tions. Of Raw's work, Holland wrote in 1903: 'The x-ray work here is of a high order, and every use is made of the apparatus. A large amount of screening is done. In lupus the results have been good, in rodent ulcer satisfactory. In addition, Dr. Raw has treated a large number of cases of pulmonary phthisis and a number of cases of malignant disease, the latter chiefly inoperable breast cases, and he reports that in both these sets of cases the result has been disappointing . . .'[25] The Stanley Hospital acquired a complete x-ray apparatus in 1900 which, in the absence of a medical electrician, was operated by a house surgeon. The David Lewis Northern Hospital installed apparatus in 1902 for diag-nostic and therapeutic work, and about 200 patients were examined each year, nearly all of them surgical cases and the majority being screened. Soon these hospitals acquired their own medical electrician, who gradually restricted his work to diagnostic and therapeutic radiology – Dr. W. C. Oram.

WALTER CHARLES ORAM, M.D.(Dublin) (1874–1926) came to Liverpool in 1904 and practised there as a radiologist up to his death. Born in Windsor, Nova Scotia, Canada where his father was a professor at King's College, Oram returned to Ireland to be educated. He qualified in medicine at Trinity College, Dublin in 1903 and proceeded to M.D. two years later. Engineer-ing was his first choice as a career, and he is said to have studied medicine in order to apply electricity to medicine.

Oram in 1904 became the Medical Officer in charge of the Electrical Department of the David Lewis Northern Hospital, Stanley Hospital and St. Paul's Eye Hospital, and later Radiologist to the Southport Infirmary.[30] In 1912 he served as the local Secretary to the Section of Electro-therapeutics at the Annual Meeting of the British Medical Association which was held in Liverpool.[31] In the First World War he spent six months in France as a radiologist to the 57th General Hospital. After the war he confined his practice in Liverpool to radiology.

CHARLES THURSTAN HOLLAND (see page 37), the Liverpool master, never ceased to experiment, to innovate and to enrich the status of the new medical specialty which he helped to create. A fellow experimenter, A. E. Barclay, recalled how he had paid Holland a visit in 1906 and found that the x-ray department of the Liverpool Royal Infirmary was 'already quite considerable . . . far in advance of any other in the country'.[32]

Holland's work at the Royal Infirmary, like that of Barclay and a few others elsewhere, was seminal in creating the scientific infrastructure of diagnostic radiology. He helped to establish clinical criteria, teaching standards and diagnostic variations which formed the basis of modern radiological practice. In no small way he helped to write the first radiological literature, contributing a total of 105 papers to medical and scientific journals. His first paper was published in 1899, thereafter his name was seldom absent from the radiological journals until he retired in 1931.

Lifelong collaboration with clinicians such as Robert Jones smoothed the path of Holland and his fellow-radiologists to achieve improved status for the new specialty. His success in this task was given substance by the University of Liverpool who in 1922 conferred on him an honorary Mastership of Surgery. A few years later he was elected as Honorary Fellow of the Royal College of Surgeons. These honours – unique distinctions for a British radiologist – rewarded his lifelong enthusiasm for teaching trainee surgeons in Liverpool. He is remembered as a doctor who enjoyed teaching his younger colleagues in the course of a day's work.

Many national honours came to Thurstan Holland:

President of the Röntgen Society, 1904–5, 1916–7
President of the Electro-Therapeutical Section of the Royal Society of Medicine, 1916–7
President of the British Institute of Radiology, 1929–30.

Undisputed leadership of the profession came in 1925, when he served as President of the first International Congress of Radiology in London.

Thurstan Holland had the vision to see the possibilities which Röntgen's discovery opened up in medicine, and he also possessed the will-power and doggedness of character required to overcome the obstacles which always lie in the path of the pioneer. His young colleague in Liverpool, Robin Roberts (see below), ascribed Holland's success to one particular characteristic – shrewdness. 'His gift of immediate estimation of values was almost uncanny. Time and again has his foresight, regardless of the opinions of others, been proved to be sound.'[33] Of such substance are pioneers made.

ROBERT EDWARD ROBERTS, B.Sc., M.D., F.R.C.P., F.F.R. (1890–1946) succeeded Thurstan Holland in Liverpool in 1931 and became a respected radiologist in his own right. One of the 'Lancashire triumvirate', he assumed leadership of the Northern radiologists after the early deaths of Paterson and Twining.

Born and bred on Merseyside, Robin Roberts qualified with distinction at Liverpool University in 1914. He served in the Army in the First World War, spending three years in India and being mentioned in despatches. After the War he returned to Liverpool and was one of the first to take the Liverpool Diploma in Medical Radiology. He then entered a radiological partnership with Dr. J. H. Mather which lasted for over 20 years.

As Thurstan Holland became less active Roberts took his place in Liverpool – as honorary radiologist of the Infirmary, lecturer in radiology in the University, a luminary of the Medical Institution. Nationally he also upheld the Liverpool tradition established by Holland, serving as:

President of the Section of Radiology of the Royal Society of Medicine, 1937–8
Vice-President of the British Institute of Radiology, 1938–9
President of the Faculty of Radiologists, 1939–40
Honorary Consultant Radiologist to the Army in the Second World War
Section Contributor to the British Authors' *Textbook of Radiology*

He died prematurely at the age of 57.[34]

EDINBURGH ROYAL INFIRMARY

'The Staff of the Edinburgh Royal Infirmary are all suffering more or less from dermatitis,' wrote Dawson Turner in 1909.[35] He attributed these injuries to the fact that 'formerly cases were almost as a matter of course examined with the screen, now a screen examination is an exception, and to be made only in special cases'.

A Medical Electrical Department was established in the Edinburgh Royal Infirmary in 1896 by Robert Milne Murray, and an x-ray service was commenced as an additional function of the Department three years later.[36] Murray was an obstetrician and gynaecologist, an unusual individual who died in 1904 at the early age of 49 years. He had wide interests, apart from his special subjects, and these included the arts, chemistry, mineralogy and electricity – in short, a typical example of the type of colleague whom Allpress Simmons described as the most likely to be recruited into the new specialty (see head of Chapter 5). In addition to Dr. Murray, a second appointment was made in November 1896, that of Assistant Medical Electrician. This latter appointment was to prove the more important, because Murray in 1901 withdrew to wholetime gynaecological practice and the incumbent of the second post was the pioneer, Dawson Turner.

DAWSON FYERS DUCKWORTH TURNER not only introduced x-rays into clinical practice in Edinburgh, as described in Chapter 3 (page 40) – but he was probably the first doctor to provide a regular radiological service in Edinburgh Royal Infirmary. Until he withdrew from diagnostic x-ray and other electrical work in 1911 through ill-health, he was an active publicist of the new photography on the local and national scenes.[37] He served as:

Vice-President, Röntgen Society, 1903
Editorial Committee, *Archives of the Roentgen Ray*, 1904
On the first Council of the Electro-Therapeutical Section of the Royal Society of Medicine, 1907–8.

He was a prolific contributor to the early literature, most of his papers describing innovations or the results of radiotherapeutic endeavours. His first book, *A Manual of Practical Medical Electricity*, which described methods of radiation treatment practised in the Edinburgh Royal Infirmary, was highly successful; a fourth edition was published in 1904. He also wrote a student's guide to the treatment of skin diseases.

From 1911 to 1925 Dawson Turner was physician in charge of the radium department, being styled Extra Medical Electrician to the Infirmary. He early recognised the possibilities of radium in the treatment of malignant lesions and initially hastened introduction of the new modality by purchasing a small quantity of the element himself and placing it at the disposal of the Hospital.[36] During this period he published a further book, *Radium, Its Physics and Therapeutics*.

Dawson Turner's early retirement from diagnostic work was a result of radiation injuries which blighted the rest of his life. He suffered from severe dermatitis, and lost several fingers of his right hand and an eye. His is one of three Edinburgh doctors whose names appear on the Martyrs' Memorial in Hamburg.

The first Electrical Department was sited in makeshift accommodation in the surgical house of the Infirmary, beneath the operating theatre of the professor of clinical surgery. A splint room and a plumber's workshop were converted into four small rooms. The examination room – at that time x-rays were used only for diagnostic purposes – and the dark room were situated in the basement, and reached only by an ill-lit and precipitous staircase. The equipment and apparatus cost only £500; and these cramped and ill-furnished rooms served as temporary home of the young department.[36] The first x-ray photograph was taken in this basement on 14 October 1898.

The impact of the new photography was immediate. In the following year, 600 examinations were made and each year thereafter clinical demand increased – and was so to continue for the next two decades. Better accommodation was soon a matter of urgency, and in 1903–4 the whole of the basement of the South-East Pavilion of the Infirmary was rebuilt and adapted as an electrical department consisting of 12 rooms.[35] This wing had served for most of the 19th century as the residential quarters of the Steward and the Dispenser, and after that date these officials were no longer required to live in the Infirmary.

Dawson Turner's tenure as the head of the Department lasted from 1901 until 1911, when he embarked on a career as the country's first specialist radiotherapist. His assistant during this early period was another martyr pioneer, J. W. L. Spence. In 1911, when both Spence and Dawson Turner left the Electrical Department, a joint directorship was embarked upon, Archibald McKendrick and William Hope Fowler being given combined charge. This arrangement lasted until both men retired in 1926. These four men, Dawson and Spence, and McKendrick and Hope Fowler, were the founders of the Edinburgh School of Radiology.

JOHN WEBSTER LOWSON SPENCE, L.R.C.P., L.R.C.S.(Edinburgh), L.F.P.S.(Glasgow) (1871–1929) was the second doctor in Edinburgh to devote his life to radiation medicine and to pay the pioneer's penalty. A graduate of the University, he was a general practitioner in Edinburgh at the time of Röntgen's discovery, and early began experimenting with x-rays. From 1901 he was Dawson Turner's assistant and in 1907 took charge of the Electrical and X-ray Department of the Royal Edinburgh Hospital for Sick Children. There he remained until he retired in 1928.

Spence by 1909 – the year in which Dawson Turner made his observation about dermatitis – suffered severely, and later his injuries became worse. In 1910 a finger was amputated from his right hand, but the spreading ulceration and destruction did not cease and led in 1916 to a below-shoulder amputation of his right arm. Spence soldiered on in hospital practice, but in 1922 his left hand became affected and just before he died he lost it also by amputation. With Hall-Edwards he was the recipient of a medal and annuity from the Carnegie Hero Fund for his services to x-ray work.[37] Spence's is one of the original British names on the Martyrs' Memorial in Hamburg.[38]

WILLIAM HOPE FOWLER, C.V.O., M.B., Ch.B., M.R.C.P.E., F.R.C.S.E. (1876–1933), the co-director of the Electrical Department for 15 years until 1926, was the third Edinburgh martyr to have his name inscribed on the Hamburg Memorial.[39]

Graduating from the University of Edinburgh in 1897, Hope Fowler soon interested himself in the new photography and in 1901 when in general practice in the city became a clinical assistant to Dawson Turner at the Infirmary. After assuming joint charge of the Department with McKendrick in 1911, he became the leading radiologist in the city – lecturer in radiology in the Royal College of Surgeons, examiner in radiology in the Royal College of Physicians of Edinburgh, and honorary consultant to several institutions. An important early contribution to the literature was Hope Fowler's paper, 'Ortho-radiography of the Heart and Aorta', which appeared in the *Edinburgh Medical Journal* in 1912. During the First World War he served as Consultant Radiologist to the Royal Navy and as a member of the War Office X-Ray Committee. Partly in recognition of this service, he received near the end of his life, the award of Commander of the Victorian Order.[40] By this time he was a leader among the radiologists. Hope Fowler was one of the

11 members of the profession who attended the important meeting at MacKenzie Davidson's house in London 1917 to organise the profession.[41] Towards the end of his life he took the lead in Scotland by founding the Scottish Radiological Society in 1930, and he was the first President.[42]

Hope Fowler's injuries were aggravated by the enormous amount of screening involved in fracture diagnosis and foreign body localisation during the First World War. He had received his first burn as early as 1899, when almost nothing was yet known of the harmful effects of x-rays. Although excised, other injuries followed from more powerful apparatus which was still inadequately protected. Ill-health forced his retirement from hospital practice when only 50 years old. His right arm was amputated a few months before his death at the age of 57 years. Scotland, wrote his obituarist in 1933,[40] had by his premature death lost its most distinguished figure in radiology.

By the 1920s the Electrical Department of the Infirmary faced a severe crisis. The accommodation which had been makeshift and cramped in 1903 had become totally inadequate to meet the demands of the medical and surgical staff, which still continued to increase. Plans to build a modern pavilion had been discussed in 1914 but shelved during the War, and they were now reconsidered. In 1923 a special subcommittee of the Hospital Board met under the chairmanship of Sir James Hodsdon, and the efforts of this body were rewarded in the opening of the New Radiological Department in October 1926. Several parallel events in Edinburgh at that time gave impetus to this project and helped to make a new department a landmark in the growth of British radiology. Doubtless there was concern that the three part-time radiologists, Dawson Turner, McKendrick and Hope Fowler, were approaching the end of their careers, two of them partly disabled by their radiation injuries; clearly a fresh beginning were required – and one which would cope with a speciality that had come of age.

In 1923 the Hospital managers approached the Court of the University of Edinburgh with important proposals. They suggested that a lectureship in medical electro-therapeutics and radiology should be established, and that the lecturer should be the doctor chosen by the hospital as the radiologist to the Infirmary. Two departures from the existing position were implied by these proposals, namely that the doctor appointed would be paid a salary by the University to teach radiology, and that he would devote all his time to the combined task of directing the x-ray department and instructing students. In Edinburgh the use of radiographs in clinical teaching was then already established, and these measures were intended to strengthen this practice. When the medical student Richard ('Uncle Fungus') Fawcitt in 1910 fractured his wrist, Hope Fowler showed him the fracture. Radiographs were already forming part of the clinical surgery *viva* examination, being usually shown to distinction or borderline candidates.[43] Agreement was reached between hospital and University in 1925, and Dr. J. M. W. Morison, then A. E. Barclay's assistant at the Manchester Royal Infirmary, accepted the dual appointment as Head of the Radiological Department and Lecturer in Radiology. The University took the next logical step in the following year, when it established a postgraduate diploma course in radiology.

JOHN MILLER WOODBURN MORISON, M.D., F.R.C.P.(Edinburgh), D.M.R.E., F.F.R. (1875–1951) was the torchbearer of academic radiology in Scotland. Not only did he occupy the first paid academic post in this specialty, but in 1930 was chosen as the first professor of radiology in Britain, tenable at the Royal Cancer Hospital in London.

Born into a doctor's family in Ayrshire, Morison was approaching middle age while serving in India during the First World War when he developed an interest in radiology. He was a friend of Thurstan Holland, and after training in Liverpool he was sent to France as the radiologist of the Liverpool Merchants' Mobile Hospital. After the War he was appointed as Honorary Radiographer to the District Infirmary at Ashton-under-Lyne, and from here he went to Manchester Royal Infirmary as Assistant Radiologist to A. E. Barclay when the new radiological department opened in 1922.[32] From this post he returned to Edinburgh.[44]

The New Radiological Department of which Dr. Morison took charge was described as the most modern in Europe.[45] It was situated in a building erected on vacant ground between the medical and surgical houses on the east side of the long corridor connecting these two sections of the infirmary, so that it was readily accessible to both houses. It was 160 feet long and 60 feet wide, and consisted of three floors. The basement contained the engineers' workshop and all the heavy (and noisy) machinery – 3 generators, the largest being of 42 kilovolts supplying alternating current to the building and 3 high-tension transformers with rotating rectifiers, supplying current to the screening rooms above. The ground floor comprised waiting rooms and administrative offices; a diagnostic radiographic room; two diagnostic screening rooms for chest and barium studies respectively; dark rooms and a large demonstration room; and deep x-ray therapy (maximum 125 kV) and superficial therapy apparatus. The first floor housed the non-radiological remains of the electrical department – massage and physical therapeutics; a gymnasium; rooms for electrotherapy; heat and light therapy; and a section for radium treatment.[46]

Robert Knox, the radiologist to King's College Hospital, acted as honorary adviser in planning the internal arrangements, which in several ways were innovative. Therapy radiographers during treatments were totally protected in lead-lined cubicles containing lead windows. All partition walls were built of barium cement slabs and the floors and ceilings were similarly protected by barium cement, to an equivalent of 4 mm of lead. Controlled ventilation was achieved by a system of exhaust fans in the roof of the building. The novel idea of siting the generators on the floor below necessitated electrical precautions – aluminium conductors, high-tension switches and tube connectors ran overhead in the rooms and out of reach. The massive insulators conducting the high-tension supply through the floors were enclosed in metal cages.[45] As the final innovation, the old name 'Medical Electrical Department' disappeared, and was superseded by the new one, 'Radiological Department'.

At the opening ceremony on 9 October 1926, performed by the Duke of York (later King George VI), the platform party consisted of distinguished Scottish and City officials and members of the medical and surgical staff of the Infirmary. Also present were Robert Knox and Thurstan Holland, the latter being not only Morison's original mentor but also at that time the acknowledged leader of British radiologists. In declaring the Department open, the Duke made a pointed reference to the great work done by the pioneers in radiology and to the sacrifices which some had made as a result of their research: to such an audience in Edinburgh, it was not necessary to mention Dawson Turner, John Spence and Hope Fowler by name.

Dr. Morison's five-year tenure as the departmental head heralded a new team to replace the old Medical Electricians, Dawson Turner, Hope Fowler and McKendrick. His assistant was W. C. Fothergill, and others first appointed at this time were J. B.

King and G. C. Allan. Continuity with the *ancien régime* was provided by a radiographer, William Law, an apprentice electrician under Dawson Turner who became a radiographer and then Radiographer in Charge, before falling victim to his injuries.[45] His distinguished successor was Neil Longden, M.B.E., Hon.F.S.R., who began working in the Infirmary as a dark room assistant in 1929 and retired 42 years later from his post as Group Superintendent Radiographer; he died shortly afterwards. Longden's father was the chief electrical engineer of the Infirmary from 1900 to 1935, and his family's service to the Infirmary totalled 150 years.[47]

ANCOATS HOSPITAL AND THE ROYAL INFIRMARY, MANCHESTER

The seeds of a radiological service in Manchester were probably sown by Professor Arthur Schuster when he suggested to the Manchester Medical Society in 1896 that rooms and a technician should be provided for this purpose, as described in Chapter 3. Before 1900 efforts had succeeded to introduce an x-ray service at the old Royal Infirmary in Piccadilly, and a place was found for the apparatus in the gallery of the chapel which had been partitioned off. Medical control was given to the directors of the clinical laboratory, Dr. C. H. Mellar and later Dr. E. B. Leech, to whom doctors sent their requests. The apparatus was operated by a firm of Manchester chemists who attended by contract to take radiographs. A technician, F. E. Doran spent each morning at the Infirmary and in the afternoons worked for the chemists, who had a monopoly of the private practice.

Intent on breaking this monopoly and changing radiology from a chemist-shop commodity to a branch of clinical medicine, there now returned to his home town a young man who became one of the founding fathers of the profession – A. E. Barclay.

In 1906 in partnership with an anaesthetist at the Manchester Royal Infirmary, W. J. S. Bythell, Barclay boldly fixed his brass plate and set up as a specialist in radiology and electrology in the City. It was a venture of faith, he recalled later,[32] and their gross takings for the first year amounted to less than half the rent of their rooms, but it was to be successful. Two decades later both men had been elected to the honorary medical staff of their hospitals and radiologists had been accepted as members of the medical team.

The great question was, wrote Barclay,[48] 'Could a medical man make a living by the practice of radiology when, for practical purposes he could look only to the fracture work to provide an income? It was a doubtful venture even in London, where most of the specialist work of the country was at that time still centred . . .' Barclay and Bythell's apparatus consisted of a coil which gave a 12-inch spark, operated by a mercury jet break equipped with a Morton rectifier – the latter was a device for cutting out the pernicious inverse current so fatal to gas tubes. In order to provide the direct current required for the coil, a transformer was acquired which, despite mounting in a soundproof box, filled the consulting rooms with noise.

Early success came to the partnership in the form of an invitation to Barclay to join the honorary staff of Ancoats Hospital, which had received an x-ray apparatus in 1907 as a gift. He accepted it, and soon created a clinical x-ray department there – the first to be established in Manchester. The opening of this department had two important results, one being to provide Barclay with clinical case material for his celebrated experiments with the bismuth subnitrate meal for studying the oesophagus and stomach, which now are a classic of radiology. At Ancoats he first identified a case of pyloric obstruction correctly, and news of this case and other successes soon spread among Manchester doctors. Late in 1908 he was invited, at the suggestion of Dr. Leech, to organise an electrical, x-ray and massage department in the new Royal Infirmary.

The new Manchester Royal Infirmary, rebuilt in Oxford Road at a distance from Piccadilly and planned to be the most modern and up-to-date hospital in the country, opened in 1908 without any provision having been made for an electrical department.[49] Barclay accepted the invitation and signed a contract to attend on six mornings a week for a salary of £50 a year, starting on 12 January 1909.

ALFRED ERNEST BARCLAY, O.B.E., M.D.(Cantab.), D.M.(Oxon), D.Sc.(Hon. Oxon. and Manchester), F.R.C.P., D.M.R.E., F.F.R. (1876–1949) was perhaps the greatest of the pioneer British radiologists. When he died, 'Uncle B' (as his friends called him) had outlived his contemporaries and was called 'The Grand Old Man of British Radiology'.[50]

His professional achievements are prodigious: between 1908 and 1948 he wrote over 100 original papers and several books on radiological subjects; he served as President of the Electro-Therapeutical Section of the Royal Society of Medicine (1919–20), the Röntgen Society (1924–5), and the British Institute of Radiology (1932); he helped to establish and for seven years personally taught the Cambridge D.M.R.E. course, one of the first courses of academic instruction in the world for radiologists; and at Oxford he pioneered the use of radiological methods in clinical research.

Born in Manchester to the wife of a merchant, Barclay first heard of x-rays at the breakfast table. His father always read the *Manchester Guardian* and during the Christmas season of 1896 a paragraph caught his eye and he announced to the family: 'A man claims to have discovered

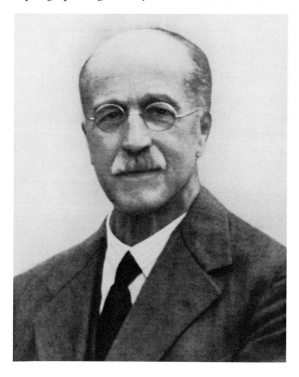

49. A. E. Barclay

a new kind of light that will penetrate solids and show the bones in the hand. How absurd!'[49] Young Barclay was educated at the Leys School and Christ Church, Cambridge and went to the London Hospital for his clinical studies, qualifying in 1904. From the start of his career he was drawn into radiology and in 1906 he returned to Manchester.

Barclay's unique standing and reputation rests on the 22 years which he spent in Manchester as a radiologist. They were the formative decades of the young specialty, and a description of Barclay's Manchester years tells the story of early British radiology.[51]

For the rest of biography, see pages 183–184.

WILLIAM JAMES STOREY BYTHELL, M.D.(Victoria) (1872–1950), Barclay's partner, was one of Manchester's three pioneer radiologists. Unlike Barclay, he never tore up his Manchester roots, playing a less prominent part in national affairs.

A Cambridge and Manchester graduate and an anaesthetist at the old Royal Infirmary, Bythell in 1906 joined Barclay in a partnership in radiology and electrology. He took charge of the electrical department at Ancoats Hospital in 1908 when Barclay moved to the new Infirmary, and later he was also the radiologist to the Manchester Children's Hospital and the Salford Royal Hospital.

Co-authorship with Barclay on the textbook, *X-ray Diagnosis and Treatment* in 1912 marked the productive period of Bythell's career. In that year he was elected to the Röntgen Society, and from 1913 he served for five years on the Council of the Electro-Therapeutical Section of the Royal Society of Medicine. Before the latter Society he was a forceful exponent of the value of radiography in the early diagnosis of lung tuberculosis, participating in the celebrated 1913 debate, see Chapter 8. Soon after this date he led a discussion on the x-ray appearances of benign and malignant bone tumours.[52]

Bythell served as a captain in the Royal Army Medical Corps throughout the First World War and continued to practise in Manchester in the 1920s. Thereafter he retired to Shropshire where he died at the age of 78 years after the Second World War.[53]

Barclay's first task in the rebuilt Manchester Royal Infirmary in 1909 was to find space for a department. Experience at Ancoats Hospital had convinced his clinical colleagues of the benefits of screening patients with gastrointestinal disorders, and they supported his demand for two diagnostic x-ray rooms, one for radiographic work and the other for screening (*see* 50). A third room was needed for treatment, as well as a dark room and an office. After a prolonged search, Barclay found that the basement space beneath the Receiving Room had been allocated in the new hospital plans to use for Russian and mud baths but, because – as he pointed out[32] – nobody seemed to know what these were, this area was given over to him. Equipping the department was an even greater problem, because the hospital rebuilding scheme had swallowed up all the money. Barclay turned to George Webb, the hospital carpenter, and together they built an upright screening stand and a couch in the carpenter's shop. Both items of apparatus served their purpose well, and the screening set remained in regular use until the basement department was abandoned in 1921. The stand had 4-inch square wooden uprights with a 3-ply insert against which the patient stood – the insert was the side of an old tea chest, according to Cuthbert Andrews.[54] The tube was raised and lowered by a ratchet, and the diaphragm was operated by curtain-ropes with tassels.

The gas tubes caused the most trouble. Their unreliability remained the Achilles heel of the new science, and their management was an art which was not widely understood. Each cost less than £2, and most early radiologists kept a supply in reserve. When Barclay demanded nine new x-ray tubes, an outraged hospital secretary asked, 'What have you done with the one we bought last year?'

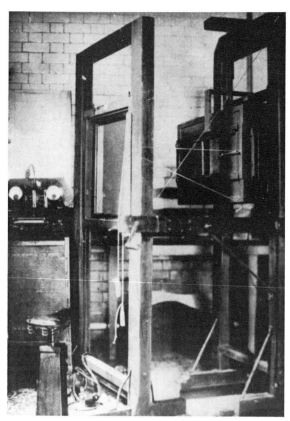

50. The upright screening stand built and installed for A. E. Barclay by George Webb, the hospital carpenter in the basement of Manchester Royal Infirmary in 1909. The stand remained in regular use until 1921

In this primitive department, unsatisfactory because it was cramped and not readily accessible for bed patients, Barclay pioneered and described the opaque meal. This method of examination was a routine practice in Manchester long before it found general acceptance in many parts of the country.[32]

Barclay's pre-1914 career in Manchester represented his missionary years – and probably his most enjoyable. His prime task and that of his partner Bythell in those early days, was to publicise the advantages of radiology in internal diagnosis, and to establish its reliability. Their early textbook, *X-ray Diagnosis and Treatment* (1912) reflected their zeal. Barclay devoted his life to the x-ray study of the gastrointestinal tract, and the foundation of his knowledge was the systematic screening of patients and his routine attendance in the operating theatre, first at Ancoats Hospital and then in the Manchester Royal Infirmary. In 1909 he read a paper before the Röntgen Society in London entitled 'The Value of X-rays in Diseases of the Digestive System'.[55] Four years later when his first book on the subject was published, *The Stomach and Oesophagus*, he noted with satisfaction that he was no longer told when his diagnosis was successful, but only when it was wrong!

In Manchester – as in Birmingham and Glasgow and other major British centres – the First World War halted the progress of radiology, which up to 1914 had been a story of steady advance and development.[48] Within months 25,000 beds had to be found in the hospitals, schools and public buildings of Manchester and Stockport, and soon the casualties arrived to fill them. The difficult access to the basement department in the Infirmary ruled out its use for the large numbers of cases of fracture and foreign body localisation that were suddenly demanded of the radiologists. Barclay, now a captain in the Royal Army Medical Corps, immediately established a temporary department in the main military hospital in Manchester, which occupied a large high-school building in Whitworth Street. This department, which was on the third floor of the building, was organised to operate at speed. With the help of volunteers from the city's business community, relays of stretcher bearers carried the injured up and down the stairs, and others prepared them for the radiologist at one couch while he was busy examining at the other couch, and yet others took down notes and the radiologist's report of the screen examination. So rapid was this service, Barclay recalled,[32] that on one occasion he examined about 80 cases in little over an hour. Later as apparatus became available for installing in the surrounding military hospitals, the demand on ambulances and the central x-ray department was reduced. Eventually, the sergeants did most of the x-ray work in the military hospitals in Manchester.

When the War ended, clinical demands on the basement x-ray department of the Manchester Royal Infirmary had become so intense that they could no longer be met. The one diagnostic room, devoted to screening and other medical examinations and serving also as the plate-viewing room, was responsible for 2,100 examinations a year, or seven examinations each working day. The other room was used for routine radiography of the surgical cases, and about 9,300 plates a year were made. It was obvious that something had to be done to rehouse not only the x-ray but also the electrotherapeutic and massage departments in more accessible portions of the hospital. Then in September 1918 an event occurred which was to hasten the arrival of a new department; Barclay, having already worked in the Infirmary for nine-and-a-half years, was elected to the honorary medical staff. He wrote: 'It was extraordinary what this change in title brought about. The status of the department seemed to change overnight. The honorary radiologist was suddenly accepted by his colleagues, who with the lay board, at once backed his campaign in working for a new and more adequate department.'[32]

In 1921 the space became available in the Infirmary which is still occupied by the x-ray department. At last the basement could be vacated. At the same time electrotherapy and massage was separated from the x-ray department and located elsewhere. In the next year, the contract with the firm of Manchester chemists to supply technical x-ray assistance was terminated. One of the measures taken to provide clinical support for the new department was the appointment of a second honorary radiologist in that year, Dr. J. M. W. Morison. As has already been noted, Morison spent little more than two years in Manchester as Barclay's assistant, before taking charge of the x-ray department of the Edinburgh Royal Infirmary.

Whatever aspirations Barclay and Morison possessed in designing and equipping the new department, they were hedged by severe constraints. The most serious of these was the need to fit the entire department into the space available, which had ferroconcrete walls that were two feet thick and unalterable, and yet to do so in a way that would allow for a large increase in the volume of work. When Barclay described the departmental plan at a meeting of the Röntgen Society in January 1923,[1] envy and admiration were expressed by his London colleagues at the 'formidable list of rooms' that had been acquired. X-ray treatment remained in the department for the time being, but it was confined to two rooms and three treatment cubicles. Nonetheless, for the 1920s the diagnostic facilities were positively lavish – three examination rooms (two for screening including a tilting couch), a properly-equipped dark room, a plate-viewing and store room (soon to be adapted for the use of films only), a secretary's office, a room to examine patients, a demonstration room, and other facilities such as a waiting hall, workshop, nurses' staff room and lavatories – in all about 20 rooms.

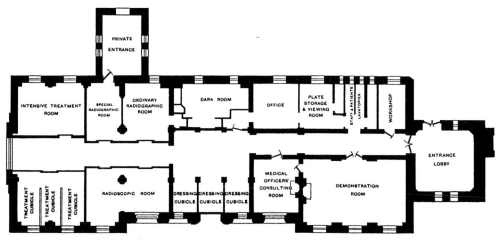

51. Ground plan of the new x-ray Department, Manchester Royal Infirmary, 1923

Several of Barclay's planned innovations were frustrated. The most important was his wish to have all the transformers on the floor below. When the department was found to be only partly cellared, this revolutionary arrangement had to be abandoned, and it was first introduced by Dr. Morison in the Edinburgh Royal Infirmary. In order to achieve radiation protection, Barclay planned to line the walls with sheet lead. However, a plaster mixture of barium sulphate and cement was found to be cheaper and more satisfactory, and the admixture of commercial barium sulphate, Portland cement and sand in equal parts applied to $\frac{3}{4}$-inch thickness on one side of a wall provided a minimum lead equivalent of 3.5 mm, as tested with radium. This was perhaps the first use of a technique which is now a standard method of radiation protection. Another successful innovation was the fitting of lead-lined sliding doors. High-tension transformers and Coolidge tubes were used throughout, replacing the coils and gas tubes on the grounds of greater reliability of output. Barclay's comment indicates how painful progress can be to the innovator: 'They may not be quite so brilliant as the very best work on the old type of outfit,' he wrote.[1]

Morison's departure to Edinburgh in 1924 brought R. S. Paterson to the honorary staff as Assistant Radiologist, and when Barclay himself went to Cambridge in 1928 (see page 183), E. W. Twining joined the department.

RONALD SIMPSON PATERSON, M.D., F.F.R., D.M.R.E. (1894–1939), who succeeded Barclay as Honorary Radiologist of the Infirmary in 1928 (at the age of 34), had an exceptional gift for organisation. For the next 11 years up to his early death, he performed pioneering work in developing a large and tightly organised department.

A son of Lancashire and a graduate of Manchester University, Pat Paterson one day shortly after the War went down the steep steps of the basement department with his Alsation dog

Bosh to ask after x-ray work. Barclay took him on as Registrar, and in 1924 promoted him to succeed Morison. He took charge of the department four years later when Barclay resigned.[56]

In the 1930s he was one of the 'Lancashire triumvirate' (Roberts and Twining being the other two) who exerted an unusually powerful influence on pre-war British radiology. In 1933, as President of the Section of Radiology of the Royal Society of Medicine, he was a prime mover in forming the British Association of Radiologists, the forerunner of the Faculty of Radiologists (now the Royal College of Radiologists). In 1926 he succeeded Dr. Brailsford as the Association's second President. He died suddenly aged 45 years, only a few weeks before his partner, Edward Twining, see below.[57]

EDWARD WING TWINING, M.R.C.S., M.R.C.P., F.F.R., D.M.R.E. (1887–1939) was a man with an original and innovative mind and great manual dexterity, who was able to translate his thoughts into reality in his own workshop. In some respects he was Barclay's successor – a writer of textbooks and a developer of techniques, a practical man of ideas whose national and international reputation brought recognition to him and Manchester and British radiology. Paradoxically, his mental energy probably sprang from his lifelong physical disability, which was a result of chronic osteomyelitis following a trivial infection of the skin acquired when a dresser as a medical student.

He was the son of a Salcombe doctor who had been tragically killed by a fall from his horse, and Twining owed his education to a foundation scholarship from Epsom College. He qualified at University College Hospital in 1913 and went into general practice in Hampshire. Although rejected for War service on account of his lameness, Twining in 1915 was placed in charge of the X-ray and Electrotherapeutic Department at Netley Hospital on Southampton Water, with the rank of captain in the Royal Army Medical Corps. Here he developed his interest in radiology, taking instruction from Dr. Norman Aldridge and attending meetings in Southampton. He remained at Netley after the War, working for the Ministry of Pensions, and then in 1922 he resigned and went to St. Thomas's Hospital to study for the newly-instituted Cambridge diploma in radiology. Barclay was the examiner when he sat the examination in 1923, and he immediately offered Twining a post in Manchester. Twining joined Barclay and Paterson as a partner and became Honorary Radiologist to Ancoats Hospital and to the Christie Hospital and Holt Institute. In 1928 when Barclay left for Cambridge, Twining was elected to the honorary staff of the Manchester Royal Infirmary.[58]

Twining's lectureship in radiology in the University and his hospital appointment for 15 years provided the ideal soil for his original seeds, and he and his successors reaped a rich harvest. During this period he wrote many papers and made three contributions of outstanding importance to diagnostic radiology. The first of these grew out of his lectures to the medical students on the radiographic anatomy of the lungs,[59] which culminated in his monumental work on the radiology of the respiratory system. It occupied most of the particular volume of British Authors' *Text Book of X-ray Diagnosis* which he edited jointly with Cochrane Shanks and Peter Kerley in 1938. For this work, which has been described as 'probably the finest account of the radiology of the chest that has ever been written',[58] he was awarded the M.R.C.P. (London) in 1938. His second contribution was the product of his workshop – a simple add-on attachment for the standard Bucky couch which brought tomography to departments all over the country and extended its applications from diseases of the chest to cerebral diagnosis.[60] His third field, and unquestionably his greatest contribution to medicine, was his study of the ventricles of the brain. It brought him a Hunterian professorship of the Royal College of Surgeons in 1936 and recognition from many authorities, including Erik Lysholm,[61] as a pioneer neuroradiologist. Nowadays the position of the fourth ventricle of the brain continues to be measured by 'Twining's line', and the medal which British neuroradiologists bestow upon presidents of their Society bears a picture of Edward Twining. He was a founder of the Faculty of Radiologists and shortly before his death he was chosen as President-elect of both the Faculty and the Section of Radiology of the Royal Society of Medicine – a fitting climax to his career. The Twining Medal of the Royal College of Radiologists commemorates his unique contribution to the profession.

ROYAL VICTORIA INFIRMARY, NEWCASTLE-UPON-TYNE

A primitive diagnostic x-ray service existed in the Infirmary as early as July 1898, when two competing firms of chemists in the City, Brady and Martin, and Proctor Son and Claque, attended at the request of the surgeons to take radiographs of patients. The clinical impetus for this service may have come from Dr. William Martin, the Newcastle doctor who made radiographs of his patients for the surgeon, Rutherford Morison. Early in 1898 the *Archives of the Roentgen Ray* published two of his cases, both illustrated with radiographs. One showed a bullet in a foot (exposure time, 90 seconds), and the other a coin in the oesophagus of a young boy who had swallowed a half-penny 25 days before (exposure, 7 minutes).[62] Twenty years later, Dr. Martin still practised radiology from his home, West Villa, Akenside Terrace in Newcastle. His teacher may have been Dr. (later Professor) Stroud of the Newcastle-upon-Tyne College of Science, who is known to have produced a radiograph of a patient's hand containing a lead bullet using home-made equipment on 21 April 1896 – less than four months after the news of Röntgen's discovery reached England.[63]

In 1899 the old Infirmary at Forth Banks acquired x-ray equipment of its own for examining patients, which was installed on Ravensworth Ward. An assistant surgeon, Mr. H. Brunton Angus was put in clinical charge of the apparatus and a technician, Mr. Dodd was appointed to operate it and to keep a record book. Thomas Dodd (died 1929), the older brother of the head porter and the first member of the x-ray staff, was associated first with the old Infirmary and then with the new Infirmary for over 20 years. He was severely burnt and lost three fingers, and ultimately died as a result of radiation damage;[65] his name is inscribed on the Martyrs' Memorial in Hamburg. Record-keeping commenced on 14 March 1899, the first patient to be examined being a case of fracture of the tibia (exposure time, 15 minutes). The second was a patient with a dislocation of the knee. The annual total number of diagnostic examinations carried out in the years 1899, 1900 and 1901 were 164, 157 and 201 respectively. These figures show that the anticipated increase in clinical demand for radiographs did not materialise, contrary to experience elsewhere in the country. The reason appears to have been the poor results, as one of the contemporary house surgeons recalled: 'The apparatus was housed in a small room at the south end of the old Ravensworth Ward and consisted of a coil, a Röntgen tube and accumulators. It was mostly very hopeful but disappointing in performance. . . . Screening was satisfactory for fractures of the hand, but when you came to the knee, shoulder or hip the results were like a foggy night at the coast!'[64]

The new Royal Victoria Infirmary opened in July 1906 with an Electrical Department which included apparatus for x-ray and electrotherapeutic work and massage. As in Manchester and elsewhere, this department may have been omitted from the original plans, and only an unsatisfactory basement site was provided beneath Ward 1. The department consisted of an x-ray room, a dark room and two rooms for massage and electrical treatment. The x-ray equipment was the standard gas tube clamped to a wooden retort stand and powered by a coil and interrupter. There was no protection. The x-ray plates when developed were viewed against a ground-glass window facing Ward 8. Slatted wooden bars were fixed across the window and into these the plates were slid. The window and its bars were found undisturbed long after the x-ray department had moved elsewhere, when the basement was refurbished in the 1960s.

The House Committee of the Infirmary at this time made two decisions which guaranteed the future of the x-ray service. By the first, it ruled that all cases of fracture or suspected fracture would henceforth be radiographed. The second was the appointment in June 1906 of a medical officer to take charge of the Electrical Department – Dr. W. D. Arnison.

WILLIAM DREWETT ARNISON, Hon.M.A., M.D.(Dunelm), Hon.F.F.A.R.C.S. (1865–1950), an early radiologist in Newcastle-upon-Tyne, was an interesting personality. He came from a long-established Northumbrian medical family – great-grandfather, grandfather and father practised at Allendale Town, and his uncle was a professor of surgery at Durham – and he attended the College of Medicine in Newcastle-upon-Tyne, qualifying in 1886 and proceeding to M.D. four years later. In 1891 he was appointed to the Royal Victoria Infirmary as the first anaesthetist, then the only one in the city. He held this post for 15 years, and his pioneering work was recognised 40 years later, when at the age of 84 he was elected an honorary Fellow of the Faculty of Anaesthetists.

In 1907 Dr. Arnison gave up anaesthetics and became the Infirmary's first medical electrician, starting in the basement room with primitive apparatus. With the aid of Mr. Dodd, he gradually built up the electrotherapeutic department over the next 18 years.

Dr. Arnison retired with the title of 'Consultant Radiologist', and served the medical community of Newcastle in many ways for another 25 years. One of his achievements in retirement was the preparation of a book, *History of the Newcastle School of Medicine*, published to commemorate the centenary of the school. He also served on the Senate of Durham University, and received an honorary Master of Arts degree.[66]

For 13 years the basement department beneath Ward 1 provided the only x-ray service in Newcastle. Continued success is reflected in the work totals, which increased annually:

1906	–	1,135 plates,	983 screenings
1909	–	2,974 plates,	474 screenings
1911	–	4,196 plates	
1915	–	7,603 plates,	960 screenings
1918	–	12,905 plates,	1,061 screenings.

The First World War forced the pace. In 1914 the War Office requisitioned Armstrong College and used the buildings as a hospital, the First Northern General (Military) Hospital, and obliged the Infirmary to find 200 additional beds for injured servicemen. This great influx of patients, many of whom required radiographs for suspected fracture or foreign body localisation, strained the x-ray department to the limit and increased the pressure to find more space elsewhere.

In 1918 following a public appeal the Military Orthopaedic Centre was built, later called the War Pensions Hospital and then the Leazes Hospital (now part of the Infirmary), and the Electrical Department moved into new quarters within this building in the following year, to a site still occupied by the x-ray department of the Infirmary. More space and new equipment produced a radiological department that would be recognisable today, although certain rooms such as the patients' waiting area continued to be shared with the electrical and massage sections, and radiotherapy had still not been hived off. The accommodation included an office and plate library where the reports were issued and stored; a radiographic room; a fluoroscopy room; dark room;

radiographers' room; the medical officer's room where Dr. Arnison saw patients mainly for massage and electrical treatment.

The latest x-ray equipment was installed, a Wappler rotary converter unit (*see* 52). Gas tubes were still used, and the fluoroscopy room had a large coil with a mercury interrupter. The chamber of the interrupter had to be filled with coal gas to expel all the air, and once in 1925 there was a serious accident. The coal gas supplier was also used to charge the interrupter of the ward mobile unit, the fluoroscopy room interrupter being temporarily disconnected whenever this operation took place. On this occasion, whoever was responsible failed to ensure that the fluoroscopy room interrupter was fully recharged when reconnected. When the radiographer innocently switched on for screening after lunch, the cast iron chamber of the interrupter exploded. Large fragments were embedded in the ceiling and walls of the room. For the radiographer it was a lucky escape. Soon afterwards a second Wappler unit was installed in the department, but mercury interrupters ceased to be used.

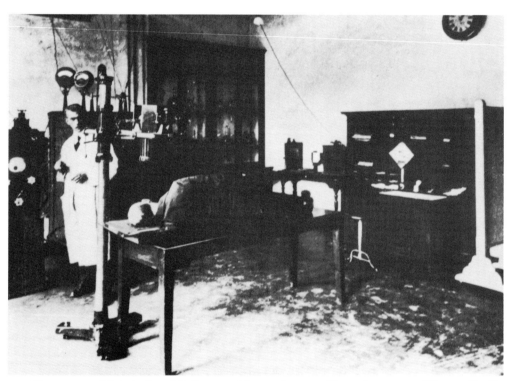

52. *X-ray room, Victoria Royal Infirmary, Newcastle-upon-Tyne about 1920. Thomas Dodd, the first radiographer, stands by the Wappler interrupter then recently installed*

When Arnison retired in 1925 he was succeeded by Dr. Harold Gamlen, a colourful Northern personality who was himself a pioneer martyr of British radiology, and when Gamlen abandoned hospital practice in 1931, he was succeeded by Dr. Whateley Davidson. The Infirmary's radiographers helped to provide continuity. Thomas Dodd's first assistant was Cornelius McMeekin who was engaged before the First World War and returned after it and worked in the Infirmary throughout the 1920s. During his war service in France, McMeekin had been a radiographer in a hospital which had the American neurosurgeon Harvey Cushing on the staff. Dodd's second assistant was Joseph Ridley (died 1957), who found work in the Infirmary at the end of the First World War and joined the x-ray staff in 1925. From 1935 onwards, he was the head of the technical staff, the Superintendent-Tutor of the Department until his retirement.[67] In the 1920s, Dodd, McMeekin and Ridley performed most of the screening themselves, including the barium meals, and Whateley Davidson recalled the neat diagrams that they drew of what they had seen on the reverse of each patient's x-ray form!

HAROLD ERNEST GAMLEN, M.B., B.S., D.P.H. (1871–1943) was an experienced radiologist aged 52 years when he came to the Infirmary, and his hands already bore the scars of radiation mutilation.

Gamlen came from Hartlepool where as a boy he had been encouraged by a local doctor, Rutherford Morison, later the surgeon in Newcastle. It was Morison who sent Gamlen into medicine. He qualified in 1893 and immediately returned to general practice in West Hartlepool. Here in August 1896 he bought his first x-ray set and thereafter radiology became his main interest. Within a decade he was an experienced radiotherapist, having visited the Finsen Institute, Copenhagen and having published a number of papers on his experience of treating skin lesions and neoplastic conditions by x- and other rays.[68] In 1904 he demonstrated a patient with an epithelioma of the tongue at a Newcastle medical meeting, whom he was treating with radium. During the First World War he was commissioned a Major in the Royal Army Medical Corps and served as a radiologist to the Italian Expeditionary Force. In 1916 he devised a foreign body localiser known by his name ('Gamlen's frying pan').[69] He was mentioned in dispatches on several occasions, and he was once congratulated by Harvey Cushing on his excellent skull radiographs.

In 1920 Gamlen moved to Newcastle. Three years later he became Arnison's assistant, and succeeded him in 1925 as head of the Electrical Department of the Infirmary.

Gamlen's early use of radium left its scars, particularly since he professed total ignorance of handling the substance correctly. He stored it in a glass tube in an empty thermometer case which he kept in his waistcoat pocket. The case also served as the applicator, being held against the patient's affected part! By 1930 he was disabled from dermatitis, at first continuing with private work in Newcastle but soon retiring to live in Somerset.[70] Gamlen's was one of the British names added to the Martyrs' Memorial in Hamburg. His brother, Thomas Gillies Gamlen, was a veteran radiographer, and T. G.'s daughter was Sophia Cleather Gamlen, M.S.R. (1891–1953), a radiographer in Harley Street before the Second World War.[71]

SAMUEL WHATELY DAVIDSON, M.D., F.R.C.P., F.F.R., F.R.C.R.A. (1896–1977), the physician in charge of the department of radiology in the Infirmary from 1930 to 1961, was the radiologist who bridged the decades between the primitive early days and modern diagnostic radiology in Newcastle.

He graduated at King's College, Newcastle, in 1920 and proceeded to M.D. and M.R.C.P. three years later, intending for a career as a physician. But in 1925 his chief, Dr. (late Sir) William Hume suggested that he became assistant physician to the electrical department. There he was to spend 36 years, devoting his professional life to the Infirmary and establishing a diagnostic unit of lasting quality. A monument to his vision and drive is provided by the present department, which was planned and built between 1948 and 1952. Many hospitals in the North-East of England owe the design of their first x-ray department to his advice.

Beyond his department, Davidson was much in demand. He served as a radiology examiner regionally and nationally, once visiting Australasia on behalf of the Faculty of Radiologists. He was a strong committee man, serving the University, Health Service and the national radiological bodies. In the 1930s he helped to unite the College of Medicine and Armstrong College to form the Newcastle division of the University of Durham, which later became the University of Newcastle. In course of his career he served as:

President, Faculty of Radiologists
President, Section of Radiology of the Royal Society of Medicine
President-Elect, British Institute of Radiology
President, North of England Branch of the British Medical Association.[72]

ROYAL SOUTH HANTS HOSPITAL, SOUTHAMPTON

An x-ray apparatus was installed in the Royal South Hants Hospital in 1901, the gift of a benefactor, and it remained in use for almost 30 years.[73] The moving force behind this gift was undoubtedly Dr. Norman Aldridge, the Southampton physician who introduced the new photography to Hampshire soon after news of the discovery reached England.

Although Dr. Aldridge was designated as 'Röntgen ray expert' by his colleagues in 1907, a hospital department was not established until 1911. In that year an outpatient block was added to the Hospital, consisting of a waiting hall and two adjoining corridors. The west corridor was used to house the Electrical Department which consisted of a large room for x-ray treatment, an x-ray photographic room, and a dark room. These rooms still form the nucleus of the present diagnostic Department of Radiology, which occupies the same site as well as adjoining premises.

NORMAN ELLIOTT ALDRIDGE, M.B., C.M.(Edinburgh) (1862–1933) was the pioneer of x-rays in the Southern counties of England, and Aldridge Ward in the Royal South Hants Hospital, Southampton commemorates the fact that he established the first x-ray service there – at great personal cost.

The Aldridges were an old Hampshire family, and his father, J. H. Aldridge was a family doctor in Southampton. Local records[74] show that Norman as a young man attended the Hospital as a student, a medical apprentice, for some years before gaining the Edinburgh M.B. in 1884, and then returning as a house surgeon. Subsequently he served for 36 years on the medical staff of the Hospital:

Honorary assistant physician, 1893–5
Honorary physician, 1895–1929
Honorary physician in charge of Electrotherapy Department, 1907–29.

Aldridge took his first radiograph in 1896 in his home at 7 Cumberland Place, and from here he practised until his retirement in 1929. After about 1900 he devoted himself entirely to x-ray and electrical practice. His election in 1907 as 'Honorary Medical Officer in charge of the Electrical Department' of the Royal South Hants Hospital confirmed him in the work which he had already performed for nearly a decade. He continued this work and in 1913, at a meeting in London, he gave details of a large series of patients with lymph-node tuberculosis whom he had successfully treated with radiotherapy between 1908 and 1913.[75]

During the First World War, he served as a major in the Royal Army Medical Corps and as Inspector of Radiology, Southern Command, having charge of the electrical department at the Royal Victoria Hospital, Netley. It is said that his war work aggravated the dermatitis from which he suffered for the rest of his life. A finger was amputated in 1922, and he lost more fingers prior to his death at Alton in 1933.[76] His name is one of the British names added to the Martyrs' Memorial in Hamburg in the 1950s.

Aldridge played his part in local medical affairs, and in 1921 served as the first chairman of the Wessex Branch of the British Association of Radiology and Physiotherapy (now the British

Institute of Radiology). He also helped to establish x-ray departments at the Southampton Infirmary and the Royal Hampshire County Hospital, Winchester. By the 1920s he was nationally known, having served on the Council of the Electro-Therapeutical Section of the Royal Society of Medicine and having participated in the attempt mounted by British radiologists to define standards for the barium meal.[77]

ROYAL VICTORIA HOSPITAL, BELFAST

The Belfast medical community quickly sensed the importance of the new photography. At the old Royal Hospital in Frederick Street, the medical committee as early as July 1896, only six months after Röntgen's announcement, considered the purchase of x-ray apparatus. In November they acquired an Apps eight-inch Rühmkorff coil, a Crookes tube, accumulators and a fluorescent screen, and arranged a contract with a firm of Belfast chemists, John Clarke and Company, to take radiographs on medical demand. This arrangement was similar to that made in Manchester, Newcastle-upon-Tyne, and several other cities, and Clarke's staff produced a total of 50 radiographs in 1897. After the first year the contract was renewed with another firm of chemists, Lizars of Wellington Place, who held it for five or more years. One of Lizars' employees, J. C. Carson, became a successful practical radiographer who took plates and gave treatments; he even carried out domiciliary radiography in the suburbs of Belfast in his jaunting car at ten shillings a time![78]

When patients were transferred from the old Royal Hospital to the new building in September 1903, the Royal Victoria Hospital was said to represent 'the last word in design and construction . . . all wards are accessible off the main corridor. . . . There is also a room for the Electrical Department where a brilliant young doctor, J. C. Rankin, takes x-ray pictures . . .'.[79]

JOHN CAMPBELL (JOHNNY) RANKIN, M.D.(Royal University of Ireland, 1906) (1876–1954), the pioneer radiologist of Belfast, qualified with first-class honours in 1900 and almost immediately became concerned in the new photography. In November 1903 he was appointed as Medical Electrician to the new hospital, and in the same month he treated his first case – a patient with lupus.[80] An early exponent of the radiotherapeutic method of treating such lesions and other skin cancers, he spent several months in Copenhagen with Finsen to learn his methods, and in 1903 he travelled to Vienna and attended dermatological and therapy clinics there for six months, in order to equip himself for this work. In a paper printed in *Archives of the Roentgen Ray* in 1906 he reported the results of treatment in 17 patients with breast cancer, 12 with sarcoma (nine of whom died) and 30 with rodent ulcer.[81]

Rankin was an enthusiastic proponent of utilising radiographs to teach anatomy, and his M.D. thesis in 1906, entitled 'Research on X-rays', is believed to be one of the first academic dissertations devoted to the new science. His work arose from a fruitful collaboration with the professor of anatomy in Belfast, Johnson Symington, F.R.S. Together they prepared a radiographic record of the developmental anatomy of the human teeth, Symington and his assistant Crymble preparing careful dissections of cadaver jaws and Rankin making radiographs of the specimens in his private house. The results were published in 1908 as Symington and Rankin's *Atlas of Skiagrams illustrating the Development of Teeth*, a slim volume of high-quality plates which was to enjoy a high reputation. Several plates were reproduced in Gray's *Anatomy*, being reprinted in successive editions.

Dr. Rankin was elected to the visiting staff of the Hospital in 1911, and remained actively associated with it until the eve of the Second World War as the venerealogist. He retired to Larne in 1944. A bachelor, he lived with his sister and died there 10 years later, aged 78 years.

For the first two decades Rankin singlehandedly provided an electrical service for Belfast. The medical committee minutes record that he received a new vacuum tube in September 1904 at a cost of £3! In 1912 new x-ray apparatus was installed and a dark room equipped, costing over £400. Demand for diagnostic radiographs then began to rise: in 1912 – 895 patients; 1913 – 1,347 patients. The rise was accelerated by the First World War, and by 1919 6–8 patients were dealt with each day – mainly for the diagnosis of fractures but also the occasional barium meal. By that time, Rankin's equipment was hopelessly out-of-date: gas tubes and glass plates were still used, and the massive coil outfit was noisy and had a low output. All radiographs were prepared using a primitive dose-measuring device: flash exposures were made by the dropping of a weight down a tube, the exposure being controlled by the distance through which the weight dropped.[82]

Major changes came during 1919 and the next four years. The Electrical Department was re-equipped and modernised, and gained the appearance of a modern x-ray unit. Double-coated x-ray film replaced the glass plates and Coolidge hot-cathode tubes the vacuum tubes, and a wax-insulated high-tension transformer the old coil (the last-mentioned change being made possible after the electrical mains supply of the Hospital was converted to alternating current). A Potter-Bucky grid was acquired soon after it was marketed. Clinical demand for radiographs now soared: 4,812 patients were examined in 1923 – more than double the total in 1919. This increasing demand had two results: more space had to be found, and more staff engaged.

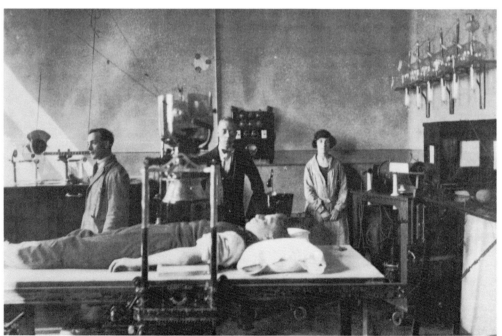

53. X-ray room, Royal Victoria Hospital, Belfast about 1924, with the three x-ray pioneers of Northern Ireland, Sister Millar, Dr. Johnny Rankin and Ralph Leman

In 1923 the Department was moved to the main floor of the Hospital into accommodation providing space for a second x-ray unit. A photograph of the x-ray room at this time shows Dr. Rankin with his veteran assistant, Sister Millar, and the new man R. M. Leman, who joined them at Easter 1919. Ralph Leman, M.B.E., F.S.R. (1894–1978) was an East Anglian who won his spurs at the Anglo-American Hospital at Wimereaux in France during the First World War. His work there as a military radiographer caught the eye of two Belfast surgeons who persuaded Rankin to employ him after the War. Leman made Belfast his home and served the Royal Victoria Hospital for 40 years. He trained his first radiographer in 1926 and founded the School of Radiography in Belfast in 1930, and achieved personal distinction in wider fields – twice winner of prizes for essays on radiographic techniques, a medallist of the Royal Photographic Society for radiographs of plants and flowers, and an Honorary Fellow of the Society of Radiographers.[83]

Other newcomers to the staff in the 1920s were Dr. R. M. Beath and Dr. Frank Montgomery.

ROBERT MAITLAND BEATH, M.B., Ch.B.(Queen's University, Belfast), M.B., B.S.(London), F.F.R. (1886–1940) joined the staff of the Royal Victoria Hospital in 1921 as Rankin's assistant, and he served it up to his death at the age of 56. An Ulsterman born and bred, he was the most brilliant medical student of his day at Queen's University. His interest in radiology was awakened while serving in the Royal Army Medical Corps in the First World War. Demobilised in 1919 with a rank of major, he took the London M.B., and then sat at the feet of Dr. Stanley Melville for a year or more before returning to practise in Belfast. Here he soon made his mark as a radiologist and as a man of unusual charm and commonsense. These qualities singled him out for higher office. As a member of the Council of the British Institute of Radiology – and one who would almost certainly have been its president, had he lived – he was one of those radiologists who foresaw the need for the British Association of Radiologists, which he helped actively to establish. In 1938–9 he served as the Association's fourth President. In 1939 the Association merged with the Society of Radiotherapists of Great Britain and Ireland to form the Faculty of Radiologists – a time when the tasks of consolidation and of harmonising conflicting interests put a heavy burden on the President. Beath's wisdom and his willingness to travel back and forth from Ireland evoked much praise and brought Belfast to the notice of the radiological world.[84]

SIR FRANK P. MONTGOMERY, M.C. and Croix de Guerre, Hon.Ll.D., Hon.F.F.R. (R.C.S.I.), M.B., B.Ch., B.A.O., D.M.R.E. (1892–1972) was Beath's assistant who took charge of the x-ray department on his death. Montgomery was a son of the manse and like Beath a graduate of Queen's University, Belfast, who joined the Royal Army Medical Corps upon qualifying in 1915. He served on the Western Front and received British and French decorations for bravery. After the War he spent four years in Cairo in the Egyptian public service, before returning to London to study radiology. He obtained the Cambridge Diploma in 1924. He returned immediately to Belfast and was appointed assistant radiologist to the Royal Victoria Hospital, and in 1929 was elected an Honorary Consultant.

Montgomery made the radiotherapy of cancer his special concern and became the architect of the cancer services in the Province. In later years his qualities as an administrator and decision-maker came to the fore. In 1948 when the National Health Service was created, he was chosen as the first Chairman of the Northern Ireland Hospitals Authority, a post which he held for eight years. In 1952 the Northern Ireland Radiotherapy Centre, established at Purdysburn, was called 'Montgomery House'. In the following year he received a knighthood for his services to medicine in Northern Ireland.[85]

Chapter 8

RADIOLOGICAL JOURNALS BEFORE 1930

'The *British Journal of Radiology* is the oldest radiological journal in the world. It is in the direct line of descent from *Archives of Clinical Skiagraphy*, through *Archives of the Roentgen Ray* and *The Journal of the Röntgen Society*.'

Allsopp (1964)[1]

Four months after the news of Röntgen's discovery reached London, a medical journal appeared which was devoted to the new science, entitled *Archives of Clinical Skiagraphy*. It was the first radiological journal to be published in the world, and it has remained continuously in print to the present day, being known since 1924 as the *British Journal of Radiology*. Other publications followed in Britain which were devoted partly or wholly to the clinical application of x-rays, and the editors of existing medical publications such as the *British Medical Journal* and *The Lancet* began to accept radiological material. The table on page 145 lists the early British radiological journals and the lineage of descent of the current publications.

The curiosity of the London medical community to learn more about x-rays and their possible clinical uses grew steadily during the first three months of 1896. This process was fuelled by the demonstrations mounted by the early experimenters and the enthusiastic accounts appearing in the medical press, which have been described in Chapters 2 and 3. By 30 March, the day on which Professor Silvanus Thompson delivered the lecture which seems finally to have won over medical opinion in London, the *British Medical Journal* had already printed several reports from its Special Commissioner, Sydney Rowland, on the clinical uses of x-rays.

ARCHIVES OF CLINICAL SKIAGRAPHY (1896–7)

1. *Archives of Clinical Skiagraphy. A Series of Collotype Illustrations with Descriptive Text, Illustrating Applications of the New Photography to Medicine and Surgery*
The new journal was launched on the crest of the wave of enthusiasm about x-rays that swept London and the rest of the country during the first few months. The first number appeared in April or early May 1896. The title page carried the sub-title printed

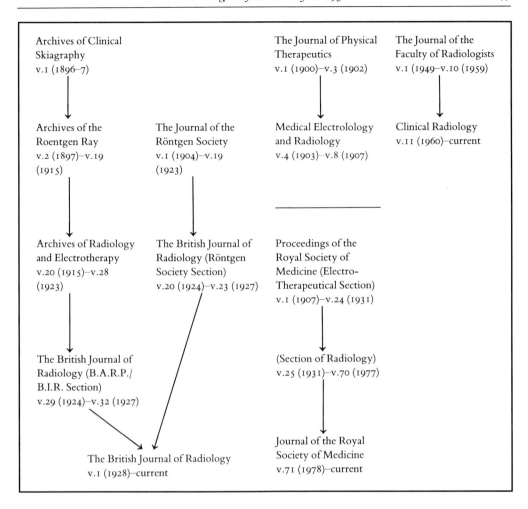

above, in addition to the names of the editor, Sydney Rowland, and the publisher, The Rebman Company. The aims of the venture were explicitly explained in the Preface, which was written by Rowland on 2 April 1896:

'The object of this publication is to put on record in permanent form some of the most striking applications of the New Photography to the needs of Medicine and Surgery. The progress of this new Art has been so rapid that, although Prof. Röntgen's discovery is only a thing of yesterday, it has already taken its place among the approved and accepted aids to diagnosis. At the first moment, the statement that it had been found possible to penetrate the fleshy coverings of the bones, and to photograph their substance and contours, seemed the realization of almost an impossible scientific dream. The first essays were of a rough and ready character; week after week, however, improvements have been made in the practical application of the Art, which I venture to call Skiagraphy; and, at the present time, we are in a position to obtain a visible image of every bone and joint in the body . . .'

The first number of *Archives* consisted of 16 printed pages, six plates of radiographs and several other illustrations. It was issued in green wrappers in a quarto format, and the back wrapper carried advertisements for a variety of x-ray apparatus. The preface

Archives

— of —

Clinical Skiagraphy.

BY

SYDNEY ROWLAND, B.A., CAMB.,

LATE SCHOLAR OF DOWNING COLLEGE, CAMBRIDGE, AND SHUTER SCHOLAR OF
ST. BARTHOLOMEW'S HOSPITAL.
SPECIAL COMMISSIONER TO "BRITISH MEDICAL JOURNAL" FOR INVESTIGATION OF
THE APPLICATIONS OF THE NEW PHOTOGRAPHY TO MEDICINE AND SURGERY.

*A SERIES OF COLLOTYPE ILLUSTRATIONS WITH DESCRIPTIVE
TEXT, ILLUSTRATING APPLICATIONS OF THE NEW
PHOTOGRAPHY TO MEDICINE AND SURGERY.*

London:
THE REBMAN PUBLISHING COMPANY, LIMITED,
11, ADAM STREET, STRAND.
1896.

ARCHIVES

— OF —

THE ROENTGEN RAY.

(*Formerly* ARCHIVES OF SKIAGRAPHY).

THE ONLY JOURNAL IN WHICH THE TRANSACTIONS OF THE ROENTGEN
SOCIETY OF LONDON ARE OFFICIALLY REPORTED.

VOLUME II.

EDITED BY

W. S. HEDLEY, M.D., | SYDNEY ROWLAND, M.A.,
M.R.C.S., *in charge of the Electro-Therapeutic Department, the London Hospital.* | M.R.C.S., *etc.*

London:
THE REBMAN PUBLISHING COMPANY, LIMITED,
129, SHAFTESBURY AVENUE, CAMBRIDGE CIRCUS, W.C.

AMERICAN AGENT:
W. B. SAUNDERS, 925, WALNUT STREET, PHILADELPHIA, PA.

1898.

ARCHIVES

— OF —

RADIOLOGY AND
ELECTROTHERAPY

VOLUME XXI.
JUNE, 1916, TO MAY, 1917

LONDON:
WILLIAM HEINEMANN (MEDICAL BOOKS) LTD.
1917

54. Title pages of early radiological journals, the precursors of the British Journal of Radiology. *Left Top* Archives of Clinical Skiagraphy, *1896–7. Right top* Archives of the Roentgen Ray, *1897–1915. Left bottom* Archives of Radiology and Electrotherapy, *1915–23* was followed by Rowland's Introduction, an 11-page essay in which he described the cathode tube, offered an account of Röntgen's experiments and reviewed his own three-month experience of radiography. This state-of-the-art report was the only article in the journal and the rest of the contents was made up of x-ray case descriptions.

The moving spirit of this venture was undoubtedly Sydney Rowland, the youthful editor, who provided all 16 pages of copy in the first number and most of the radiographs. For him, this sprouting of an independent journal devoted to radiology was the logical outcome of his journalistic efforts for the *British Medical Journal*, which published the first of his weekly reports earlier on 8 February. However, Rowland was no mere scribe of the early days of radiology – he was a working radiographer, who himself took many radiographs during the formative stages of the new profession.

SYDNEY DOMVILLE ROWLAND (see page 19) was the x-ray pioneer who coined the word 'skiagraphy' in 1896 when as a 24-year-old medical student he served as editor of the world's first radiological journal. His interest in radiology did not last long beyond his undergraduate years, but his brief career as a practical radiographer and 'Special Commissioner to the *British Medical Journal*' earned him a permanent place among the British pioneers.[2]

Directly after qualifying with the Conjoint Diploma in April 1897, Rowland abandoned radiological work and commenced a career in laboratory medicine. Even election to the Council of the Röntgen Society in November 1898 failed to deflect him from his purpose,[3] and in that year he was appointed Assistant Bacteriologist at the Lister Institute. He devoted the rest of his professional life to medical research. In 1905 he went to India with the Plague Commission, and at the outbreak of the First World War he joined the Royal Army Medical Corps and served in France in charge of a laboratory. In 1917 he died there of cerebrospinal fever.[4] A bronze plaque in the Lister Institute commemorates his work as a micro-biologist.[2]

The second and third numbers of *Archives of Clinical Skiagraphy* – issued in June and December 1896, respectively, ran to seven pages and consisted of x-ray case reports, except the last page of the second number, which was filled with 'Answers to Correspondence'. Both numbers were thinner than the first because Rowland could not contribute as fully as before; early in 1897 he was preparing for his final examinations and probably had no time. Of the seven cases in the third number, only one was Rowland's; and his name did not appear at all in the inside pages of the fourth number, issued four months later. Other medical contributors were found. Albert Morison, one of the doctor brothers in West Hartlepool, reported a fractured olecranon process in a 16-year-old boy which was secured by internal wiring on 16 June 1896. James MacKenzie Davidson in Aberdeen described the case of a 20-year-old girl with six toes on each foot. J. Lynn Thomas, assistant surgeon to the Cardiff Infirmary, contributed a radiograph of a double monster, giving details of the congenital skeletal fusion. The most important contribution came from Dr. John Macintyre in Glasgow, entitled 'Skiagraphy of the Soft and the Hard Tissues' including a chest radiograph showing the human heart which he claimed to be the first ever produced of the heart.

2. *Archives of Skiagraphy*

The fourth number (April 1897) bore this abbreviated title – the only number to drop the word '*Clinical*'. This alteration might have reflected a deliberate change in editorial policy because, although all contributors to the issue were doctors, several articles dealt with non-clinical aspects of x-ray work. The longest was entitled 'Skiagraphy in

Zoology', and was unconnected with clinical medicine. The author, R. Norris Wolfenden, was a London doctor with an interest in natural history who spent his holidays on field expeditions. In the autumn of 1896 he travelled to the Orkney Islands to collect specimens from the shore waters of Scapa Flow. These he preserved in surgical spirit and posted south to Glasgow, and in February 1897 he followed them there and made radiographs of the collection in the laboratory of Dr. Macintyre. Three examples were printed in *Archives* – exquisite radiographs of an edible crab, a hermit crab, and a rock lobster. These plates are the earliest instance of utilising x-rays to study the anatomy of invertebrates. Another author was W. S. Hedley of the London Hospital, who presented two radiographs of skeletal lesions; his was a significant contribution which may have been solicited, see below. The last six lines of the final printed page of the issue carried an important message: It announced the formation of a Skiagraphic Society in London (on 18 March 1897), whose fortunes will be described in the next chapter.

The shortage of contributions and Sydney Rowland's impending departure into laboratory medicine was a threat that the publishers of *Archives of Skiagraphy* could not afford to ignore. The publishers were also the owners, two members of a German family, F. J. and A. J. Rebman, who had established and managed a small business in London. The Rebman Publishing Company, then at 11 Adam Street, Strand, specialised in marketing the translations of Continental medical textbooks. The Rebmans took the original risk and for 17 years owned and published the first international journal of radiology in the English language. Both men were founder members of the Röntgen Society in 1897.

ARCHIVES OF THE ROENTGEN RAY (1897–1915)

The mounting interest provoked in London medical circles by the new photography gave rise to two events which served as a lifeline to the Rebmans and their ailing journal. The announcement by several doctors in March 1897 of their intention to form a Skia-graphic Society led three months later to the creation of the Röntgen Society with Silvanus Thompson as its President. One of the first acts of the new Society was to reach agreement with the Rebmans to publish its proceedings quarterly and to provide each member with a copy of their journal. The legal agreement was drawn up by the brother of Thomas Moore, the Society's treasurer, who was a solicitor.

This agreement blew new life into *Archives of Skiagraphy* and guaranteed the survival of the journal. It enabled the Rebmans to expand the contents, and thereby to attract non-medical readers such as physicists and engineers. In keeping with the fashion of the moment to honour the discoverer of the new rays, the words 'Roentgen ray' were substituted for 'skiagraphy' in the title.[5]

1. *Archives of the Roentgen Ray (formerly Archives of Skiagraphy)* (1897–1903)
Number 1 of Volume 2 appeared in July 1897. An announcement from the publishers, printed at the head of the first page, read: 'This journal now appears as a quarterly record of all that appertains to the Roentgen ray. . . . It is chiefly as a pictorial record

that "The Archives" has hitherto won its way. This feature will be steadily adhered to. . . . But there will be added a certain amount of useful letterpress. This will record the proceedings of the recently formed Röntgen Society, and will consist of original communications, "notes" and correspondence. . . . In other words, the "Archives of the Roentgen Ray" offers itself, not merely as a journal of the new photography, but to some extent as the exponent of the important discovery.'

Archives was never the official journal of the Röntgen Society, and remained the commercial responsibility of the Rebman family. The special relationship that they established with the Society was defined in a phrase which became the sub-title of the journal. It read: '*The Only Journal in Which the Transactions of the Roentgen Society of London are Officially Reported*'. This phrase remained on the title page until the Society and the Rebmans parted company in 1904 and the Society began to publish its own journal (see below). It was then removed, although *Archives* continued to report the meetings of the Röntgen Society.

With Volume 2 and the altered title in 1897, *Archives* for the first time began to assume the appearance of a scientific journal. The content, features and range of topics are instantly recognisable to readers of present-day journals such as the *British Journal of Radiology*. The large quarto format – chosen purposely to avoid having to reduce the size of the radiographic plates when printed – was not abandoned until later. But the subjects discussed at that early stage, scarcely 18 months after the discovery of x-rays, have a familiar ring and topicality in our own time. Original articles began to appear which were written by physicists and early manufacturers of x-ray apparatus, in addition to practising radiologists. Regular features were book reviews, summaries of articles written by Continental and early American pioneers, and detailed reports of meetings of the Röntgen Society.

Sydney Rowland's successor was the key to the future success of *Archives*. As soon as the publishers became aware that his professional interests lay elsewhere, they sought a new editor. Rowland agreed to continue to serve as the junior co-editor of Volume 2. The senior co-editor chosen by the Rebmans was W. S. Hedley, the medical electrician of the London Hospital. A distinguished group of collaborators joined the Editorial Committee, including the radiologists MacKenzie Davidson and John Macintyre, surgeons Thomas Moore, Lynn Thomas and Norris Wolfenden, scientists Campbell Swinton and Silvanus Thompson, and two pioneer American radiologists, W. J. Morton of New York and W. White of Philadelphia.

During the early years of *Archives* and until Deane Butcher started his decade of service to the journal in 1905, several editors came and went. The longest serving of these in the first decade was the Sussex physicist, Ernest Payne, who edited Volumes 3–8. The editors before 1904 were:

Sydney Rowland	April 1896	– May 1898
W. S. Hedley	July 1897	– May 1898
Ernest Payne	August 1898	– October 1903
Thomas Moore	August 1898	– September 1900
C. Mansell-Moullin	November 1900	– December 1902
F. Harrison Low	December 1902	– July 1903
J. Hall-Edwards	August 1903	– September 1905.

The first article in the first issue of Volume 2 was a brief paper entitled appropriately, 'On the Nature of Roentgen's Rays' and the author was Professor Silvanus Thompson. The second article, which covered six full pages, written by the senior editor, W. S. Hedley, was entitled 'Roentgen Rays – a Survey, Present and Retrospective'. It was the first clinical review of the value of the new diagnostic method to be published in England. The paper was unique also, in containing footnote references – a practice that did not take root in medical literature until the First World War. Hedley quoted 52 sources, mostly papers describing the experiences of pioneer German workers in using x-rays to examine patients, but also those of Macintyre and other British authors.

Already – Hedley wrote[6] – x-rays had gained a place in surgery. They had revealed a bullet in the brain, a dilated oesophagus (this had been done by feeding nitrate of bismuth cream to the patient), urinary tract calculi, and skeletal lesions such as fractures, scoliosis, bone necrosis and tuberculous dactylitis. With improved apparatus, he believed, the time would come soon of undoubted profit to medicine: aortic aneurysm, pleural effusion and empyaema, and diaphragmatic movements would be studied by plates or on the fluorescent screen.

ERNEST PAYNE, M.A.(Cantab.), A.I.E.E. (died 1936) was a gifted lay pioneer who devoted a decade of his life to radiography during its seminal period. He was a founder member and a strong supporter of the Röntgen Society. For five years he jointly edited *Archives*, serving successively with the surgeons Thomas Moore and Mansell-Moullin and then with Dr. Hall-Edwards, until the Society withdrew its support early in 1904.

Payne lived at Haywards Heath and later at Hove in Sussex, and soon after 1896 he was appointed honorary radiographer of the Royal Alexandra Children's Hospital and the Royal Sussex County Hospital in Brighton. Almost certainly using home-made apparatus, he took radiographs of patients including a young child which were published in 1897;[7] and he performed many experiments. One of these, entitled 'Localisation and Measurement of Hidden Bodies by the Aid of Roentgen Rays', involved making two exposures on the same film: by moving the film between the exposures, the foreign body could be localised by a graphic measurement. Payne's method first appeared in print at the end of 1897[8] – at the same time as Mackenzie Davidson and Hedley published their method.

Payne wrote a dozen or more papers during the next decade, which appeared in *Archives* and after 1904 in *The Journal of the Röntgen Society*. They describe other personal inventions such as a double-dipper contact breaker and his experiments and clinical results with fluoroscopy. In 1898 Payne after election to the Council of the Röntgen Society persuaded his colleagues to collect information on x-ray-induced injuries, and by November six cases had been reported and five more were mentioned. In December 1899 he and Dr. Walsh presented their findings on x-ray deaths to a meeting of the Society.[9] Payne's work laid the ground for others in Brighton, where at least one doctor, Percy Lake Hope, used mains electricity and short exposures to produce radiographs of good quality before 1905.[10]

After 1906 Payne played no further part in the development of x-rays, but his original experiments and publications ensured him an honoured place in its history. Russell Reynolds named him as one of the six pioneer physicists in the United Kingdom and an obituarist correctly described him as 'one of the earliest pioneers of x-ray research'.[8] His was one of the British names added to the Martyrs' Memorial in Hamburg in the 1950s.

CHARLES WILLIAM MANSELL-MOULLIN, C.B.E., M.D., F.R.C.S. (1851–1940), the second President of the Röntgen Society, served as co-editor of *Archives* for about two years after 1900.

Mansell-Moullin was an outstandingly brilliant student at Oxford who became a guiding light in the surgical world of London after 1882 when he was appointed assistant surgeon and lecturer on surgery at the London Hospital. He remained there for the rest of his professional life, identifying with many technical advances, such as the start of abdominal surgery and the introduction of x-rays. He published scholarly papers on many subjects, e.g. the treatment of malignant disease, the surgery of gastric ulcer and the biology of tumours, and he remained mentally active to the end of his long life. At the age of 80 years he learnt Russian and visited Moscow to examine the Soviet medical services.[11]

At the London Hospital in 1896 he played a leading part in convincing more conservative colleagues to accept the clinical x-ray service started by Dr. Hedley. He also cooperated with Dr. Hedley in the Röntgen Society, which they both helped to found in 1897, and he was chosen to succeed Silvanus Thompson as President when MacKenzie Davidson declined the office in 1898. After completing his year of office the sudden death of the surgeon Thomas Moore deprived *Archives* of a medical editor and Mansell-Moullin took the post for two years.[12]

Although subsequently serving as a Vice-President of the Society, Mansell-Moullin played no further leading part in radiological affairs. A quarter-century later, when aged 74 years, he was elected to Honorary Membership of the British Institute of Radiology.

Early in 1904 a rift developed between the publishers and the Society over the control of the journal. Hitherto the Rebmans' management of *Archives* followed the policy of the Society, which was to maintain a balance between medical and lay interests. For example, the two co-editors whom they chose after 1898 were, respectively, always a doctor and a physicist and both were members of the Society. This approach, while pleasing to the Society, did not always ensure the smooth running of the journal. Sufficient material was not always available to fill it and to publish on time. The Rebmans themselves may have aggravated these difficulties in 1902 by their decision to issue *Archives* monthly. A crisis arose when the editors were unable to find enough copy for the additional numbers, and the eight issues of Volume 7 came out irregularly. In July 1903 the publishers took corrective action: in effect, they sacked the editors. 'In the face of these difficulties' – their announcement read[13] – 'we have been forced to make more effective arrangements for the future. With our August issue we shall commence a new era. The general arrangement of the journal will not be altered, but we intend to enlarge its scope so as to cover the whole area of electrotherapeutics, and to issue it monthly. . . . We crave the help of our readers, and of the members of the Roentgen Society in particular, in supplying us with original articles. . . . It is our aim and wish to make the 'Archives' indispensable to x-ray workers. . . .'

The next paragraph announced the appointment of Dr. John Hall-Edwards as the sole editor, with a number of prominent contributors to assist him. A 'preliminary list' of twelve names was published in the following year. One of these was Leopold Freund, the celebrated Austrian pioneer radiologist, and the remaining 11 were British pioneers including H. E. Gamlen, John Macintyre, David Morgan, Dawson Turner, Hugh Walsham, Lewis Jones, Edward Shenton and Norris Wolfenden.

While none could dispute the publishers' claim that the new team contained 'names which are almost "household words" to every electro-therapeutic worker',[14] their measures did not satisfy the Röntgen Society. Hall-Edwards was not a member of the Society, nor were five of his contributors. When the Society met, it condemned the appointment of a non-member as editor as well as 'some further proposed alterations' which were not defined. As a result, the Council decided to terminate their agreement with the Rebmans on 30 June 1904 and to publish a house journal.[15] The first number of *The Journal of the Röntgen Society* appeared a month later, see below.

2. *Archives of the Roentgen Ray and Allied Phenomena (formerly Archives of Skiagraphy).*
   An International Monthly Review of The Practice of Physical Therapeutics (1903–11)

This new title, introduced in July 1904 (Number 2, Volume 9), was necessitated by the expanding nature of the journal and the need to cater for readers interested in aspects of electrotherapeutics apart from radiology. Each of the four corners of the title page had one of the following words inserted diagonally across it: Electrotherapy, Radiotherapy, Phototherapy, Thermotherapy; and all four words appeared as a sub-title on the first page of the text.

W. Deane Butcher was appointed editor in 1905. The first years of his long tenureship saw *Archives* alter from a house journal for British radiologists into an international journal for electrotherapeutists. In an editorial commemorating the 100th number in 1908, Butcher announced that the aim of the editors was 'to make it a journal of physical therapeutics in all its branches . . . although Roentgenology will remain, as heretofore, the chief interest of the Journal'.[16] For several years by that date, the 'International Monthly Review' had had an American editor and a French correspondent, and by 1909 foreign editorial collaborators outnumbered the British ones. Initially the Rebmans cultivated the American market and they opened an office on Broadway, New York. However, by 1909 American radiologists were served by their own publications and the publishers had redirected their thrust to cultivate Continental readers. In that year, the countries of origin of the 22 collaborators were: Britain – 10, France – 5, Austria – 2, Germany – 2, Holland – 2, and Belgium – 1.[17]

WILLIAM DEANE BUTCHER, M.R.C.S., F.P.S. (1846–1919) edited *Archives* single-handedly for a decade – longer than any other man except Robert Knox.

Butcher was a grammar school boy who gained a scholarship to St. Bartholomew's Hospital and qualified in 1868. After serving as house surgeon to Sir James Paget, he spent 25 years in general practice, successively in Calcutta, Reading and Windsor. In 1895 he settled at Ealing, and thereafter devoted the rest of his life to applying Röntgen's discovery to clinical diagnosis and therapy. He held an appointment as surgeon to the London Skin Hospital, and is credited as being the first Briton to repeat the experiments of Schiff, of Vienna, on epilation by x-rays.[18] As a result of these and other early studies, he was named by Finzi as one of the 11 pioneers of radiotherapy in the United Kingdom.[19]

Butcher understood the physical basis of radiology better than most of his medical contemporaries and he made an important contribution to early attempts to measure and standardise the x-ray dose. He also pioneered the introduction of radium and measures to protect x-ray workers. In 1906 he delivered a lecture entitled 'On the Rationale of Radiotherapeutic Treatment'.[20]

Deane Butcher was an early leader of the radiological profession:

Editor, *Archives of the Roentgen Ray,* 1905–14
Member, British Electrotherapeutic Society, 1902–7
First President, Electro-Therapeutical Section of the Royal Society of Medicine, 1907–8
President, Röntgen Society, 1908–9

He was one of the first British radiologists to attend conferences abroad, and represented each of the three Societies at Continental gatherings between 1905 and 1910. He was a linguist and translated several French textbooks of dermatology and electricity into English.

3. *Archives of the Roentgen Ray. A Review of Physical Therapeutics* (1912–3)

The third alteration to the sub-title of the journal was made in June 1911 at the start of Volume 16. At the same time, the familiar banner, '*(Formerly Archives of Skiagraphy)*', was finally dropped from the title.

Archives in the previous year had altered in form, abandoning after 14 years the large size of page in favour of a smaller format which was, the editor wrote,[21] less awkward – the new journal would go into a letter box, fit onto a shelf. The original quarto size – chosen by Sydney Rowland in 1896 to permit full-size reproduction of radiographs – was no longer necessary because technical advances had improved them so much that they could be reduced to half-size with satisfactory results.

ARCHIVES OF RADIOLOGY AND ELECTROTHERAPY (1915–23)

'Today the English School of Radiologists is severed from its colleagues on the Continent, the Pioneers and Masters of our art,' wrote Deane Butcher in September 1914 at the outbreak of the First World War.[22] This event, which heralded the greatest disaster yet to overtake Europe, soon forced the scientists on opposing sides to alter their traditional friendly attitudes to one another. For the duration of hostilities, cross-frontier co-operation and international goodwill were suspended.

The effects of the break with Germany were felt immediately and with particular severity by British radiologists, who were cut off from their traditional source of supply of glass tubes and apparatus, as well as from contact with leaders of the profession such as Albers-Schönberg, Freund and Holzknecht. They had no quarrel with their German and Austrian colleagues, and the break when it came was not of their making: but gradually during the winter months of 1914–5 the national attitude hardened against the militant face of Germany, and they were forced to follow suit.

Deane Butcher himself was a casualty. In September 1914 he confined himself in an editorial to lamenting the declaration of war, and gave the impression that *Archives* would continue unchanged. In December the names of the five distinguished German and three Austrian radiologists still appeared among the 27 collaborators who assisted the editor at that time. He wrote:

'The brief frenzy of war should not cause any lasting breach between radiologists of different tongues. . . . We have no intention whatever of retaliating by altering the title of our paper. No temporary insanity of a military caste should allow us to forget the debt which we owe to German science.'[23]

The ink had scarcely dried on these words when Butcher was forced into retirement by ill-health, and public opinion compelled his successors to take the very measures which he had eloquently rejected. Volume 20 in June 1915 appeared without the names of the eight editorial collaborators in Germany and Austria and – in keeping with the mood of the country to drop all German names and titles – *Archives* received a new title:

1. *Archives of Radiology and Electrotherapy (Archives of the Roentgen Ray)* (1915–6)
Professor Röntgen's support of the German war effort incensed his British colleagues, and especially his decision to donate his Rumford Medal when the German Red Cross Society appealed for gold objects in 1914.[23] This gesture, which Röntgen viewed as

a patriotic one, they saw as provocative, and it provided the owners of *Archives* with a further reason to dispense with the words 'Roentgen Ray' in the title. The new editors in their first statement referred to the great shortage of clinical material as a result of severing the German connection, but also pointed to the opportunity it offered 'of consolidating and extending the school of *British Radiology and Electrotherapy (sic)* . . .'.[24] Writing under this new title in June 1915, they emphasised more strongly their intention to include the electrotherapeutists. 'If this journal is to continue . . . there must be a closer and more intimate co-operation of those readers interested in radiology and medical electrology.'[25]

Commercial anxieties may have prompted the owners to force changes upon the radiologists. *Archives* had changed hands in 1913 when after 17 years the Rebman Company sold the journal to William Heinemann (1863–1920), who thereby established William Heinemann (Medical Books) Limited, the London medical publishing house which still flourishes. A Rebman associate, Hugh Elliot, became the managing director of the new Company.[26] The Rebman family withdrew from publishing in London but remained the American agents of *Archives* in New York until at least 1923.

William Heinemann, in persuading the radiologists to share *Archives* with their fellow medical electricians in the place of their German colleagues, altered more than the title of the journal. In January 1915 three co-editors replaced Deane Butcher; after a 12-year interval non-radiologists and scientists were again appointed as editors. The editorial triumvirate was Robert Knox, the radiologist of King's College Hospital; E. P. Cumberbatch, the medical officer in charge of the Electrical Department at St. Bartholomew's Hospital; and Sidney Russ, the physicist of the Middlesex Hospital. Together they were to edit six volumes, and all three men continued to serve the journal almost up to the time of amalgamation with *The Journal of the Röntgen Society*, which produced *The British Journal of Radiology (New Series)* in 1928.

2. *Archives of Radiology and Electrotherapy* (1916–8)
The sub-title '(Formerly Archives of the Roentgen Ray)' disappeared at the end of Volume 21 in May 1916.

3. *Archives of Radiology and Electrotherapy. The Official Organ of the British Association of Radiology and Physiotherapy* (1918–23)
The final alteration in title was introduced with Volume 23 in June 1918. The need to provide training for radiologists had been emphasised by the bitter experiences of the War, and the medical men who met in the home of Sir James MacKenzie Davidson in 1917 decided to form themselves into a body to undertake teaching, the British Association of Radiology and Physiotherapy; the details are described in Chapter 9. One of the clauses of the agreement which they signed declared *Archives* to be the official journal of the Association, of which each paid-up member would receive a free copy. The editors believed that this official link with the Association would increase still further the proportion of original papers they received from British readers, which had risen steadily during the War.[27] All three editors were officers of the Association: Knox and Cumberbatch served as joint honorary secretaries and Sidney Russ was a member of the Council.

This decision sealed the fate of *Archives* and numbered its days as an independent mouthpiece of radiologists and electrotherapeutists. A logical and early step for the profession, after establishing a representative body, was to gain control of its official publication. Outright purchase of *Archives* from its owner was financially impossible in 1918, but this step remained the Association's aim. A not unrelated matter at that time was the future of *Archives*'s competitor, *The Journal of the Röntgen Society* and of its parent body, which many radiologists supported. Through the foresight and diplomacy of Sir Archibald Reid and his colleagues, these difficulties were overcome and the early 1920s proved to be the formative years of modern British radiology. During those years not only did the two bodies unite but the two radiological journals assumed the same name – *The British Journal of Radiology* as a prelude to complete amalgamation. The last issue of *Archives* (Number 7, Volume 28, December 1923), carried the following announcement on its final page:

IMPORTANT NOTICE.

THE ARCHIVES will appear in the first issue of the New Year in another form and with a change of name.

This is the outcome of negotiations between the Röntgen Society and the Council of the B.A.R.P. regarding an amalgamation of the respective Journals. The Editor has pleasure in announcing that from January, 1924, the ARCHIVES will assume the name of THE BRITISH JOURNAL OF RADIOLOGY (formerly the *Archives of Radiology and Electrotherapy*).

"The Journal of the Röntgen Society" will in like manner become the BRITISH JOURNAL OF RADIOLOGY, RÖNTGEN SOCIETY SECTION.

The two Journals will be published separately, each maintaining its individuality. The ARCHIVES will be altered in size of page, type, etc., to conform with that of "The Journal of the Röntgen Society." There will be a close collaboration by the Editorial staff of both Journals.

It is hoped that this step will ultimately lead to complete amalgamation.

Before following the details of this process, it is necessary to turn back the clock 20 years, in order to view the vicissitudes of the other early radiological journals.

THE JOURNAL OF PHYSICAL THERAPEUTICS (1900–2) *MEDICAL ELECTROLOGY AND RADIOLOGY* (1903–7)

When the disruption took place in the Röntgen Society in 1901 and the medical members left to form the British Electrotherapeutic Society (see Chapter 9), they decided to publish a journal of their own. Accordingly, they took over an existing magazine which was then in its third year, and this journal became the official organ of the Society.

1. *The Journal of Physical Therapeutics. An International Quarterly Review*
This journal made its appearance in 1900, edited by Dr. W. S. Hedley and an American lady doctor, M. A. Cleaves. A preliminary announcement justified the new journal on

the grounds that it would embrace all the various physical 'therapies' then practised, namely electro-, hydro-, vibro-, photo-, radio-, balneo- and aerotherapy. Clinical applications of electricity and the Roentgen rays would also be reviewed.

Soon after the British Electrotherapeutic Society was founded, important radiological articles began to appear in the journal, being the papers read by members at the monthly meetings. In February 1902 Edward Shenton spoke on 'A Diagnostic Line about the Hip Joint', and in April Hugh Walsham gave a lecture on 'The Diagnosis of Thoracic Aneurysm', and illustrated his paper by plates of abnormal chest radiographs.[28]

2. *Medical Electrology and Radiology. An International Monthly Review (with which is incorporated 'The Journal of Physical Therapeutics')*

Once the Society was established, the journal became its official organ. With Volume 4 in the following year the title was altered, the new name being described as 'more indicative of (the journal's) role as the official organ of the Society'. After Hedley was elected President in 1904, there were two more editors:

Archibald Reid   January–June 1904   H. Lewis Jones   July 1904–July 1907

Both men – the 33-year-old Reid of King's College Hospital just starting his career and Lewis Jones, the doyen of British electrotherapeutists reaching his peak – were able to fill the journal's pages with clinical radiological material, because the monthly meetings of the Society were well attended by practising London radiologists – unlike those of the Röntgen Society – and their discussions yielded ample copy to choose from.

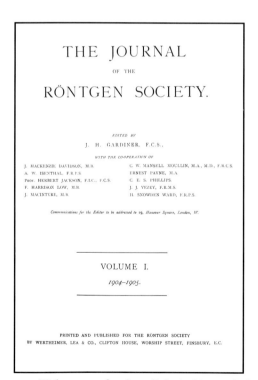
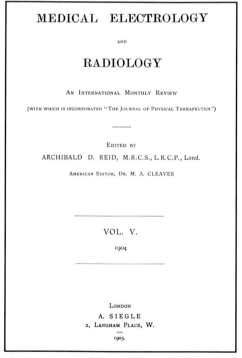

55. *Title-pages of early radiological journals.* Left The Journal of the Röntgen Society, *1904–23*. Right Medical Electrology and Radiology, *1903–7*

This ready source of supply made the editor's burden much lighter than the editors of *Archives of the Roentgen Ray* or *The Journal of the Röntgen Society*.

For the four years after January 1904 until it ceased publication, *Medical Electrology and Radiology* was the best radiological journal in Britain. The following titles are examples of its contents:

W. S. Hedley (1903): 'Medical Electrology and Radiology in 1902' (Presidential Address).

E. W. H. Shenton (1904): 'X-rays in the diagnosis of joint conditions'.

H. E. Gamlen (1904): 'The treatment of some skin diseases by X-rays, Finsen and other light rays'.

A. D. Reid (1905): 'A case of achondroplasia'.

R. Higham Cooper (1905): 'The treatment of leucaemia (*sic*) and lymphadenoma by x-rays'.

W. Deane Butcher (1905): 'On the rationale of radiotherapeutic treatment'.

Chisholm Williams (1906): 'X-rays in the treatment of carcinoma and sarcoma'.

J. Hall-Edwards (1906): 'Ten years' experience in localisation of foreign bodies by means of X-rays'.

H. Lewis Jones (1906): 'Cervical ribs and their relation to atrophy of the intrinsic muscles of the hand'.

W. Ironside Bruce (1906): 'The extended uses of the Röntgen ray in the diagnosis of disease'.

G. Harrison Orton (1907): 'The x-ray diagnosis of thoracic aneurysm'.

G. Batten (1907): 'Some practical points respecting the x-ray treatment of ringworm of the scalp'.

A. Howard Pirie (1907): 'Treatment of tubercular glands by x-rays'.

The British Electrotherapeutic Society was one of the medical groups in London in 1907 which amalgamated to form the Royal Society of Medicine, and *Medical Electrology and Radiology* was a casualty of the new arrangement. The last number was published in December 1907, when the first parts of *Proceedings of the Royal Society of Medicine* had already appeared. Members of the old Society became members of the Electro-Therapeutical Section of the great new Society, and henceforth sectional *Proceedings* took the place of their journal.[29]

THE JOURNAL OF THE RÖNTGEN SOCIETY (1904–23)

'The time (has) come for the Society to publish its proceedings in a Journal that should be entirely under its control'.[30] With these words, the Röntgen Society in July 1904 announced the first number of a journal, the title of which was to survive independently for two decades under this title, and which was destined to exert a powerful influence on British radiology. The differences between the Society and the Rebman Publishing Company which precipitated this step, have already been mentioned and will be outlined in more detail in Chapter 9. The Society's venture in publishing required courage, because *The Journal* appeared only six months after the first number of *Medical Electrology and Radiology*, as a competitor to it and to the other monthly radiological journal, *Archives of the Roentgen Ray*. Thus at birth *The Journal of the Röntgen Society* had the appearance of being a sickly child with a poor chance of a long life. However, it possessed several advantages which enabled it to stand alone and to survive to respected maturity. First, it was published only quarterly and in slim numbers and, since the Society held monthly scientific meetings, adequate material was always available to fill the pages. Secondly, a copy was issued free to each member of the Society, consequently the circulation was satisfactorily large. The third advantage stemmed from its unique nature as the mouthpiece of the scientific and commercial following of the new science, which attracted the financial support of the x-ray apparatus makers and other suppliers.

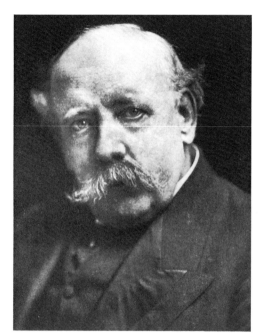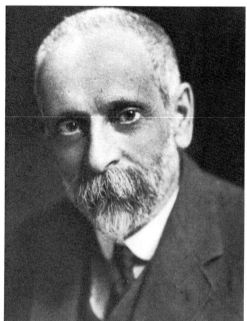

56. Early editors. Left *William Deane Butcher.* Right *James Gardiner*

The editorship was entrusted to a founder member of the Society who devoted his life to *The Journal*; and the high level of editorial workmanship and selection achieved must be attributed to him. He was the physicist, J. H. Gardiner. Lay and medical collaborators drawn from the ranks of the Society's stalwarts were selected by the Council to assist the editor. The original medical collaborators were John Macintyre, Charles Mansell-Moullin and James MacKenzie Davidson, each of them a past or future President, and F. Harrison Low, the secretary.

JAMES H. GARDINER, F.Inst.P., F.C.S. (died 1946) edited *The Journal of the Röntgen Society* for 14 years. For much of this time he served also as librarian and curator of the Society, offering a personal service to members from his home in Balham.

Gardiner was assistant to Sir William Crookes for nearly 40 years after 1881 and after his death he joined the board of Crookes' company, Powell and Sons, as technical director. He contributed significantly to the national effort during the First World War by devising methods of manufacturing high-quality glass for laboratory apparatus.

Gardiner joined the Röntgen Society in 1897 and loyally served it as Council member, Editor and President (1915–6). In the early days he frequently contributed new ideas at the monthly meetings or in the pages of *The Journal*. His article entitled 'The Origin, History and Development of the X-ray Tube', published in 1909, was on several occasions reprinted.[31] In 1938 he was mentioned as one of the four great non-medical x-ray pioneers still alive (the others being Sir Oliver Lodge, C. E. S. Phillips, and R. S. Wright).[32] He outlived them all, reaching nearly 90 years.[33]

The subject matter of *The Journal* matched the contents of *Archives* and *Medical Electrology and Radiology* except in one respect: very few clinical papers were printed. Society reports, abstracts of foreign papers and book reviews appeared regularly, in addition to the transcripts of lectures delivered at the monthly meetings. Several special features enhance *The Journal*'s value for the radiological historian: to a degree achieved nowhere else, it printed a continuous record of contemporary happenings in the x-ray world between 1904 and 1919, such as novel apparatus, important conference and society news, and the death notices of pioneers. An attractive feature was the practice of including a full-page rotogravure portrait of a former president of the Röntgen Society in each volume.

Articles with a clinical content appeared only rarely, since very few medical men attended the monthly meetings. A review of the first ten volumes shows that medical contributions comprised presidential addresses – the Society tried to fill its highest post alternately with radiologists and scientists – and articles which may have been solicited by the editor, such as John Macintyre's recollections of 'Early X-ray Photographs'.[34] *The Journal of the Röntgen Society* was a scientific journal of high quality which printed occasional medical articles.

The Tenth Annual Report of the Society provided a summary of the 1906–7 scientific programme. The speakers and lecture titles give an indication of the contents of *The Journal*:[35]

C. V. Boys, F.R.S. (November 1906): Presidential Address.

Lord Blythswood and W. A. Scoble (December 1906): 'A comparison of the sensitiveness of photographic plates to light and Röntgen rays'.

Dr. Deane Butcher: 'On the comparative practice of Röntgen techniques in England and abroad'.

Geoffrey Pearce: 'Reduction in exposure. Demonstrated'.

Lord Blythswood and W. A. Scoble (January 1907): 'The relations between the measurements from a focus tube, with a view to determining which are proportional to the intensity of the Rays'.

T. Thorne Baker (February 1907): 'An x-ray plate and tube tester'.

C. E. S. Phillips: 'A short preliminary note on some work to be described in April'.

Dr. G. B. Batten showed a new form of stereoscope, etc.

Dr. E. S. Worrall (March 1907) gave a lantern demonstration of radiographic work.

C. E. S. Phillips (April 1907): 'The measurement of radioactivity and x-rays'.

C. E. Kenneth Mees (May 1907): 'The theory of the photographic process'.

A. A. Campbell Swinton (June 1907): 'Some recent investigations in connection with Crookes tubes'.

The year 1919 brought a new editor to *The Journal*. In that year several numbers of Volume 15 were delayed through the illness of Dr. Gardiner. Eventually they appeared with the help of Sidney Russ, then recently appointed the physicist to the

Middlesex Hospital. Although Gardiner recovered, he retired as editor, and the Röntgen Society chose his successor from its own close ranks. Their choice was Dr. G. W. C. Kaye, a physicist who identified his life with British radiology and who during his career acquired an international reputation. Dr. Kaye oversaw the remaining years of *The Journal*, continuing to edit it after the 'closer-working' arrangement in 1923 which altered its title to *The British Journal of Radiology (Röntgen Society Section)*. The last number to appear under the old name, *The Journal of the Röntgen Society*, was Number 4 of Volume 19, in October 1923.

PROCEEDINGS OF THE ROYAL SOCIETY OF MEDICINE (now JOURNAL OF THE ROYAL SOCIETY OF MEDICINE) (1907–current)

1. Electro-Therapeutical Section (1907–31)

Volume 1 of *Proceedings* appeared in 1908, and a preliminary note explained the contents as 'Comprising the Report of the Proceedings for the Session 1907–08'. The individual sections had been issued in the course of the Session and they were bound together and published as the first annual volume. The report of the Electro-Therapeutical Section, which was numbered pages 1–138, found a place in the second half of Volume 1. The immediate success of the Section's monthly meetings ensured that the editors of *Proceedings* received copy which was recent and relevant to clinical radiology. The journal became in reality as well as by design the successor to *Medical Electrology and Radiology*, which in its final years had proved the most useful journal for radiologists to read. *Proceedings* now took its place. The contents of the Electro-Therapeutical Section of each volume, although including many papers not connected with x-rays (electrotherapy remained linked to radiology until the 1930s), covered the whole field of diagnostic and therapeutic radiology of the day.

Before the First World War abruptly halted all development, numerous valuable papers appeared in *Proceedings*, and they formed the ground substance of the new science. By 1908 radiological practice and technique had advanced beyond the original surgical field of fractures and foreign bodies to the point as W. S. Hedley had prophesied, where it was the turn of medicine to benefit. Physicians interested in the heart and lungs and in diseases of the alimentary tract now were drawn by the benefits of the new investigative method. Many pages of the journal were filled with lectures and reports on pulmonary tuberculosis and the investigation of the gastro-intestinal tract, but other topics were also considered, e.g. Snook's high-tension generator replacing the induction coil; radium and x-rays for treating deeply-seated malignant processes; radiological descriptions of diseases such as arthritis, syphilis and acromegaly. Inevitably also, the toll of radiation injury was chronicled, the most dramatic presentation being given by a lecturer who was himself a victim, Dr. Hall-Edwards.

Notable papers in *Proceedings* before 1916 were:

Chest Diseases:

1907: Dr. Stanley Green (Lincoln): 'The diagnostic value of the Röntgen rays in some diseases of the chest'.[36] A pioneer user himself, Dr. Green after 1902 strongly pleaded the use of x-rays in detecting early tuberculosis, and he helped to define the radiological signs.

1913: Sir Richard Douglas Powell, K.C.V.O., the eminent physician, led a discussion on the use of x-rays in the diagnosis of pulmonary tuberculosis at the February meeting of the Section. Two members, Stanley Melville and W. J. S. Bythell, delivered important lectures on the same evening. Powell, representing the more conservative of his colleagues, was provocative: 'Are x-ray findings facts?' – he asked[37] – 'I have always regarded them as shadows which have to be rightly interpreted.' He implied that he could never accept 'shadows' as possessing the same coinage as clinically detectable signs of tuberculosis. Bythell and Melville made spirited replies in their lectures which followed, quoting from their experience to prove that radiography offers the earliest evidence of the disease. It often starts not at the apex but centrally in the lung as enlarged mediastinal lymph nodes, Melville pointed out, which only radiography will reveal.

Alimentary Tract:

1909: A. E. Barclay: 'The value of x-rays in diseases of the digestive system'.[38]

1910: Franz M. Groedel (Germany): 'Examination of the intestines by means of Röntgen rays both under normal and pathological conditions'.[39]

1910: Alfred C. Jordan: 'The Röntgen ray examination of the oesophagus'.[40]

1913: Jordan and Barclay: 'Gastric ulcer'.[41]

Dr. (later Sir) Archibald Reid in his Presidential Address to the Section in October 1911 referred to intestinal contrast studies, the so-called 'bismuth breakfast', as a particular activity pursued by radiologists such as Hertz and Jordan at Guy's Hospital and Barclay and Holland in Lancashire.[42] This activity prompted Thurstan Holland, the Section's President in 1913, to nominate a sub-committee to advise on the technique and standardisation of barium studies, consisting of Hertz and Jordan, Barclay, Gilbert Scott and Reginald Morton.[43] Eighteen months later it made the following simple recommendations: the meal should consist of bread and milk or porridge to half-a-pint in volume; to which was added two ounces of barium sulphate or two ounces of bismuth oxychloride; and the patient was to have an empty stomach and to have received no aperients or other medicines. While less opaque than the bismuth mixture, barium sulphate was cheaper and Dr. Hertz thought it equally good. The report doomed the bismuth breakfast, first introduced in Munich by Rieder in 1904 and used in Britain since 1908, and established the barium meal as the standard means of radiological examination of the alimentary tract.[38,44]

Apparatus:

1907: Archibald Reid: 'An abdominal compressor for intravenous pyelography'.[45]

1909: George B. Batten: 'A photographic plate rocker'.[46]

1910: Reginald Morton: 'The relative value of various types of high-tension transformers (including coil) used in the production of x-rays'.[47]

1910: Stanley Melville: 'A new tube stand'.[48]

1914: R. W. A. Salmond: 'Experiments in x-ray filtration'.[49]

1915: Sir James MacKenzie Davidson: 'A new commutator attachment for rectifying the current supply to the x-ray tube'.[50]

Deep Radiotherapy:

1908: W. Ironside Bruce: 'The treatment of leukaemia, exophthalmic goitre, sarcoma etc. by x-rays'.[51]

   1909: N. S. Finzi: 'Radium in the treatment of malignant growths'.[52]

   1910: A Howard Pirie: 'The disappearance of enlarged glands in lymphadenoma under treatment by x-rays'.[53]

   1910: J. Hall-Edwards: 'Notes on the treatment of cancer by means of the x-rays and radium'.[54]

Radiation Injury:

1908: J. Hall-Edwards: 'On x-ray dermatitis and its prevention'.[55] Dr. Hall-Edwards delivered his lecture shortly after his hand had been amputated after an illness which is described in Chapters 3 and 11. The lecture received such wide publicity that it is viewed as a landmark in the struggle to introduce adequate protective measures against radiation damage.

After 1915 the Electro-Therapeutical Section of *Proceedings* gradually lost the appearances of a radiological journal. As the War disrupted radiologists' lives, attendances at Society meetings became sporadic and the meetings themselves became irregular. *Proceedings* mirrored this disruption by a reduced thickness and an altered content. Sir James MacKenzie Davidson heralded the change in subject matter in October 1914 when he led a discussion on 'The localisation of foreign bodies (including bullets etc.) by means of x-rays'[56] – a topic to which the Section was to return again and again during the next three years. Other novel subjects were: the radiological appearances of war injuries such as gas gangrene and compound fractures; descriptions of electrical departments in military hospitals; and electrical methods of treating the wounded.

Proceedings never regained its pre-war position as the leading radiological journal. During the War years and afterwards, it lost ground to its competitor *Archives of Radiology and Electrotherapy*, which began to print more articles on subjects relevant to clinical radiologists. *Archives* from its inception in 1896 pursued a policy of publishing the lectures or proceedings of societies irrespective of whether they had previously appeared in print elsewhere. Lecturers not infrequently found their papers printed in *Archives* as well as *Proceedings* or *The Journal of the Röntgen Society*, and this practice continued to the 1920s. However, after 1915 the editors of *Proceedings* seem to have become more selective in the material they chose to accept for publication from the electrotherapeutists – and *Archives* gained in radiological stature. *Proceedings* lost further ground after 1923 when *Archives* became the property of the British Institute of Radiology, and thus the mouthpiece of British radiologists.

2. *Section of Radiology* (1931–current)

In 1931 the radiologists in the Royal Society of Medicine under their President, Professor J. M. W. Morison, parted company with the electrotherapeutists, and created a new section of practising diagnostic and therapeutic radiologists. The Section of Radiology still exists.

   In 1977 the format and name of *Proceedings of the Royal Society of Medicine* was abandoned, which became the *Journal of the Royal Society of Medicine*.

THE BRITISH JOURNAL OF RADIOLOGY (1923–current)

1. *The British Journal of Radiology (Röntgen Society Section). The Journal of the Röntgen Society* (1924–7)

The Röntgen Society in agreeing during the latter half of 1923 to establish a closer relationship with the British Association of Radiology and Physiotherapy, moved with extreme caution. It did nothing which could not have been undone later. The agreement concerning the journals of the two bodies consisted of two clauses. The first clause established a joint editorial committee to advise both editors. The second clause altered the name of *The Journal of the Röntgen Society* to '*The British Journal of Radiology, Röntgen Society Section, incorporating The Journal of the Röntgen Society*'. The first number of Volume 20 appeared in January 1924 under this title, minus the word 'incorporating'. A preliminary note from the editor, Dr. Kaye, assured his readers that the journal would continue to preserve its individuality and financial independence. Only if and when complete amalgamation between the Society and the Association came about, he assured them, would the new arrangement be altered.[57]

The first members of the Joint Editorial Committee were:

Röntgen Society: Dr. Kaye (Editor of Röntgen Society Section), Cuthbert Andrews, Dr. F. L. Hopwood, Dr. E. A. Owen, Geoffrey Pearce, and Captain C. E. S. Phillips.

B.A.R.P.: Dr. Knox (Editor of B.A.R.P. Section), Dr. H. A. Colwell, Dr. A. E. Barclay, Dr. E. P. Cumberbatch, Dr. Thurstan Holland, Dr. G. Harrison Orton, and Professor Sidney Russ.[57]

The Journal survived the transition unscathed internally, only the title and covers were altered. Dr. Kaye remained at his post, and he continued to be an editor of the new journal after the full amalgamation at the end of 1927. Indeed, he was an editor for the rest of his life, serving x-ray journals in this capacity for nearly 20 years, and he deserves to be credited here. But Kaye, like his medical *protégé*, Robert Knox, was first and foremost a man of his Society, a begetter of British radiological institutions, and his biography appears more appropriately in Chapter 11.

2. *The British Journal of Radiology (British Association of Radiology and Physiotherapy Section). Archives of Radiology and Electrotherapy* (January–April 1924)

In January 1924 a preliminary announcement greeted readers of this section of *The British Journal of Radiology*, which was the first number of Volume 29 of the journal which had been born in 1896 as the *Archives of Clinical Skiagraphy* and which had appeared continuously since that date. The title was announced as '*The British Journal of Radiology, British Association of Radiology and Physiotherapy Section, incorporating the Archives of Radiology and Electrotherapy*'. However, as happened with the *Röntgen Society Section*, the word 'incorporating' was omitted from the titlehead.

The preliminary announcement, using the words agreed between the Röntgen Society and the British Association of Radiology and Physiotherapy, gave the same cautious welcome to the Joint Editorial Committee and to the promise of future amalgamation. It also described additional changes in page size, printing type and general appearance, which were introduced to achieve conformity with the Röntgen Society's journal, 'thus bringing both sections of *The British Journal of Radiology* into line with the journals of other scientific societies in this country'.[58] These changes were largely cosmetic, and subscribers of the old *Archives* found their journal to be not greatly altered inside.

3. *The British Journal of Radiology (British Institute of Radiology Section). Archives of Radiology and Electrotherapy* (May 1924–7)

When the British Association of Radiology and Physiotherapy transferred its incorporation as a limited company to the British Institute of Radiology in April 1924, its property, *The British Journal of Radiology (B.A.R.P. Section),* became the property of the Institute. This transfer necessitated the alteration of its sub-title to the words shown above. Robert Knox, an editor of *Archives* for nine years, remained at his post. Like Dr. Kaye of the Röntgen Society, he was destined three years later to steer his journal through complete amalgamation. Knox ranks with Butcher, Gardiner and Kaye as one of the great editors but, since he was first and foremost a man of his organisation, his biography belongs to Chapter 9.

4. *The British Journal of Radiology (New Series)* (1928–current)

'On the face of it, it looks as if an amalgamation of the two British Journals has a great deal to be said for it, not only as regards the value of the publication itself, but more especially on the financial side,' Dr. A. E. Barclay told the Röntgen Society in his Presidential Address on 4 November 1924.[59] However, Barclay's logic did not convince his audience, and the marriage between the Society and the Institute was not immediately arranged.

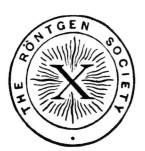 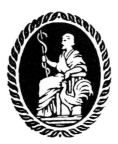 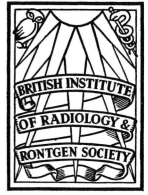

57. *Publishers' colophons.* Left *The Röntgen Society.* Middle *William Heinemann (Medical Books) Limited.* Right *British Institute of Radiology*

Three years were to pass before the 'closer-working' arrangement bore fruit in the amalgamation of the two Sections of the journal into a single publication. Finally in January 1928 the first number of Volume 1 of the *British Journal of Radiology, New Series* made its appearance. The familiar 'rising sun' emblem, incorporating the words 'British Institute of Radiology and Röntgen Society', was printed for the first time on the title page in 1929 (Volume 2), when it replaced the colophon of William Heinemann (Medical Books) Limited, the previous owners who had continued to publish the journal for the Association (and later the Institute) after 1923. *The British Journal of Radiology* continues to be issued monthly, the series reaching Volume 57 in 1984.

Chapter 9

SOCIETIES, SECTIONS AND THE INSTITUTE

'Before the first meeting Dr. Walsh sent a note to the *British Medical Journal* announcing that the new society (i.e. The Röntgen Society) would have a mixed medical and lay membership. . . . It is clear that he was none too happy that the society was to be formed on satisfactory lines from a medical man's point of view. The history of fifty years has confirmed his fears, on the other hand, the constitution has ensured a Society that has performed a wider range of usefulness, bringing together workers in the diverse fields of medicine, physics, engineering and photography, which was envisaged by those who decided against purely medical membership'.

Barclay (1947)[1]

THE RÖNTGEN SOCIETY

The climate was ripe in the Spring of 1897, both in the medical and scientific circles of London, for establishing a society to study the Röntgen rays. Professor Silvanus Thompson in March of the previous year had mobilised the doctors' enthusiasm for the new clinical method, and this idea arose directly out of his lecture.[2] The first three numbers of *Archives of Clinical Skiagraphy* as well as reports in the medical and popular press helped to keep the subject of x-rays before the eyes of the medical profession. The fourth number of *Archives*, published in April 1897, carried the following announcement:[3]

'A Skiagraphic Society has been formed in London by some of the leading men interested in the study of the X rays both in their medical and general scientific applications. That such combination is greatly needed, is well recognised by all those engaged in working at the subject. All interested are requested to communicate with D. Walsh, 5, Pump Court, Temple, E.C.'.

The meeting reported was attended by only three medical men – David Walsh, F. Harrison Low and F. E. Fenton, F.R.C.S. It took place on 18 March 1897 in the offices of the Medical Defence Union at 20 King William Street, Strand. Low presided, and after the three men decided to proceed, Walsh undertook to canvass the support of prominent members of the medical profession for the new society, which they named 'The X-Ray Society'.

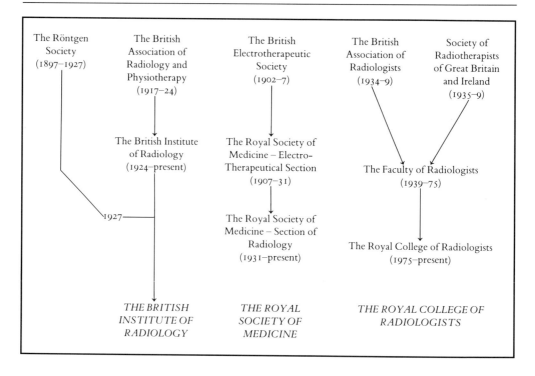

The burning question, over which argument was joined immediately, was whether non-medical men were to be admitted to the Society. How could confidentiality be preserved, it was asked, if doctors were obliged to discuss clinical matters before an audience of apparatus makers and photographers? The announcement in *Archives* and Walsh's note to the *British Medical Journal* reflected the medical founders' dilemma. 'The difficulty of discussing medical matters before a mixed audience will probably be got over by forming a medical sub-section', he wrote.[4] On 2 April he and eight other doctors met and made the crucial decision: membership of the Society was not to be restricted to medical men, but instead it would be offered to scientists and laymen who wished to join. Thus was devised the only qualification for admission – 'That candidates must have shown some scientific interest in the Roentgen rays'. During April and May a provisional committee under the chairmanship of Thomas Moore, F.R.C.S. wrote the rules, appointed officers and prepared to launch the Society.[5,6,7] At this point, the selection of a President became necessary, and the provisional committee invited Professor Silvanus Thompson, who accepted the office.

'Silvanus Thompson was the man who first made the medical man feel the necessity for a society where he could meet the physicist and others interested, to discuss the properties of the new rays and to see how the discovery could best be harnessed to the service of medicine. It was fitting and proper that the first President should be the man whose lecture had been its inspiration'. These words, written by A. E. Barclay in 1930,[2] explained the choice of Thompson as the first president, perhaps also the decision – unique in the medical world – to admit laymen to a body concerned with clinical affairs. No other man, lay or medical, had ever drawn an audience of 400 doctors and won their acclamation, as Thompson succeeded in doing on 30 March 1896 before the

Clinical Society of London. Over 30 years later his performance was recalled in *The Lancet* by their secretary, Sir William Hale-White:[8] 'Silvanus Thompson was a prince among lecturers. I have never heard a better demonstration or attended a more memorable medical meeting'. It was for this success, his skill as a lecturer which showed him to be the man of the hour, that he was chosen as President of the Röntgen Society, rather than other, better-known physical scientists such as Sir William Crookes or Professor Herbert Jackson.

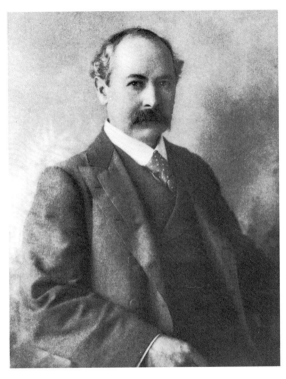

58. Silvanus P. Thompson

SILVANUS PHILLIPS THOMPSON, Ll.D., D.Sc., F.R.S., F.R.M.S., M.I.E.E. (1851–1916) was one of the three experimenters in London who are known to have verified Röntgen's experiments on the very day that the news reached England (the others being Campbell Swinton and Russell Reynolds, see Chapter 3). Although an academic physicist by profession, Thompson's intellect was so brilliant and diverse that he can be viewed as a Victorian example of the Renaissance man – he knew about everything, and everything he attempted he excelled at. Combined with this God-given gift and serving as a vehicle to apply it, was Thompson's greatest talent, by which he is chiefly remembered – his ability to communicate knowledge.

Silvanus Thompson was born in York, the son of a Quaker schoolmaster and his wife, whose two uncles were Fellows of the Royal Society. He himself grew up as a Quaker, and later was an Elder of the Society of Friends. He chose to read chemistry at university but so wide was his learning even as a young graduate that, when at the age of 25 he applied for the chair of chemistry in the new University College at Bristol and failed to get the post, he was offered and accepted the post of lecturer in physics instead! In Bristol his qualities as a teacher soon inspired his students, one of whom was a youth from Bridgwater in Somerset, Thurstan Holland.

He moved to London in 1885 as Professor of Applied Physics tenable at the City and Guilds College, Finsbury, pursuing his interests in electricity and optics; a post that he held until his death. These were decades of prodigious achievement in many directions, as the following list shows:

Electrical engineer – he was President of the Institute of Electrical Engineers in 1899;

Experimental physicist of phenomenal industry – Professor Sidney Russ classified 166 of his papers as 'important';[9]

Writer of popular scientific textbooks, including *Elementary Lessons in Electricity and Magnetism*, a book which ran to over 40 editions, and *Calculus Made Easy*;

Biographer of Lord Kelvin, Faraday, and Philip Reis, the inventor of the telephone;

Linguist, a master of five languages – he lectured in German in Berlin, and translated William Gilbert's *De Magnete* from the original in Latin;

Competent artist, whose paintings were hung in the Royal Academy

University administrator, who helped to remodel the University of London as a teaching centre;[10] and

Musician and naturalist.

In 1896 Thompson was established and known as a master in the art of lecturing, skilled in conveying the meaning of a difficult subject to an audience unversed in the subject. At the Royal Institution (to which Sir William Crookes had introduced him), his reputation always drew a large crowd to his evening lectures. In May 1896 his discourse, when he repeated Röntgen's experiments, was an exciting demonstration for the audience which included distinguished scientists such as Sir William Crookes.[11]

After completing his term as President of the Röntgen Society, Thompson made little further contribution to x-rays, moving to perform research in other fields of pure science. He was elected an Honorary Member of the Society in 1897, after Röntgen and Crookes; a distinction not accorded to all his successors. On his death the Society established an eponymous annual lecture to honour his memory and Lord Rutherford delivered the first Silvanus Thompson Memorial Lecture in 1918.[12,13]

Thompson chaired the first Annual General Meeting on 3 June 1897 in the rooms of the Medical Society of London, Chandos Street. The provisional committee had prepared their work thoroughly, and the 20 persons attending the meeting approved their proposals for rules, officers and members of the Society, which now emerged in its final form. In only one important respect were the original intentions reversed. In deference to the discoverer, the name of the Society was altered to 'The Röntgen Society'.

The objects of the Society were defined as follows:[14]

'1. To discuss the Röntgen rays in relation to Medicine, the Arts, and Sciences.
2. To discuss and exhibit apparatus and methods in connection with the rays.
3. To hold periodical meetings for the reading of papers and discussions thereon; with exhibition of clinical cases, skiagrams and all matters bearing on the Röntgen rays.
4. To provide a museum, library and Röntgen ray appliances.
5. To publish transactions in a convenient form.'

One of the most far-reaching rules was clause 10 which stipulated that no new rule could be introduced or existing rules altered except by a three-fourths majority at a general meeting. Although it was probably agreed without demur, little could those who acquiesced have realised – Barclay reflected 50 years later[1] – of what fundamental importance this clause would prove to be. On several occasions it was to save the Society from becoming the platform of sectional interest.

The first President, Officers and Council, all of whom except the secretary were elected to hold office for one year, were:[15]

President: Professor Silvanus P. Thompson, F.R.S.

Vice-Presidents: Professor David Ferrier, F.R.S.; Professor J. Hall Gladstone, F.R.S.; Dr. John Macintyre; C. W. Mansell-Moullin, F.R.C.S.; Fletcher Moulton, Q.C., F.R.S.; and Dr. Dawson Turner.

Council: Dr. J. MacKenzie Davidson; F. E. Fenton, F.R.C.S.; J. E. Greenhill; Dr. W. S. Hedley; Dr. F. Harrison Low; Thomas Moore, F.R.C.S.; Dr. Sydney Rowland; A. A. Campbell Swinton; H. Snowden Ward, F.R.P.S.; William Webster, F.C.S.; Dr. Norris Wolfenden; and subsequently completed by election of A. W. Isenthal and John J. Vezey.

Treasurer: Thomas Moore, F.R.C.S.

Secretary: Dr. David Walsh.

The choice of the first officers reflected the fine balance between doctor members and others that the Society was to maintain throughout the 30 years of its independent existence. Of its 127 members at the end of the first year, about half were doctors including several in overseas countries. The non-medical members were a interesting group, representing diverse interests and levels of British society but united in complying with the single criterion of membership, namely, of having shown a scientific interest in the x-rays. Some contributed significantly, others hoped for reward from their membership. At the head of the list were several nobles of the realm who dabbled in science, such as the Duke of Newcastle and the Earl of Crauford. The most influential group were the professional scientists – chemists and physicists of the calibre of the President, such as William Webster and Oliver Lodge. The embryo x-ray manufacturing industry was represented by men such as Cox, Cossor and Isenthal. More controversial was the membership of professional photographers like Snowden Ward and editors of the photographic magazines, who were prominent in the early life of the Society before the medical profession secured a monopoly over the taking of clinical x-rays. Finally there was the large body of amateur experimenters, wholly without self-interest, such as the Reverent Walter of Norfolk, Colonel Gifford of Chard and the Crimean War veteran, Lord Blythswod, who are mentioned in Chapter 3.

FLETCHER MOULTON (later BARON MOULTON), K.C.B., C.B.E., P.C., M.P., Q.C., F.R.S. (1844–1921) was the most remarkable of the amateur experimenters attracted to membership of the Society. Moulton came from Wesleyan stock in Shropshire and read mathematics at Cambridge, where he was President of the Union in 1868. Thereafter he was admitted to the Middle Temple and began his career at the London bar, at the same time pursuing his interest in scientific matters: when he took Silk in 1885 his electrical researches had already won him an F.R.S.

This astonishing record continued throughout his life as he applied his quite exclusive knowledge of scientific matters to his legal practice and the affairs of state. In 1897 when he joined the Röntgen Society, he was said to be the most successful patents lawyer and the barrister with the highest income in London. For six years after 1906 he was a Lord Justice of Appeal. During the First World War he chaired the committee responsible for producing high explosives and propellants, which controlled all chemical manufacture in Britain. For this service he was honoured further and received a life baronetcy. Moulton was the first chairman of the Medical Research Council.[5,16]

DAVID WALSH, M.D.(Edinburgh), the Society's first secretary and the author of one of the earliest textbooks of radiology in the English language, must be credited with Harrison Low

for taking the initiative in establishing a skiagraphic society in London. He served as secretary
for two years. In 1899 he resigned after a difference with the Council over the question of a
fee for a photographic exhibition mounted by the Royal Photographic Society at the Crystal
Palace. Walsh demanded payment for medical exhibits and when the Council disagreed, he
went.[5] Thereafter his name does not appear in the Society's affairs. He lived to a ripe age, and
was elected an Honorary Member of the British Institute of Radiology in 1928.

FRANK HARRISON LOW, M.D., C.M.(Aberdeen, 1876) (died 1912) might have claimed
to be the Father of the Röntgen Society since he chaired the exploratory meeting of doctors
who decided to form a skiagraphic society in London. He was a medical practitioner in Henrietta
Street, off Cavendish Square and an early radiographer at the Children's Hospital, Paddington
Green and the Poly Clinic.

A stalwart of the Röntgen Society, he succeeded David Walsh as secretary in 1899, and continued to hold the post up to his death.[17] In 1902–3 he served briefly as the medical editor of
Archives of the Roentgen Ray.

Silvanus Thompson defined the aims of the Society in his introductory remarks at the
June meeting. 'The position of the Society' – he stated[14] – 'is between those devoted
purely to medicine, to physics, and to photography. In ourselves we focus a number
of interests provided for by no other existing bodies, such as, for example, the Royal,
the Physical, the Photographic Societies or the Institute of Electrical Engineers. *There
is a very definite place to occupy and a function to fulfil*'. He announced that the first meeting
of the Society would take place in the Autumn of 1897.

The inaugural meeting or *conversazione* held on the evening of 15 November 1897,
was a grand and glittering occasion, patronised by the rich and famous, the curious
and the interested of the metropolis. Over 300 were present, of whom 130 were ladies,
and they included several nobles with their wives and other fashionable folk. No less
than 12 journalists attended, including the editor of *Queen* magazine, who it must be
presumed were grateful to be admitted to a public demonstration of the scientific
phenomenon that had captured the curiosity of the nation. However, the audience had
its serious side, and physicists, apparatus makers and photographers were there in force.
About 40 doctors attended, but only a few of the early medical experimenters and not
all the members of the Council of the Society.

The meeting was held in St. Martin's Town Hall, Marylebone – a building since
demolished – because the Society required a suite of rooms for exhibitions and demonstrations as well as a hall to seat a large audience to hear the President's Address.
Silvanus Thompson rose at 9.00 pm and spoke for 40 minutes. Purposely adapting his
remarks to the various elements in his audience, he traced the history of the search for
x-rays, described Röntgen's experiments (see the head of Chapter 1) and outlined the
developments that had taken place in the 23 months since the discovery. With studied
courtesy he praised the contributions of the most eminent scientist in the field, who
sat in the audience – Sir William Crookes – and of 12 other Britons, most of whom
were Society members and several present.

The programme continued in the adjoining rooms. In a large hall was mounted an
'Exhibition of Photographs', which consisted of 600–700 x-ray prints arranged by Snowden Ward and others. *Archives* reported the display as follows:

> 'Dr. Gladstone, F.R.S., showed photographs of aluminium and other metals
> in order of the power of absorbing the Röntgen rays.

Mr. F. C. Abbott, F.R.C.S. exhibited photographs of bullets taken at the seat of the recent Graeco-Turkish War.

Mr. Gifford – early work.

Mr. Gardiner and Dr. Norris Wolfenden – natural history objects.

Mr. Greenhill – illustrated short exposures.

Numerous other photographs of general and special interest by Messrs Glew, Ogston, Ernest Payne, A. A. Campbell Swinton, William Webster, Sir Gervas Glyn, Bart., and Drs. Barry Blacker, Hall-Edwards, W. Cotton, F. S. Low, Newman, Nathan Raw and others'.[18]

Webster's prints showed head and arm radiographs taken with exposures varying from 1/25 to one second in duration, and an adult abdomen and chest exposed for three minutes.

In another room Dr. Hedley had charge of an exhibition of apparatus:

'Mr. MacKenzie Davidson and Mr. Hall-Edwards each demonstrated new methods of localizing foreign bodies.

Dr. Hedley – a stereoscope, showing among other objects an injected human brain.

Dr. Barry Blacker – a motor interrupter, etc.

Mr. Ernest Payne – coils, interrupter, and apparatus.

Dr. Walsh – transparency: plates to illustrate book, *The Röntgen Rays in Medical Work*.

Mr. A. C. Cossor – tubes of own manufacture'.[18]

The most exciting exhibit was the 'Demonstration of the Living Body', arranged by Thomas Moore and William Webster of the Miller Hospital. Using Webster's 20-inch spark Apps-Newton coil, pulsations of the human heart were demonstrated on a fluoroscopic screen 'for the first time in public' to small groups of the audience herded into a dark room. In another room – and also ignoring the radiation dose – x-rays were produced by Dr. Fenton and Mr. Isenthal, during demonstrations on the behaviour of different gases *in vacuo*. The evening ended with a programme of vocal and instrumental music. Among the performers, William Webster sang '*Il Sogno*' by Mercadanto, Miss Cordelia Grylls followed with songs by Schumann, and a Mr. Webbe rendered Liszt's '*Liebestraum*' in a masterly way. The last items had to be abandoned 'owing to the lateness of the hour'.[18]

After this auspicious start, the serious work of the Society began. Eight monthly meetings were held between November and June of each year, at which papers were read and discussed, and occasionally inventions were shown. The shortage of clinical material was felt from the beginning, and the need for it was recognised. The first Annual Report called for meetings at which apparatus and x-ray photographs could be exhibited, and 'for the interchange of views and experiences'.[15] However, the strong non-medical slant shown by the papers of the first session (1897–8) did not alter in succeeding years. This programme was:

5 November 1897 – President's Address on the Aims of the Society.

December 1897 – A. A. Campbell Swinton: On adjustable focus-tubes.

January 1898 – W. Webster: Practical work with the x-rays.

February 1898 – Dr. David Walsh – Periosteal and other soft-tissue shadows. Dr. J MacKenzie Davidson: Localisation.

March 1898 – J. H. Gardiner: Photographic activity and penetration of Roentgen rays at different vacua. Wilson Noble: Some observations on various makes of tube, and varying conditions of vacua.

April 1898 – James Wimshurst, F.R.S.: The influence machine and its advantages for lighting x-ray tubes.

May 1898 – A. Apps, M.I.E.E.: Notes on the description of a new induction coil. J. Macintyre: Some notes on contact-breakers.

June 1898 – T. C. Porter: Work on the x-ray. A. A. Campbell Swinton: A pinhole Roentgen ray camera and its applications. Drs. Forbes and Wolfenden: A preliminary communication on the action of the x-ray on micro-organisms.

The non-clinical bias of the Society's meetings reflected the greater activity of its physicists and lay members – or, to put the matter in another way, the lack of support that it received from its medical members. For the doctors, the problem of discussing patients' diseases and radiographs before a mixed audience – a thorny question which had been optimistically minimised by the medical founders – proved to be an insurmountable barrier to wholehearted medical participation. An analysis of the Society's membership list in 1901 shows that only 25 doctors out of 100 medical men who belonged, possessed addresses in the London postal district; whereas almost all of the 110 non-medical members lived in London. Therefore, the most likely attenders at the monthly meetings were the physicists and lay members rather than the doctors.

In 1901 a group of the medical members, which included the leading x-ray specialists of London, announced their wish for a society devoted exclusively to medical matters. They invited the Council to consider their request. The Society was torn by conflicting views, and when after much procrastination the doctors were offered their own meetings – in effect, a medical sub-section from which other members of the Society were excluded[19] – the proposal came too late. Fifteen members resigned and in 1902 the dissident doctors formed the British Electrotherapeutic Society, see below. They included W. S. Hedley, Lewis Jones, Chisholm Williams, Reginal Morton, Howard Pirie and Cecil Lyster, who collectively formed the radiological 'establishment' of the metropolis. This controversial step was deplored by the small group of medical men who did not resign – MacKenzie Davidson, Mansell-Moullin, Batten, Low, Walsh and Deane Butcher – almost all of whom served as Presidents of the Society.[20,21]

A second setback befell the Society early in 1904 when the Council and the publishers of *Archives of the Roentgen Ray* disagreed over the editorial control of the journal. This difference has been outlined in Chapter 8. At the root of the matter was the secession of the doctors, whose new society, comprising leading radiologists and electrotherapeutists, was an immediate success. It opened the eyes of the publishers to the wider medical market for *Archives* beyond the confines of the x-ray world. The Röntgen Society's original agreement with the Rebman Publishing Company in 1897 had been a less preferred solution, entered into only after the Royal Society rejected its overtures and declined to publish its proceedings;[5] now the Society boldly revoked this agreement and decided to publish its own house journal, *The Journal of the Röntgen Society*. These two setbacks stunted the growth of the Society by isolating it permanently from the body of the medical profession. The London radiologists, who collectively guided the growth of the young clinical specialty, actively transferred their patronage to the British Electrotherapeutic Society. From the viewpoint of the medical man, the Röntgen Society no longer served his needs; and the less scientifically-minded of his colleagues might have wondered why it continued to exist at all.

But the Society did survive, and even continued to recruit medical members. It was financially secure and intellectually vigorous, a model of the ideal scientific society. In 1904 it acquired the lease of a property in Hanover Square, and for the first time the Society had a permanent home. Hitherto it endured a peripatetic existence, first holding meetings in the premises of the Medical Society at 11 Chandos Square, and later in the rooms of the Royal Medical and Chirurgical Society at 20 Cavendish Square. Dr. David Walsh worked from his rooms in the Temple, and the honorary librarian stored the Society's collection of books in his home at Balham, whence members could borrow them. A permanent home in town, overseen by volunteers such as A. W. Isenthal, allowed the library to expand, and by 1914 it consisted of 100 volumes and the files of a dozen journals. A collection of early x-ray tubes and apparatus was started in 1898 by Wilson Noble's gift of a 10-inch spark coil and a battery,[15] and these items also could be accommodated.

The pre-War decade (1905–14) saw the Society grow a little but chiefly consolidate the pattern of cooperation between radiologists, physicists and manufacturers. The mainspring of the Society's success remained a small band of loyal volunteers who were mostly Londoners; dedicated members who readily gave help at all times and who never deserted it. These were the medical faithful, Walsh, Low, and MacKenzie Davidson, George Rodman and George Batten, and non-medical members such as Gardiner, Isenthal, and Vezey, C. E. S. Phillips and Geoffrey Pearce.

JOHN JEWELL VEZEY, F.R.M.S. (died 1906), the retired City businessman who became the practising radiographer of the Miller Hospital, was a pillar of strength to the Society at a critical stage of its existence. He served on the Council after 1898, and remained the Treasurer up to his death. His paper, 'The Röntgen Society: It's Past Work and Future Prospects',[19] the first article to be printed in the new journal in 1904, was a dignified but spirited defence of the Society in the wake of the defecting doctors. Vezey's City experience equipped him to give a lead. He virtually deputised for the President, Lord Blythswood, who seldom left Scotland and only rarely attended meetings. On Vezey's death the Council decided to honour him as the President, by adding his portrait to the Presidents' portraits hanging on the walls of the Council chamber.[22]

GEORGE HOOK RODMAN, M.D., F.R.P.S. (1862–1933) was a family doctor in East Sheen who was an early user of x-rays. In middle age he developed a severe dermatitis which obliged him to retire from practice, and he spent the latter half of his life in scientific pursuits. He joined the Röntgen Society in 1900, and soon thereafter began contributing case material to the radiological journals. With Norris Wolfenden he pioneered the radiography of shells and molluscs, and he made microradiographs of skeletal tissue which were used to illustrate Lawford Knaggs's textbook of bone diseases. In 1909 Rodman catalogued the x-ray tubes in the Society's possession and published an important description of the collection.[23] He served as:

President, Röntgen Society, 1910–1.
President, Royal Photographic Society, 1920–1.[24]

Rodman is chiefly remembered as a photographer; in 1917 he was one of the four radiologists to exhibit at the Salon of the Royal Photographic Society, the others being Thurstan Holland, Robert Knox and F. S. Worrall. He was elected an Honorary Member of the Röntgen Society in 1927.

GEORGE BECKETT BATTEN, M.D., C.M.(Edinburgh), Hon.D.M.R.E.(Cantab.) (1860–1941) joined the Röntgen Society in 1899 and served on the Council for 23 of the 30 years of its existence. He was a family doctor in Dulwich, who began x-ray work in October 1896 with a 6-inch spark Miller coil and a Jackson focus tube. He was one of the first to use x-rays as a therapeutic agent, and by 1904 had treated 3,000 cases of ringworm of the scalp by x-ray epilation. He is named as one of the eight medical pioneers and one of the 11 radiotherapy pioneers in Britain.[6,7]

Batten was a great meeting-goer and debater, who remained active until deep in his seventies. His name first appeared in *Archives* in 1901, and he published his last paper in the early 1930s. He served as:

President, Röntgen Society, 1918–19
President, Electro-Therapeutical Section of the Royal Society of Medicine, 1926–7.
Batten's daughter, Dr. Grace Batten, was also a respected London radiologist.[25]

Throughout its existence the Röntgen Society never ceased to promote scientific developments, and its Annual Congress became an outstanding event. Many of the major advances of British radiology owed their origin to impetus or encouragement from within the Society. Such milestones were: the Cambridge D.M.R.E. (1920); the founding of the Society of Radiographers (1920); the formation of the British X-Ray and Radium Protection Committee (1921); and the first International Congress of Radiology (1925).

When A. E. Barclay was elected President of the Society in 1924, the process of amalgamation with the British Institute of Radiology had already begun. For example, the Society's meetings during the 1925 session were held in the Institute's house and, as described in Chapter 8, the journals of the two bodies had adopted a uniform format in January 1924 as a preliminary step to possible amalgamation. Pressure now mounted on the Society to throw in its future with the Institute.

Barclay's Presidential Address on 4 November 1924 contained a clear message.[21] He prefaced his remarks with the quotation, 'I come to bury Caesar, not to praise him', and then proceeded to review the state of the Society and its future prospects. The Röntgen Society had been formed, he said, to function in the words of Silvanus Thompson, as 'a liaison between the medical profession and the various branches of pure and applied physics – a triple alliance. But the position had changed because the doctors had reverted to their natural habitation in the British Electrotherapeutic Society, consequently the proceedings had tended towards pure physics; the balance had not been maintained. The doctors were as much to blame as any one else for the breakdown of the triple alliance. The problem was, What step could be taken which would guarantee the future of the Society? Barclay answered the question himself: 'Personally, I think the British Institute of Radiology provides the obvious solution to the problem'.

The President's advice was not heeded at once, but it did not fall on deaf ears. The Society's stalwarts, uneasy about the precarious financial position of the Institute and exhibiting a natural reluctance to surrender their independence, took no immediate action. But Barclay had sounded a requiem of the Society, and his successor, Dr. Neville

Finzi, was to be its last President. The Röntgen Society amalgamated with the Institute on 17 November 1927. On that day the membership was transferred to the new body, and the Röntgen Society ceased to exist.

THE BRITISH ELECTROTHERAPEUTIC SOCIETY (1902–7)

A. E. Barclay described the doctors' defection from the Röntgen Society in 1901 as an instance of natural reversion: 'They returned to their natural surroundings in the British Electrotherapeutic Society', he wrote.[21] The logic of their action was promptly borne out by the success of the new society.

Fifty-six doctors crowded into the rooms of the Medical Society of London in Chandos Street on 10 July 1902 to attend the inaugural meeting.[26] The two senior electrotherapeutists in the country were chosen to lead the Society, Dr. Hedley of the London Hospital who was elected President, and Dr. Lewis Jones of St. Bartholomew's Hospital, Vice-President. Chisholm Williams, the pioneer radiotherapeutist, became the first secretary. Monthly meetings commenced and in the following year the name of the quarterly publication, *The Journal of Physical Therapeutics*, was altered to *Medical Electrology and Radiology* and issued monthly as the Society's official publication. Thus was established the first national association for clinical radiologists in Britain. Within a few years 160 doctors had joined the Society, and all the radiologists in the country belonged to it. About 30 retained their membership of the Röntgen Society as well. Only a handful of the latter Society's medical members failed to join the British Electrotherapeutic Society, but they included three Presidents, MacKenzie Davidson, Mansell-Moullin and John Macintyre.

Growing approbation came from the younger generation of radiologists who unfailingly joined the Society as soon as they completed their training. For example, Bythell and Barclay when seeking a London affiliation at the start of their careers in Manchester in 1906, chose to join this Society, and they became members of the Röntgen Society only some years later. After 1903 the British Electrotherapeutic Society was *the* Society to join, and its meetings (and those of its successor, the Electro-Therapeutical Section of the Royal Society of Medicine) became the testing arena of British radiologists. Young men, and old, soon felt obliged to bring any new observation, radiographic technique or theory before the Society, where it could be subjected to the informed scrutiny of the leaders of the profession.

Notwithstanding the nationwide distribution of its members, the Society derived its strength from the 50 London members, most of whom held appointments in the teaching hospitals. The professional thrust and experience of these men guaranteed that the monthly discussions remained relevant and of a high quality. Most of the papers were published in *Medical Electrology and Radiology*, and a sample is printed in Chapter 8. The following London radiologists delivered lectures or served the Society as officers during the years 1904–5: Hedley and Morton (The London Hospital), Lewis Jones and Walsham (St. Bartholomew's), Greg (St. Thomas's), Shenton (Guy's), Bruce (Charing Cross), Reid (King's College), Simmons (later St. George's), Orton (later St. Mary's), Worrall (University College), Lyster (The Middlesex Hospital), Arthur and Chisholm Williams (West London Hospital, Hammersmith).

The Society's Annual General Meeting rivalled that of the Röntgen Society in popularity. It took the form of a *conversazione* and an exhibition of apparatus. In 1904 x-ray equipment was shown by Cossor, Harry Cox, A. E. Dean, K. Schall and the Sanitas Electrical Company.[27] All these were active supporters and members of the Röntgen Society and regularly exhibited at the annual meetings of the British Electrotherapeutic Society.

The British Electrotherapeutic Society was one of the 22 medical groups in London who chose to unite to form the Royal Society of Medicine in 1907, see below. The 46th and last meeting of the Society was held at 11 Chandos Street on 24 May 1907. A 'Committee of Reference' consisting of Deane Butcher, Reid, Morton and Lewis Jones oversaw the transfer of members and their assets to the new body, whereupon the name of the British Electrotherapeutic Society disappeared.

THE ROYAL SOCIETY OF MEDICINE (1907–present)

The movement to amalgamate the numerous medical groups in London at the beginning of the present century gained momentum in 1905 with the publication of the Report of Unions of Medical Societies in London. The report had found a total of five thousand doctors in 22 groups, and it recommended a single body to be called the Royal Society of Medicine, with its headquarters at 20 Hanover Square.[28] In the event, when these plans bore fruit two years later, 16 sections were established, the sixteenth being Therapeutics including Electrotherapy – the Electro-Therapeutical Section.

1. *Electro-Therapeutical Section* (1907–31)

The first meeting of the Section took place at 20 Hanover Square on 12 July 1907, seven weeks after the British Electrotherapeutic Society had dissolved itself. The offices of the Section for the 1907–8 session were:

President: W. Deane Butcher.
Vice-Presidents: H. Lewis Jones, Archibald Reid, Samuel Sloan.
Council: W. Ironside Bruce, A. Stanley Green, Dr. W. S. Haughton, G. H. Orton, A. H. Pirie, W. Allpress Simmons, Francis Somerville, James Taylor and Dawson Turner.[29]

Dr. Butcher introduced his Presidential Address in October 1907 by referring to the historic nature of their meeting, since it was the first occasion on which electrical medicine had been represented in the Witenagemot★ of medicine. The electrotherapeutists' struggle for recognition had, in fact, been won some years earlier, when the British Medical Association allowed a sub-section of medicine for therapeutic electricity (see below); but the ultimate professional accolade of equal status was sectional membership of the Royal Society of Medicine.

The President's Address, entitled 'The Future of Electricity in Medicine', was a survey of the entire field of clinical electrotherapeutics including the first ten years of the Rönt-

★ OED: Witenagemot = The National Council in England in Anglo-Saxon times.

gen rays and speculation about their future uses. Deane Butcher was well suited for this task, being one of the most scientifically curious and intellectually brilliant of the early radiologists. In his estimation, the discovery which transformed Röntgen's experiment into practical reality was Professor Jackson's focussed cathode. He predicted that advances of similar magnitude would be made by further reducing the exposure time, and in improving the developing and printing of the photographic image. In chest diseases, skiagraphy (or Roentgenography, as he preferred to describe the science) was rapidly overtaking conventional methods. For example, apical infiltrations and mediastinal lymphadenopathy, lesions which were not detectable by physical examination, could now be shown. The time had come, he said, for each chest infirmary to have an x-ray unit as a matter of course. Gastro-intestinal diseases, as a result of the work of Holzknecht and Rieder in Germany, also had become the province of the radiologist. The same was true of cardiac work. 'One of the most vivid impressions of my life was my first view of the beating heart, like some living creature, tranquilly breathing within its bony cage. Still more impressive was the sight of the stomach during the digestion of a bismuth breakfast. . . .'[30]

When the Royal Society of Medicine moved to its new home in 1912 at the southern end of Wimpole Street (which it still occupies), the pattern was complete. British radiologists possessed a home which served both as a professional society and as a London club; an ideal arrangement. For the next 20 years and beyond, the Royal Society of Medicine was to remain the focal point for the profession. No important event or scientific advance escaped discussion at the monthly meetings of the Electro-Therapeutical Section. Up to 1914 all the lectures, and thereafter the most important ones, were printed in *Proceedings*, as has been detailed in Chapter 8. The pattern of activity started in 1902 by the old British Electrotherapeutic Society has continued in a modified form to the present day.

Eighteen Sectional Presidents followed Deane Butcher before 1930, the majority holding office for one year only. Six of these were electrotherapeutists including Lewis Jones and Sir Henry Gauvain, and the rest were radiologists. Of the latter, all were Londoners except the two Lancashiremen, Thurstan Holland and A. E. Barclay. A better balance between radiologists and electrotherapeutists, metropolis and provinces was maintained on the Council, and the members reflected the Section's national roots. The original council included the pioneer Glasgow electrotherapeutists, Samuel Sloan and Francis Somerville, and x-ray pioneers in Dublin, Lincoln and Bristol.

2. *Section of Radiology* (1931–present)
At the end of the 1930–31 session an internal re-arrangement within the Royal Society of Medicine brought into being a Section of Radiology. The names of 159 radiologists belonging to the Electro-Therapeutical Section were transferred to the new Section which met under the Presidency of Professor J. M. Woodburn Morison.

The creation of a Section of Radiology had a salutary effect on membership and activity. Eleven months later it was reported that 70 new members had joined. The average attendance at the eight meetings of the 1931–32 session had been 61, in addition to 'a considerable attendance of visitors from other sections, showing the wide interest which practitioners in medicine and surgery generally take in the problems of radiology. The Section welcomed all these guests . . .'.[31]

THE BRITISH MEDICAL ASSOCIATION

The medical electricians' struggle for equal status with physicians and surgeons was brought to a satisfactory conclusion in the first seven years of the present century. Victory was signalled by the inauguration of the Electro-Therapeutical Section of the Royal Society of Medicine in 1907, but the campaign had started some years before, and the decisive battle was fought elsewhere, at a meeting of the British Medical Association.

The opening shots had been fired by the pioneer electrotherapeutists, W. S. Hedley and Lewis Jones, in supporting a separate craft journal in 1900 and an entirely new medical body in 1902. The success of *The Journal of Physical Therapeutics* and the British Electrotherapeutic Society might have dispelled any doubts about the need for such innovations, but they did not necessarily persuade conservative doctors to approve. In 1903 – the first occasion on which official recognition was sought – the British Medical Association rebuffed the electrotherapeutists. Meeting in Annual Congress in July of that year in Swansea, they refused their hospitality to the British Electrotherapeutic Society.[32] However, this rebuff – an anticlimax to the Society's active campaign for recognition at that time[33] – contained elements of victory, because the Association held out an olive branch. They offered the electrotherapeutists a sub-section of medicine for therapeutic electricity, which was to be formed under the aegis of the Association. The electrotherapeutists promptly accepted, voted Lewis Jones to the Chair, and held a notably successful meeting.[34]

After Swansea, the electrotherapeutists and radiologists regularly mounted programmes at each Annual Meeting of the Association. In 1904 they were much in evidence at Oxford, lectures being given by Dr. Greg of St. Thomas's, Dr. Sequeira of the London, and Drs. Morgan and Robert Jones of the Royal Southern Hospital, Liverpool.[35] It was the Association's annual meeting in Exeter in 1907 which finally saw the inauguration of a separate Section of Electrotherapy and Radiology.[36] This event took place a few months after the Royal Society of Medicine had decided to create an Electro-Therapeutical Section. Taken together, they indicated that the fight was over, and that radiologists and electrotherapeutists at last had won their battle for professional recognition. But the victory proved to be illusory, because they were to learn that sectional parity signified no more than paper recognition; the reality was very different. Professional equality was another matter: it was a blessed state to be earned in a harder school, as the radiologists were to find through bitter experience in the First World War, see below. For individual doctors dabbling amateurishly in electricity before the War, it remained a pipe-dream.

THE BRITISH ASSOCIATION OF RADIOLOGY AND PHYSIOTHERAPY
(1917–24) AND THE CAMBRIDGE DIPLOMA (1920–42)

In 1917 a group of radiologists met in London and decided to form a new body with the single aim of protecting the status of radiologists and electrotherapeutists – or, in the words of the preamble[37] – 'to promote the advancement of radiologists and physiotherapists on scientific lines under the direct control of the medical profession'. The reasons for this extraordinary step must be explained, particularly since two organised bodies already existed to represent their interests, namely the Röntgen Society and the Electro-Therapeutical Section of the Royal Society of Medicine. In order to do so, it is necessary to review the position of the medical electrician at the outset and in the course of the First World War, before radiology had come into its own as a specialist branch of the medical profession.

'Before 1914 anyone, by purchase of an x-ray apparatus, became *ipso facto* a radiologist. In private x-ray practice, the financial reward came from fractures and other bone work, with a steadily increasing sprinkling of chest and renal cases, to which gastric studies began to be added after about 1908. The radiologist, both in hospital and in private practice, was constantly wrestling with his inefficient apparatus and most of his attention was necessarily given to it. It is to the credit of the early workers that, under such conditions, they obtained observations that were of clinical value. . . .'

'In only the larger hospitals was a medical man in charge. While there were a few exceptions, the radiologist was as a rule viewed as a doctor possessing the technical ability to produce a good x-ray for the clinician to interpret; this was often regarded as the one and only function of the medical man responsible for the x-ray service. It was only slowly that his colleagues came to recognise that the radiologist's constant experience in interpretation made his opinion on x-ray plates of real value, yet by 1914 there were still very few who had attained anything approximating to consultant relations with their colleagues.'[38] A. E. Barclay was not surprised that this should have been so, the radiologists having started at a very great disadvantage, for he believed that the legacy of the basement origins of hospital x-ray work bred an inferiority complex in the early workers. Thurstan Holland, in an outspoken Presidential Address, to the Röntgen Society in 1916, spelt out the radiologists' difficulties.[39]

Holland argued that the x-ray department was the most important single department in any hospital. Experience had shown that whenever a department had been allowed to develop fully and the radiologist had the support of his colleagues, a shutdown of the department paralysed the work of the whole hospital. He and his colleague, Dr. Oram, were fortunate to enjoy such relations, but Liverpool was still a rare exception. Elsewhere in the country's teaching hospitals, the position was often very different, he claimed, and deplorably few radiologists had been accepted as full staff members. Many were paid a small honorarium − not from feelings of generosity, he asserted, but to ensure that they remained in a junior position. He blamed this state of affairs on the conservative attitude of some staff physicians and surgeons who remained unwilling to concede full staff privileges to radiologists. Holland cited the great injustice done to A. E. Barclay who, despite his international reputation, was not elected to the staff of the Manchester Royal Infirmary until 1918, ten years after he had established its x-ray department. Many early radiologists shared Barclay's experience of being undervalued and denied equality of status by their clinical colleagues.

Outside the teaching hospitals, the problem was the reverse. Too many of the persons put in charge of x-ray departments were untrained and, according to the definition advanced by Holland, unqualified. He defined a 'qualified radiologist' as *a doctor skilled in interpretation*, and spoke dismissively both of the doctor and of the non-medical man who could make good plates but did not know how to interpret them − 'the time for that sort of thing has gone by . . . the real essential for an x-ray expert (is) interpretation. The good plate can now be obtained by anybody with modern apparatus with very little training . . . interpretation can only be done by a medical man of unusual professional attainments. . . .'

All these difficulties were brought to the surface and intensified by the First World War, which suddenly placed radiology in the limelight as an urgently needed specialty. There were no medical specialists in the regular army, and the x-ray service was in the hands of army surgeons. Military x-ray preparations had been made on a small scale only, and soon they were overwhelmed by events. Early on, a War Office X-Ray Committee was established to try to avert chaos. It consisted of several radiologists including Dr. Archibald Reid and several physicists including C. E. S. Phillips, all of whom were enlisted into the Army with the rank of major and given the task of making good the gross deficiency in x-ray apparatus and manpower. To meet the national emergency, all available x-ray equipment was brought into use, and anyone with a nodding acquaintance of electricity, photography or physics was pressed into service as a radiologist.

Professional concern at the use of unqualified radiologists was voiced as early as 1915 in the editorial of *Archives*; the article was probably written by Robert Knox.[40] 'New departments have sprung into existence, as it were with the wave of a hand, and men to work these departments are urgently required. The demand exceeds the supply, and must continue to do so unless steps are taken at once to meet the need. The employment of men who have had no medical training and no special instruction is to be deprecated.' The editorial made three recommendations: (1) the need for teaching facilities and the appointment of lecturers; (2) the creation of chairs of radiology in universities; and (3) the full recognition of the radiologist and electrotherapeutist as consultants in the Army and Navy. Many informal discussions took place as to how radiology could be put on a more satisfactory footing, and Thurstan Holland's hard-hitting Address received wide publicity in the medical and lay press. It proved to be the turning point. 'Thereafter it seemed that not only radiologists but the medical profession as a whole began to recognise that radiology was not merely a question of apparatus and the ability to produce an x-ray plate, but that there was also something in interpretation, and that this required expert knowledge.'[38]

The matter came to a head in March 1917, when a letter was read to the Council of the Electro-Therapeutical Section of the Royal Society of Medicine, which requested action. However, the Royal Society of Medicine was a forum for clinical and scientific matters only, and discussion was not allowed. Similarly, a politically sensitive issue such as the status of the radiologist could not be raised in the other body concerned with radiology, the Röntgen Society, because of its mixed medical and lay membership. Therefore a private meeting was arranged.

The meeting took place on 4 April 1917 at 26 Park Crescent, the home of Sir James MacKenzie Davidson (Davidson had received a knighthood in 1912). It was convened to discuss the following matters.

1. To consider the best means by which to deal with questions concerning the status of medical men holding positions as radiologists and electrotherapeutists; and
2. To consider the steps to be taken for the promotion of the teaching of radiologists and electrotherapeutists.

Those attending were the nominees of the Royal Society of Medicine or the Röntgen Society, but the private venue was chosen with deliberation in order to emphasise that the meeting was not convened by either body. Nonetheless, those present represented the British radiologists and electrotherapeutists of the day. They were: Sir James Mac-Kenzie Davidson and Ironside Bruce (Charing Cross Hospital), Harrison Orton (St. Mary's Hospital), Cecil Lyster and Sydney Russ (The Middlesex Hospital), E. P. Cumberbatch (St. Bartholomew's Hospital), Robert Knox (King's College Hospital), W. J. Turrell (Radcliffe Infirmary, Oxford), A. E. Barclay (Manchester Royal Infirmary), Thurstan Holland (Liverpool Royal Infirmary) and Hope Fowler (Edinburgh Royal Infirmary).

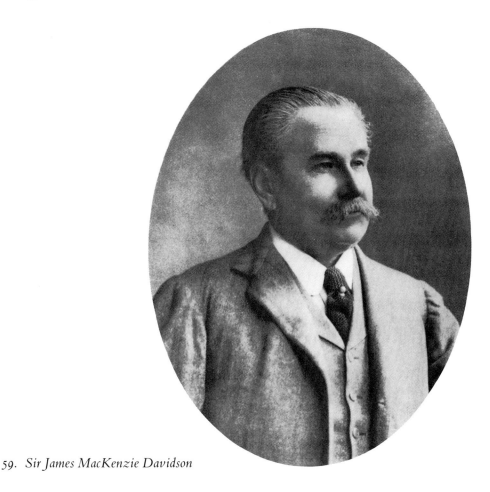

59. Sir James MacKenzie Davidson

SIR JAMES MACKENZIE DAVIDSON (see pages 41 and 98) after 1910 was the leading radiologist in the country, and his house became a centre for all x-ray activity, to which radiologists from all parts of the world journeyed. In that year he chaired a Section of Radiology at the 78th Annual Meeting of the British Medical Association, and three years later he was a President of the International Congress of Medicine in London. His knighthood in 1912 for services to medicine – the first and only pioneer radiologist to be so honoured – was viewed as much as official recognition of the x-ray profession as a personal award.[41] MacKenzie Davidson had been a founder member of the Röntgen Society, and he was one of the minority of medical members who remained a loyal supporter of the Society. He was offered the presidency after Mansell-Moullin in 1899 but declined it, believing that 'a physical man should be appointed to follow a medical President'.[5] He was a vice-president in 1902 and served as President in 1912–3. Shortly before his death he was elected an Honorary Member.

MacKenzie Davidson never lost his interest in radiology. Six months before his death he designed a table for localization work. His description of the table at a meeting of the Royal Society of Medicine was published in the April 1913 number of *Archives*, the number which announced his death; the paper was printed immediately after obituary notices.[42] Thurstan Holland in a tribute spoke of 'the circumstances which helped to render (Davidson's) position amongst British radiologists somewhat unique – there appears to be no one at the present time to fill his place'.[43] This unique status, recognised on his death, was perpetuated beyond it through the generosity of his widow and family, and his friends in several ways. Firstly, Lady MacKenzie Davidson presented her husband's medical library to the profession, as the nucleus of the reference library of the proposed Radiological Institute.[44] The MacKenzie Davidson Memorial Library remains one of the major assets of the British Institute of Radiology. Secondly, the Davidson family in 1920 endowed a lectureship with the sum of £500, the lecture to be known as the MacKenzie Davidson Memorial Lecture and to be given annually at a joint meeting of the British Institute of Radiology and the Electro-Therapeutical Section of the Royal Society of Medicine. Professor Torgny Greitz of Stockholm, in delivering the 1985 Lecture, paid tribute to Davidson's use of the principle of the Cartesian coordinates for his localisation method.

Davidson's first posthumous contribution to radiology was derived from the MacKenzie Davidson Memorial Fund, an appeal launched in 1920 to perpetuate his memory by public figures including the Prime Minister, Stanley Baldwin. The Trustees of the Fund wrote in *The Lancet*:[45] 'In this country (MacKenzie Davidson) was highly regarded as the head of his profession and throughout his career he was unsparing in his efforts to raise the status of radiology among the sciences. He was especially insistent on the fundamental value of physics to radiology particularly in regard to methods of measurement and the designing of equipment.' About £1,400 was collected and the Trustees contributed this sum towards the purchase of 32 Welbeck Street as a home for the British Institute of Radiology, see below.[44]

The meeting at MacKenzie Davidson's house reached two conclusions: '(1) that one of the universities be urged to institute a diploma course and to grant a diploma; and (2) that a new and purely medical society be instituted to deal with clinical teaching'.[46] The second conclusion was implemented immediately, in order to establish a body which could negotiate with a university. This new society was the British Association of Radiology and Physiology – or 'British Association for the Advancement of Radiology and Physiology', as it appears initially to have been named – which came into being in April 1917 with a single object, namely, 'to promote the advancement of Radiology and Physiotherapy on scientific lines under the direct control of the medical profession'. Although the Regulations restricted membership to qualified doctors and dentists, a clause was inserted which allowed the Council to elect suitable scientists to ordinary and honorary membership. This loophole was considered necessary in order to enable the Association to fulfil its immediate two aims to persuade a university to run a diploma course and to provide practical radiological instruction in London. The scientist elected to the first Council was the distinguished medical physicist of the Middlesex Hospital, Dr. (later Professor) Sidney Russ.

The first officers of the Association were chosen from the radiologists who attended the meeting at Davidson's house:

President: Sir James MacKenzie Davidson.

Vice-Presidents: Drs. Harrison Orton and W. J. Turrell.

Treasurer: Dr. Gilbert Scott.

Secretaries: Drs. Robert Knox and Elkin Cumberbatch.

Council: Drs. Barclay, Lyster, Thurstan Holland, Stanley Melville, Archibald Reid,
    Francis Hernaman-Johnson, and Sidney Russ.

Within a year 165 practising radiologists and electrotherapeutists had joined.[47]

The search for a British university to undertake a diploma course was assisted by two responses to the Association's exploratory advances – the first as negative as the second was positive. London University, despite proximity to the major reservoirs of clinical material in the country, declined to participate. The University of Cambridge, where Sir Ernest (later Lord) Rutherford was soon to succeed J. J. Thomson as Cavendish Professor of Experimental Physics, welcomed the radiologists' overtures. Two years of protracted negotiations, undertaken chiefly by Barclay and Knox for the radiologists with Dr. (later Sir) Hugh Anderson, Master of Gonville and Caius College on behalf of the University, led eventually to the regulations for the Diploma being approved by Grace of the Senate in March 1919.[38]

The regulations provided for an examination in two stages, Part I being physics and Part II radiology and electrology, thus creating a pattern which was followed by other radiological diplomas and which became an established feature of pre-Fellowship British radiology. In the early years the course lasted six months, the first three months being devoted to physics, and the remainder of the time to lectures in radiology and clinical experience in hospital x-ray departments. Later the course was extended to one academic year (nine months) and candidates for a while were required to produce a thesis; but this rule was soon abandoned. For the first years the Diploma was granted to established radiologists on presentation of a thesis, and 34 diplomas were issued on this basis including several to prominent American radiologists.

The University created two lectureships and a special committee in Cambridge to control the Diploma and supervise the course. Dr. Francis Shillington Scales of Addenbrooke's Hospital was appointed Lecturer in Radiology, and Dr. (afterwards Professor) J. A. Crowther became Lecturer in Physics as Applied to Medical Radiology. Both men served on the new University Committee for Medical Radiology which first met on 25 October 1919 and which included the Regius Professor of Physic Sir Clifford Allbutt, Sir Ernest Rutherford, and Drs. Knox, Cumberbatch and Russ.

FRANCIS SHILLINGTON SCALES, M.A., M.D.(Cantab., 1912) (1866–1927), physician-in-charge of the electrical department of Addenbrooke's Hospital, became in 1920 by virtue of his position the first radiologist to hold an honorary title in a British university.

A product of Jesus College, Cambridge and the Middlesex Hospital, Shillington Scales trained as a histologist (he was vice-president of the Royal Microscopical Society), before turning to radiology and electrology in middle age. From 1919 up to his death he served as Secretary of the Diploma Committee in Cambridge and as a member of Council of the Association and the British Institute of Radiology. He was a devoted and enthusiastic lecturer, who continued to teach students up to a few days before his death.[48]

ALFRED ERNEST BARCLAY (see page 130) was Shillington Scales's successor. When Barclay left Manchester in 1928 to be the University Lecturer in Radiology in Cambridge, he was lured by the prospect of developing a radiological department serving the biological laboratories of that great centre of scientific learning. According to one of his obituarists, his altruism in abandoning his comfortable and secure position in Manchester was never fully appreciated.[49]

Others thought that Barclay was naive for failing to obtain assurances about his future from Cambridge University. No Briton at that time was better qualified or would have filled a chair of radiology with more distinction than Barclay, and he made major personal sacrifices to enable the University to bring it about. But the initial enthusiasm for the project in Cambridge evaporated, and Barclay's vision of a great radiological institute for teaching and research remained unfulfilled. Instead, he was given a few rooms in the Department of Zoology for the Diploma teaching and sufficient only for very limited research experiments. Here he remained whilst suffering an increasing sense of frustration, until he resigned in 1937 when it was clear that the University planned to abandon the Diploma course.

Barclay was then 60, at an age when most men look forward to their retirement, and his subsequent career at Oxford was a brilliant Indian summer. He joined Dr. Franklin at the newly-established Nuffield Institute of Medical Research, and entered upon a decade of active work which was interrupted only by his national duties in the Second World War and terminated by his final illness. In many ways Oxford provided Barclay with the environment whch he had sought in Cambridge and not found. Over 30 publications were to emerge from this prolific period, many of them reflecting the impact of invasive radiological techniques upon biological research. Cinéradiology was used to study the mode of closure of the ductus arteriosus in the circulation of sheep foetuses injected with Thorotrast. This study was made possible only after Barclay had devised a horizontal couch for cinéangiography in animals using direct serial angiography. Towards the end of the War he and his colleagues began to investigate the cause of uraemia in traumatic crush injuries of limbs, and the results were published as *Studies of the Renal Circulation* in 1947. In this book, Barclay utilised microradiography to demonstrate vascular shunts of the renal circulation, a technique elaborated in his final book, *Micro-Arteriography*, which was published posthumously in 1951.

Barclay spent the War years as Adviser in Radiology to the Ministry of Health, assuming a responsibility for the organisation of the entire civilian x-ray service. He travelled the length of the country several times to visit each newly-established Emergency Medical Service hospital, helping to raise morale at the grassroots level; an exercise which brought him into contact with the entire x-ray profession.[50] The affection in which he came to be held was echoed by his colleagues in May 1951, at the Ceremony of Dedication of the Barclay Room in 32 Welbeck Street.[51] Barclay's portrait, painted by a colleague, Dr. A. A. Rackow, was hung, and his friends, 'Uncle Fungus' Fawcitt and Brigadier McGrigor spoke of the exceptional man who devoted his life to radiology.

A legacy bequeathed by Barclay enables the British Institute of Radiology each year to make two awards to authors of articles printed in the *British Journal of Radiology*. The Barclay Medal is awarded as a token of distinction to authors who have contributed notably, and the Barclay Prize is given for original work, especially in the clinical or experimental fields.

The clinical teaching of radiology for the Diploma course was organised in London by a committee of the British Association of Radiology and Physiotherapy, with Dr. Robert Knox and Dr. Stanley Melville acting as educational secretaries. The first course started on 4 February 1920 with an Inaugural Lecture given by Dr. W. J. Turrell, entitled 'The History of Electrotherapeutics'. For several years the lectures were given at 1 Wimpole Street, the house of the Royal Society of Medicine, but after 1922 they were transferred to 32 Welbeck Street. By the late 1920s the Diploma course, particularly the system of tutorial teaching of clinical radiology, was an established feature of medical life in London. Nearly all the leading radiologists gave tutorials, many of them acted as examiners for Part II, and some served on the Cambridge Committee. Dr. Cumberbatch bore the whole burden of teaching and examining in electrology up to his death in 1938.

Originally the University had intended that all the candidates should be resident in Cambridge for Part I. For many of those taking the Diploma such residence was impossible, and a parallel Part I course was arranged in London. This concession worked well educationally, but it meant that for those candidates who were never resident in Cambridge the University was acting purely as an examining body. It was this state of affairs which was inconsistent with academic policy, which finally prompted the University to abandon the Diploma and course in 1942. By that date, more than 500 candidates coming from all parts of Britain and 18 other countries had attended the course and taken the Diploma. Liverpool University at the instigation of Thurstan Holland instituted a similar course and diploma in 1921, followed by Edinburgh in 1926, and London University and the Conjoint Board in 1933. The vicissitudes of these courses are beyond the scope of this book. It suffices here to quote Barclay's epitaph on the Cambridge Diploma in 1942: 'Very shortly after the first examinations had taken place, advertisements announced that candidates for radiological posts must hold the Cambridge Diploma. At one bound the status of the radiologist as a qualified specialist had been established. Today a radiologist would have little or no chance of obtaining any radiological post if he did not hold the Diploma. *Pari passu*, the x-ray department naturally but slowly came from its cellars and took its place as a central key service. That, in a nutshell, is what has been effected by the Cambridge Diploma.'[38]

The Association, apart from its main task as the partner of Cambridge University in the Diploma course, soon began to undertake other functions for the radiological profession. After 1920 it offered facilities for teaching and examining to the Society of Radiographers who granted a Certificate of Membership (M.S.R.), see below. A special sub-committee was established to deal with political and ethical affairs affecting radiologists. In 1922 the Association sponsored a highly successful meeting of foreign radiologists in London. Initially the Association used *Archives of Radiology and Electrotherapy* as its publication, but in 1918 *Archives* became its property, as outlined in Chapter 8.[47] This move entailed a legal change because the Association was obliged to obtain incorporation as a registered company, in order to own property. Accordingly, in September 1921 the Association was converted into a limited liability company. By virtue of the fact that it was not a company working for profit, the Board of Trade granted a licence which allowed it to dispense with the word 'Limited' in its title.[21]

THE BRITISH INSTITUTE OF RADIOLOGY (1924–present)

The concept of a radiological institute was first advanced by Deane Butcher in 1907 at the time when the specialty of electrotherapeutics first achieved sectional status in the Royal Society of Medicine.[30] Butcher was a visionary, and his picture of a London headquarters for the profession was not revived until the disastrous consequences of the First World War on radiological practice had been felt. The radiologists then established the British Association of Radiology and Physiotherapy and initiated the Cambridge Diploma, as outlined above. These measures, highly effective in themselves, emphasised still further the need for a professional focal point in London – a building in which teaching, research and other activities could be undertaken under one roof.

In 1917 Dr. G. W. C. Kaye devoted a part of his Presidential Address to the Röntgen Society to restating the need for a radiological institute, and his plea was repeated by his successors in office, notably Robert Knox in 1920 and Professor J. W. Nicholson in 1921. The leaders of the Association then took up the cause. In the spring of 1923, a Committee was formed with representatives of the Electro-Therapeutical Section of the Royal Society of Medicine, the Röntgen Society and the Association under the Chairmanship, first of Knox and then of Sir Archibald Reid, with Dr. John Muir as secretary. A decision was made forthwith to found the British Institute of Radiology and to establish it in premises in central London.

The objectives of the Institute were defined as follows:

(a) to promote the advancement of radiology and physiotherapy on scientific lines under the direct control of the medical profession, protecting in every way possible the interests of those engaged in these subjects; (b) to secure legislative improvements in this connection; (c) to provide for the delivery of lectures, the holding of classes and examinations, the establishing of scholarships, and the granting of prizes, diplomas, and certificates; (d) to arrange for the publication of papers, communications, or treatises; (e) to promote and provide for research in experimental work, and to establish grants and rewards in connection therewith; (f) to establish and maintain a library and museum, and to organise exhibitions of apparatus; (g) to establish charitable and benevolent funds for the benefit of persons engaged in radiology and physiotherapy.

Sir Archibald Reid, acting with characteristic vigour, found a house two doors from his own in Welbeck Street, which had formerly been the Imperial Russian Embassy, and he secured a 50-year lease. This purchase was paid for, partly out of the MacKenzie Davidson Memorial Fund, partly out of private subscription and largely on mortgage. A bank loan of £2,000 was personally guaranteed by Reid and his friends, Barclay, Harrison Orton and Stanley Melville. 'In the last year of (Sir Archibald Reid's) life, the Institute was almost an obsession with him. It was he who found the premises, he who saw to all the details of the purchase, decoration, and preparation of the building, and so forth. In a word, he was the mainspring of the movement.'[21]

SIR ARCHIBALD DOUGLAS REID (see pages 89 and 95), the leader of men, earned his knighthood in the First World War, through his ability to mobilise radiological resources for military purposes.

The son of a Tenby doctor and his wife, Reid divided his medical career between King's College and St. Thomas's Hospitals. By the age of 40, his ability and outgoing personality had already brought him to the fore in London. Between 1911 and 1913 he served as President of the Electro-Therapeutical Section of the Royal Society of Medicine and in 1913 as Sectional Secretary of the International Congress of Medicine in London.[52]

Soon after the War broke out he was commissioned as a major and assigned to the Queen Alexandra Military Hospital, Millbank, and the Second London General Hospital, Chelsea. From 1914 to 1919 he acted as President of the War Office X-ray Committee, an important military body with responsibility for the planning, equipping and organising of x-ray services at home and on the battlefield. For these services he was twice honoured and received a knighthood in 1919. Being at the centre of military medical affairs, and concerned with the shortage of trained x-ray staff, he instituted in 1915 a course of training lectures at Millbank, assisted by Dr. Russell Reynolds and the physicist, C. E. S. Phillips.[53]

Reid's unique military experience convinced him that national training facilities for radiologists were urgently required, and he was one of those who instigated the meeting at the home of Sir James MacKenzie Davidson to establish the British Association of Radiology and Physio-

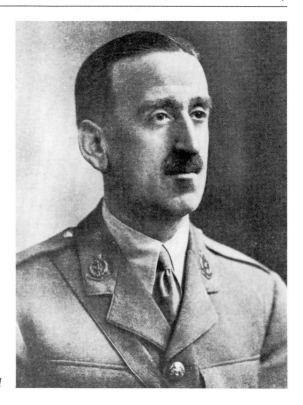

60. Sir Archibald Reid

therapy. He chaired the educational subcommittee of the Association and undertook much of the preliminary planning for the Cambridge Diploma. He himself took the D.M.R.E. by thesis in 1920.

His single-minded espousal of the cause of a radiological institute is described above. He helped to create the Society of Radiographers in 1920, and served as its first President.[54]

Reid's later years were darkened by severe radiation dermatitis which steadily worsened and contributed to his premature death at the age of 53, when in the full flood of his professional life.

ROBERT KNOX (see page 96), Reid's successor at King's and the pioneer radiotherapist at the Cancer Hospital, Fulham, was the other begetter of the Institute. It is appropriate that the meeting chamber in the Institute's House should have been called the Reid–Knox Hall to honour the two men above all others who created it. Knox was Reid's administrative *alter ego*; in the memory of one of his registrars, a Dr. Watson to Reid's Sherlock Holmes.

Born in Leith and educated at Edinburgh University and Guy's Hospital, Knox in 1894 settled in Highgate, where he built up a large practice and served on the Hornsey Borough Council. Soon after Röntgen's discovery he began experimenting with x-rays, and some years later while still in practice in North London he took rooms in Harley Street for x-ray consultations. The first of his contributions to the radiological literature appeared in 1907,[55] and two years later he took his first hospital post – honorary medical electrician at the Great North Central (now Royal Northern) Hospital. In 1911 he was appointed to the Cancer Hospital, Fulham and succeeded Archibald Reid as Medical Radiographer to King's College Hospital some time later. He then abandoned general practice to specialise in radiology, and commenced a life of total involvement in the radiological world which only ceased on his death 16 years later. Before 1920 he wrote many original papers and his textbook, *Radiography, X-Ray Therapeutics, and Radium Therapy*, which first appeared in 1915, was re-issued several times in an expanded form up to 1932. A reviewer described the book as 'the standard British treatise on radiology'.[56] In

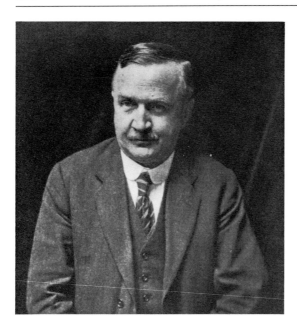

61. Robert Knox

1921 his wife, a North London family doctor, Dr. Alice Nance Knox, published a book of her own, *General Practice and X-rays. A Handbook for the General Practitioner and Student.*

After 1920 Knox served on every radiological committee (and presided over many of them), edited a journal, wrote a textbook, acted as external examiner, advised on x-ray departments and conducted a huge private practice:

> Secretary of the Röntgen Society after Harrison Low, President in 1920–1
> Editor, *Archives of Radiology and Electrotherapy* and *British Journal of Radiology,* (1915–28)
> President, Electro-Therapeutical Section of the Royal Society of Medicine, 1922–3
> President, Section of Radiology, British Medical Association Annual Meeting, Newcastle-upon-Tyne, 1921
> Examiner in Radiology, Universities of Cambridge and Liverpool
> Member, War Office X-ray Advisory Committee
> Instigator and Member, X-ray and Radium Protection Committee, 1921 onwards.

Thurstan Holland in his obituary tribute observed that it was difficult to imagine the Röntgen Society, the British Institute of Radiology, the Royal Society of Medicine or the Society of Radiographers, or the *Journal* without Robert Knox who was a moving spirit of all these bodies several of which he had helped to create.[57]

JOHN MUIR, O.B.E., M.B., Ch.B. (1874–1950), the first secretary and medical director, was the third stalwart of the Institute. He is said to have carried a chair and a cupboard into 32 Welbeck Street in 1923 – the first furniture that the Institute possessed, to replace the soapboxes and packing cases, and he withdrew from Institute work four years later after he had made it financially secure.[58]

Born in Kilmarnock and educated at Glasgow University, Muir was a family doctor in Hertfordshire until 1914 when he was commissioned into the Royal Army Medical Corps. After being injured and invalided home from France, he joined Dr. Archibald Reid at the War Office as Secretary of the X-Ray Advisory Committee. After the War he studied radiology with Dr. Robert Salmond at University College Hospital, and became the radiologist to the Hackney and Bethnal Green Hospital.

As medical director, Muir had day-to-day responsibility for the headquarters of the Institute in the days before it reached financial solvency. They were anxious years and – in the words of his obituarist[58] – while Reid and three others guaranteed the banker's overdraft, it was Muir who did the worrying! He was a born diplomat to whom much of the credit belonged for the immediate popularity and activity of 32 Welbeck Street. He organised meetings, planned timetables for the Diploma course and arranged hospital attachments for the candidates, purchased books and indexed the Library, wrestled with the finances. His tact and bluff Scots ways won friends and recruits for the Institute; it was Muir who arranged the affiliation of the Society of Radiographers and the amalgamation of the Röntgen Society with the Institute.

Muir retained his hospital appointments until ill-health obliged him to retire in 1934. In 1917 he re-wrote the second edition of David Arthur's book, *A Manual of Practical X-ray Work*, and a third edition was published under his name in 1924.[59]

The British Institute of Radiology attached its plate to the door of 32 Welbeck Street early in 1924. In April of that year the British Association of Radiology and Physiotherapy, which had so greatly enhanced the status of radiology by teaching for the Cambridge Diploma in London, altered their name and threw in their lot with the Institute – in fact, they became the Institute. Originally, therefore, the Institute was a wholly medical body funded by its members, comprising about 300 doctors. The first few years proved to be a testing time, because the Institute was not financially viable, and had to be supported with financial loans. But the officers' fear of bankruptcy through lack of support were soon dispelled because 32 Welbeck Street attracted visitors and users and the headquarters became a centre of activity. It was soon the focal point of radiologists and other persons involved with x-rays – a meeting place in London for committees, lectures, teaching and reference reading. The Röntgen Society in 1924 transferred its monthly meetings there. Within the year all x-ray activity in Britain was centred on 32 Welbeck Street.

Teaching for the Cambridge Diploma – and later the M.S.R. Certificate of the Society of Radiographers – was the most important activity in the early years. Two rooms were set aside exclusively for this purpose, and equipped with modern x-ray apparatus, and there were two dark rooms with the facilities for making prints and slides. Radiologists from the London teaching hospitals attended, and later staff radiographers were employed to instruct the students in radiographic technique, the principles of photography and other technical matters before they were sent to clinical departments.[60] Shortly after this work started in the Institute, it received a tremendous fillip from the General Medical Council, who decreed that henceforth all undergraduate medical students should be instructed in radiology and physical therapeutics. The Council's decision set the seal of approval on the efforts of the British Association of Radiology and Physiotherapy to establish the academic credentials of their members.

An unexpected development that grew spontaneously from the founding of the Institute was the first International Congress of Radiology which was held in London in 1925.[61] Soon after the doors of 32 Welbeck Street opened and the Institute began to take shape, the Council decided that the premises should be formally opened. They felt that a formal ceremony would provide appropriate publicity and stimulus for the new organisation, and that a few foreign radiologists should be invited. When canvassed, it was soon evident to the Council, from the enthusiastic response of the persons approached, that 32 Welbeck Street would be inadequate for the function. Therefore, they decided to hire the Central Hall, Westminster and advertised the event widely. No more than six months after the inception of the scheme, 500 doctors from 39 countries assembled in London for the meeting. Dr. Thurstan Holland was the President, and Robert Knox, Stanley Melville and John Muir were the organisers of the Congress. At the first session it was decided that the meeting would be the first International Congress of Radiology, and that such a congress should be held every three years. The 16th International Congress of Radiology was held in Hawaii in 1985. The fortunes of the Institute, still financially beleaguered, were immensely boosted by the success of the 1925 Congress.

The decade following the First World War seems to have seen the radiologist triumph finally in his struggle for equal status with his clinical colleagues. Thus the notion of an institution was accepted, which could offer him and his technician proper training. Financial solvency followed the amalgamation of the Röntgen Society with the Institute – a process which took two years to complete, as already mentioned in Chapter 8. This act, which involved the acceptance of non-doctors as members of the Institute, proved as controversial as it had been 30 years previously in the Röntgen Society, but the leaders of the Institute believed that amalgamation was the only option. They accepted that the risks inherent in widening the membership – described by C. E. S. Phillips as 'converting the British Institute of Medical Radiology into the British Institute of Radiology' – were the price that had to be paid for financial solvency and wider support. These latter objects were paramount, and Reid and Knox and their supporters in the Institute (which included Barclay) were determined to secure them. In 1927 the Röntgen Society finally succumbed to their invitation, and Sir Humphry Rolleston, Regius Professor of Physic in the University of Cambridge, was chosen as the first President of the amalgamated organisation, called 'The British Institute of Radiology Incorporated in the Röntgen Society'. The marriage was celebrated on 17 November of that year.[44]

This amalgamation at one stroke brought the entire British x-ray community under one roof, and it secured the future of the Institute. Membership doubled to 600 within two years, and a great influx of talented men and gifts occurred which further stimulated the Institute's activities and greatly enriched it. One of these men was Dr. G. W. C. Kaye, who succeeded Rolleston as President, and who was already an internationally respected figure in the x-ray world. Gifts included furnishings or fittings for the Institute's house, donated mostly by the x-ray suppliers – for example: oak library shelving (Messrs. Solus), library table and chairs (Messrs. Schall), lantern accessories (Messrs. Newton and Wright). Dr. Barclay presented a clock for the Reid–Knox Hall, and Sir Archibald Reid's oil portrait, painted and presented by his friend and fellow-member, C. E. S. Phillips, was hung. Dr. L. A. Rowden (1871–1953), the veteran Leeds radiologist and President in 1935–6, provided the Presidential badge of office which was made to the design of Mrs. Phillips. Dr. J. H. Gardiner presented the Museum with a collection of historical objects, including a print made by Becquerel in 1896 and a letter from Madame Curie.[62]

The amalgamation heralded the beginning of the third great activity of the Institute (its educational function and the publication of the *British Journal of Radiology* being the first two) – namely, commercial representation. Once the leaders of the x-ray industry had been included, the full weight of their financial resources became available to underwrite legitimate activities such as an annual meeting.[63] Since 1929, the Institute's Annual Congress and Exhibition has been a regular event in the calendar of the British radiologist.

THE SOCIETY OF RADIOGRAPHERS, *since 1976* THE COLLEGE OF RADIOGRAPHERS (1920–present)

A new profession arose directly from Röntgen's discovery, consisting of persons whose task it became to examine patients with x-rays. All the early experimenters were amateurs, and many of them were motivated simply by the challenge of producing x-rays and not of applying the discovery clinically. The first persons regularly to carry out the work of the modern radiographer were surgeons such as John Macintyre, Mac-Kenzie Davidson and Thomas Moore of the Miller Hospital, who pioneered the use of x-rays as an aid in the diagnosis of their patients. At first they made the radiographs themselves, but within five years 'x-ray assistants' relieved them of this chore and enabled them to concentrate on their clinical work, which included interpretation of the radio-graphic plate. In the London Hospital and other large well-regulated centres where the x-ray service was integrated into existing electrical departments, unqualified assistants, usually men, were employed to perform the radiography and apply x-ray treatments. Elsewhere such assistants were engaged by chemists and professional photographers, and others worked on their own account, as contractual x-ray takers to the medical profession and the public.

By the end of the First World War there were probably one hundred x-ray assistants employed in hospitals throughout the country. Twenty of them who staffed the major early departments are individually named in Chapters 5, 6 and 7. These 20 assistants and an additional 20 were selected in 1920 as foundation members of the Society of Radiographers without examination.[64] At least 20 radiographers worked in London, and the best known of these were Messrs. Forder (King's College Hospital), Westlake (Cancer Hospital, Fulham), Winch (St. Thomas's Hospital), Suggars and Blackall (The London Hospital), Turner (Middlesex Hospital), and Watson (West London Hospital, Hammersmith). Cyrus Winch recalled the position in 1918:[65] 'Radiographers were a scattered body through London, hardly any one of them knowing the other. We never visited each other's hospitals – we did not know how each other lived.'

Dr. Robert Knox is credited with the original idea of founding a society,[66] and his x-ray assistant, Mr. Forder in 1918 took the first step. Forder visited Winch at St. Thomas's Hospital and told him that Blackall, Westlake, Turner and he intended to meet. At that initial meeting, which was held in the summer of 1918, they agreed to form a Society and began at once to draw up Articles of Association. They were strongly influenced – perhaps pushed to proceed, by the radiologists and the electrical engineers, and the Society of Radiographers was born under the protective umbrellas of the British Association of Radiology and Physiotherapy and the Institute of Electrical Engineers. Archibald Campbell Swinton, the early x-ray experimenter, was then an influential figure in engineering circles in London, and he must be credited, together with the three radiologists, Knox, Reid and Melville, for overseeing the event. The Association and the Institute of Electrical Engineers provided the legal advice and financial support required for drawing up and printing the articles and for publicising the venture. An editorial in *Archives of Radiology and Electrotherapy* welcomed the initiative,[67] which took almost two years to bring to fruition.

On 6 August 1920 'The Society of Radiographers' was registered as a limited company by the Board of Trade, with the word 'Limited' omitted from the title. The aim of the Society was declared to be 'to give a definite professional status to those certified non-medical assistants who work in x-ray and electrotherapeutic departments'.[44] Shortly afterwards the aims were more completely defined: 'It is obviously essential that the assistants employed in the manipulation (of x-rays) shall have undergone an adequate technical training and shall receive some official recognition of the responsible position which they hold. . . . The Society of Radiographers was formed to comprise those approved persons, who are at present working (as radiographers), and to qualify new workers after due training and an exhaustive examination. . . . It appears to us that the appointment of persons who are not specially trained and qualified in radiology to important posts in the x-ray departments is fraught with danger, and we hope that hospitals will co-operate with us . . . by employing only duly qualified persons.'

The first council meeting was held on Monday, 18 October 1920, at 1 Albemarle Street, London. By prior agreement it was decided that the Council should consist of equal numbers of members representing respectively the British Association of Radiology and Physiotherapy, the Institute of Electrical Engineers, and the radiographers. The six radiologists' representatives were: Sir Archibald Reid, Robert Knox, Stanley Melville, G. Harrison Orton, Francis Hernaman-Johnson, and Professor Sidney Russ. The six engineers included Campbell Swinton. The six radiographers were: R. G. Blackall (The London Hospital), F. E. Doran (Manchester Royal Infirmary), A. O. Forder (King's College Hospital), A. Henry (Royal Army Medical Corps), H. Turner (The Middlesex Hospital) and G. F. Westlake (The Cancer Hospital, Fulham). Sir Archibald Reid was chosen as the Society's first President. George Westlake became the honorary secretary, a task which he fulfilled with fanatical loyalty for seven years, and henceforth Council meetings were held at Fulham.[64]

The Council began its work by encouraging membership. Letters were sent to assistants in all x-ray departments inviting them to seek it, and rules for admission to the Society were drawn up. Initially this invitation offered membership with and without examinations. In order to attract the old stalwarts of the profession who were in the latter category, the Council ruled that all applicants with ten years of active and continuous work experience in any x-ray or electrotherapeutic department would be admitted without examination.

All the remaining applicants were required to pass an examination. The Society's founders were determined to ensure that they and their successors should remain the arbiters of professional competence of the radiographer, and that their examination should be the sole test of theoretical knowledge. The task of preparing a syllabus for the examination, roughly to parallel the non-clinical parts of the Cambridge Diploma Course, was entrusted by the Council to Messrs. Blackall and Forder. A preliminary examination was held in February 1921 at the Royal College of Physicians in London, but the first regular batch of students were entered in January 1922; of the 45 students accepted, twenty passed the examination and received the Society's certificate (M.S.R.). One of these students was destined to write her own radiographic history: Miss K. C. (Katy) Clark, later the Society's first woman President, was the author of *Positioning in Radiography* (1939), a magisterial book which set international standards in radiographic technique. A minimal training period and age was subsequently introduced for candidates. By 1930 the M.S.R. examination was widely accepted as the radiographer's qualification, and the Society had already turned its attention to the more difficult task of dissuading institutions from appointing as radiographers persons who did not possess it – that is, persons who were not qualified.

An ethical issue faced the Society several years after its inception, which nearly destroyed it, and caused it to part company with the Institute of Electrical Engineers. The dispute concerned the legal right of the radiographer to make a diagnosis and issue a report to the doctor upon the radiograph he had taken. Although the monopoly of the medical profession over the clinical use of x-rays had grown gradually and was widely accepted by the 1920s, it relied upon commonsense for its acceptance rather than any statute. Before 1900, many early experimenters including scientists such as Campbell Swinton and C. E. S. Phillips, both later Presidents of the Röntgen Society, advertised their x-ray laboratories to the public, as mentioned in Chapter 2. Such laboratories continued to exist until the 1920s, being owned by firms of chemists.

A. J. (Jack) Walton, Hon. F.S.R., a member of the original Council and the Society's Vice-President, and one of the most respected pioneer radiographers, ran his own private practice in Taunton and accepted patients from doctors until he retired. Walton simply continued in civilian life what he had done throughout the First World War in a military hospital in France.[66] The issue came to a head in 1924 because the Articles of Association were not sufficiently specific on the issue of interpreting radiographs and issuing reports. They laid down that 'No non-medical members shall accept patients for radiographic, radioscopic, or therapeutic work except under the direction and supervision of a qualified medical practitioner, and any breach of this regulation shall be deemed conduct unfitting the member guilty thereof to remain a Member of the Society.' While it had been tacitly accepted that radiographers did not report on radiographs, this rule was not written down, and in 1924 attempts were made to modify or abolish this restriction, but they came to nothing. The General Medical Council, whose advice the Board of Trade had sought, vetoed the Society's proposals. Several stormy meetings followed, but on 23 June the modifiers accepted defeat. Mr. Blackall on behalf of the Council of the Society moved the withdrawal of the offending proposals, stating that a poll of members showed that 90 per cent of radiographers favoured this course. Members of the Institute of Electrical Engineers had supported the modifications as a matter of principle, and when Blackall's motion was carried they resigned from the society.

The loss of the engineers was mitigated by the Society's affiliation to the British Institute of Radiology. Closer co-operation was first mooted in 1923, but the Council finally took the step only in March 1928. The Society, for a rent of £100 a year, moved into its own office in the Institute's house at 32 Welbeck Street – an address which was to remain its home for the next 40 years.

The success of the Society, which became the College of Radiographers in 1976, was reflected by its rising membership. From 40 original founder members in 1920, it was to grow to 6,500 in 1970 and to nearly 10,000 in 1980. While the story of this growth to maturity can be found elsewhere,[68] it is appropriate to note that two of the four honours within the gift of the Society, the Archibald Reid Memorial Prize and the Stanley Melville Memorial Lecture, commemorate the much-loved radiologists who served as its first and second Presidents.

Chapter 10

X-RAYS ON THE BATTLEFIELD

'I maintain it is now the duty of every civilized nation to supply its wounded in war with an x-ray apparatus, not only at base hospitals, but close at hand, wherever they may be fighting and exposing themselves to injury. . . .'

Surgeon-Major W. C. Beevor (1898)[1]

'The discovery of the Roentgen rays and their use for the detection of hidden bullets has put a new weapon in the hands of the military surgeon. . . .'

F. C. Abbott (1899)[2]

'I have shown you how probing for an uncertain bullet, with its subsequent pain, is now a thing of the past in military surgery.'

Surgeon-Major J. C. Battersby (1899)[3]

Army doctors in the services of the major powers quickly grasped the importance of Röntgen's discovery in military surgery. Portable sets were soon used on the battlefield to demonstrate bullets and localise their position, and to diagnose shattered limbs. Other benefits also were found – for example, *pied forcé*, or march fracture, the hitherto mystifying swelling of the foot encountered in young soldiers after prolonged marching, was shown to be caused by fracture of the second metatarsal bone. X-rays were soon harnessed to further tasks, and by the time of the First World War, radiography of the chest was an enlistment requirement to exclude tuberculosis.

The British Army acquired its first x-ray set at the Royal Victoria Hospital, Netley in 1896, and clinical radiographs were produced in November of that year. By mid-1898 kits were being operated (or about to be installed) in the military hospitals at Aldershot, Dublin, Woolwich and Gibraltar, and portable units had been ordered for the Nile Campaign.[1]

The impetus for acquiring x-ray equipment came from Surgeon-Lieutenant-Colonel Stevenson, Professor of Military Surgery in the Royal Army Medical School at Netley. In May 1896 Stevenson persuaded the young pioneer radiographer, Sydney Rowland, to transport his x-ray apparatus to Netley to examine a man with a severe knee injury. The radiographs revealed a complicated fracture of the tibial plateau extending into the knee-joint, and Rowland described the case in the *British Medical Journal* and in the second (June 1896) number of *Archives of Clinical Skiagraphy*.[4] Early in the following year Stevenson welcomed another London visitor, when MacKenzie Davidson travelled down with his cross-thread localiser to re-examine one of the British casualties invalided home from the Tirah Campaign (see below).

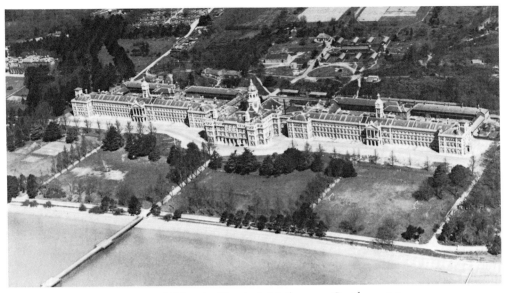

62. Royal Victoria Hospital, Netley near Southampton

SURGEON-GENERAL WILLIAM FLACK STEVENSON, C.B.(Military, 1900), B.A., M.B., M.Ch.(Dublin, 1865) (born 1844) was an Irishman who joined the British Army directly after qualifying. In 1895 he held the rank of lieutenant-colonel and the title of Professor of Clinical and Military Medicine in the Royal Army Medical School on Southampton Water. He was the author of the standard textbook of military surgery, *Wounds in War: the Mechanism of their Production and their Treatment*, of which later editions contained radiographic illustrations and a section on radiological localisation by MacKenzie Davidson.

Stevenson's enthusiasm for x-rays hastened the introduction of apparatus into the major military hospitals, and he instructed young army surgeons in its use. Throughout his career he remained interested in the apparatus required for radiography, acquiring a cross-thread localiser shortly after MacKenzie Davidson invented the device in 1896 and describing, before his retirement nearly a decade later, Cox's new platinum contact breaker in military use.[5] He was promoted Surgeon-General in 1913.

On the outbreak of the Boer War, Stevenson was appointed Principal Medical Officer of the British Forces and he spent 15 months in South Africa. He edited the official account of the War, *Report on the Surgical Cases noted in the South African War, 1899–1902*, and contributed an interesting account to the literature, illustrated by skiagrams produced in the field.[6]

The first occasion on which military casualties were examined by x-rays appears to have occurred during the Abyssinian War of 1896. This was a result of the Italian invasion of the ancient kingdom of Abyssinia, which itself was part of the European powers' scramble for colonies in Africa in the latter half of the 19th century. The Italians lost a disastrous battle at Adowa on 1 March 1896, and their casualties were evacuated home by sea to Naples. In May Lieutenant-Colonel Guiseppe Alvaro of the Military Hospital, Naples successfully took radiographs of two soldiers with fractures of the forearm bones. Alvaro, in describing the cases in an Italian medical journal,[7] gave a prophetic view of the value of radiography to the surgeon demonstrating foreign bodies in the soft tissues, internal concretions, and the form of fractures or other skeletal disease. Alvaro's examination, made only six months after Röntgen's announcement, is accepted as the first use of x-rays in military medicine.[8]

THE GRAECO-TURKISH WAR

Hostilities broke out in the Balkans in the spring of 1897, and the great European powers were divided in their support. German sympathies lay on the Turkish side, and the German Red Cross Society despatched a hospital unit to Constantinople, while British, Russian, and French help went to the Greeks. The British Red Cross Society, aided by a public appeal mounted by the London newspaper, *The Daily Chronicle*, provided two fully-staffed and equipped hospital units which were sent to Greece in the charge of a surgeon from St. Thomas's Hospital, F. C. Abbott. The equipment included a complete outfit of x-ray apparatus which was personally selected by his colleague, Dr. Barry Blacker, the medical officer in charge of the electrical department of the Hospital. The equipment was described in *The Daily Chronicle*, of 4 May 1897: 'The apparatus forwarded will consist of an absolutely complete outfit in itself, similar in every detail to the apparatus in daily use at St. Thomas's Hospital, and it will be an excellent opportunity for testing its utility in military surgery at the seat of war. It will be hard to estimate the saving of pain to the sufferers, and of time to the medical officers in the diagnosis of injured bones and the location of bullets or foreign bodies, which this new and rapid method of examination will render possible. The x-ray apparatus consists of:

(1) A large induction coil for obtaining the high-tension currents for generating the rays in the vacuum tubes.

(2) A double set of accumulators for supplying the current to magnetise the iron core of the coil, thus rendering the working of the rays possible for very many hours in succession.

(3) A sufficient number of the most efficient type of x-ray focus tubes.

(4) A fluorescent screen, capable of showing every joint and bone in the body, coated with a sensitive layer of platino-cyanide of barium on which shadows of the bones and bullets will be cast.

(5) A quantity of Eastman's x-ray paper, with developing solution capable of taking 500 skiagrams, should the operator not have the time at his command to see personally the shadows on the fluorescent screen.

The secondary winding of the coil is over 13 miles in length, and will give a heavy discharge over 10 in. of air. Strange to say, the same coils are used in another of the very latest of development of applied electricity – viz., telegraphing without wires by means of invisible rays of a much slower rate of vibration than x-rays are supposed to have.

'It is hoped that it will be possible to use the fluorescent screen to the exclusion of the photographic method, as the position of the bullet or the seat of the injury may be viewed in many positions rapidly, and the time required to develop a dry plate (although much shortened by the use of Eastman's new x-ray paper) constitutes a serious delay to a busy surgeon.

'All the apparatus is made and supplied by Messrs. Miller and Woods, manufacturing electricians of 2 Gray's Inn Road, Holborn, who have supplied most of the London hospitals with electrical apparatus.'

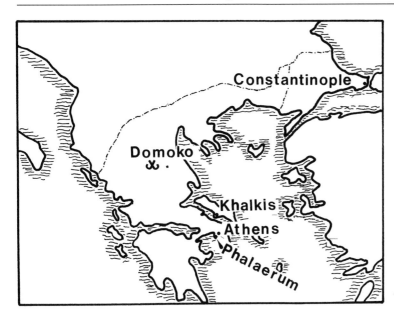

63. The Graeco-Turkish War, 1897

The Graeco-Turkish War afforded the first opportunity for evaluating the usefulness of radiography close to the firing line. The British team established two hospitals. One was placed at Khalcis, about 100 miles north of Athens, to receive Greek casualties from the battle of Domoko on 17 May. The other hospital was established on the outskirts of Athens, near the Piraeus at Phalaerum, in a villa loaned by the Queen of Greece. A surgeon, Mr. H. Moffat, had charge of the patients at Phalaerum, and a young doctor, Robert Fox Symons, manipulated the x-ray apparatus.

FRANCIS CHARLES ABBOTT, C.B.E., M.S. (London, 1896), F.R.C.S. (England) (1867–1938) was the son of a vicar and a brilliant undergraduate at St. Thomas's Hospital, a gold-medallist several times over. Early in 1896 while the resident assistant surgeon of the Hospital, he contributed a case of a curious bone lesion ('hypertrophic osteosclerosis of the fibula') to the first issue of *Archives of Clinical Skiagraphy*. In the following year he was chosen by the British Red Cross Society to go to Greece. On his return from the campaign, he recorded his surgical experiences on the battlefield, crediting his colleague, Fox Symons, see below.[2]

Abbott spent his entire professional life as a surgeon of St. Thomas's Hospital, earning a C.B.E. for his work during the First World War.[9]

SIR ROBERT FOX SYMONS, K.B.E., M.R.C.S., L.R.C.P., D.P.H. (died 1932), also a product of St. Thomas's Hospital, was a house surgeon when Abbott persuaded him to accompany his team to Greece. Fox Symons was the radiographer of the team, and probably drafted the section on x-rays which appeared in the account published under Abbott's name in *The Lancet*.[2]

When the Boer War broke out, he went to South Africa and remained on afterwards in the Transvaal for more than ten years. He occupied several important posts in Alfred Milner's administration: medical officer of health of Pretoria and the Transvaal, inspector general of Provincial Hospitals, and Member of the Transvaal Legislative Council, and he served as a medical adviser to the South African Government and the British High Commissioner. Before the First World War broke out, he returned to England and a practice in Kensington. He was knighted in 1918 for his services to the Red Cross during the War.[10]

A room in the base hospital at Phalaerum was set aside for the x-ray equipment, which Fox Symons installed and had working by 1 June 1897. Casualties began arriving soon afterwards, and the x-ray work continued for about six weeks. Despite the difficulties which were formidable and numerous, the results were successful. Abbott and Fox Symons were able to illustrate their report with several radiographs in order, they claimed, 'to record the first skiagrams taken in war time, as well as to show that even inexperienced hands working can get fair results'.[2] All the original prints were exhibited at the first *conversazione* of the Röntgen Society in London on 15 November 1897. Abbott and his colleagues treated a total of 114 patients with war wounds, and Fox Symons probably photographed about half of them.

Abbott's article is interesting – and important to read, because his account of the use of x-rays under field conditions was the first to become available to the British Army, and it influenced the provision of apparatus in subsequent campaigns. Fox Symons's list of technical difficulties included the following: the heavy weight of the coil and accumulators, the fragility of the Crookes tubes and glass plates, the danger of transporting casks of sulphuric acid for the accumulators, and the delicacy and temperamental nature of the apparatus; all factors which aggravated the problems of transportation. An amusing additional source of difficulty in Greece was the superstition of the local people, who viewed the x-ray apparatus and its use as the work of the devil. It was difficult, Fox Symons complained, to take a skiagram when the subject was constantly crossing himself to ward off the evil spirits!

The most serious obstacle to field radiography – the one which Abbott and Fox Symons were unable to overcome satisfactorily – was the lack of a reliable source of electrical power. It prevented them from siting the x-ray apparatus where it would have been most useful, namely at Khalcis in the hospital nearest to the front line. Even Phalaerum on the Piraeus was beyond the reach of a mains supply, and they were obliged to depend on a peripatetic source – a warship of the Royal Navy, H.M.S. *Rodney*, to recharge their wet batteries.

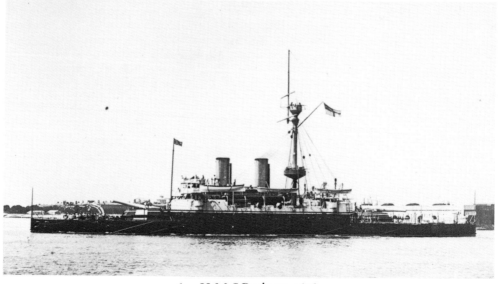

64. H.M.S Rodney, *1898*

The casualties examined with the x-rays were cases of fracture or suspected retained bullets, which in several patients had penetrated the body cavities. The radiographic findings, apart from aiding in the immediate surgical treatment of the patient, helped to write a new chapter in military medicine. During the 1890s the major European powers were equipping their armies with magazine rifles such as the Martini-Henry and the Mauser, which fired a high-velocity bullet possessing great penetrative power; the bullet made a small entrance wound and frequently passed through the body. The gaping entrance wounds formerly seen, which were enlarged and infected by pieces of clothing being driven into the tissues, soon passed into history.

Coinciding with the introduction of the new rifle into the armies of the Queen's enemies, a new breed of doctor replaced the traditional regimental surgeon in the British Army. They were properly qualified young men trained in Listerian concepts of antisepsis and attracted to a professional career in the newly-established Royal Army Medical Corps. For them and for the War Office, Abbott's experience in Greece of the new type of war wound pointed the way forward. It could not have been more timely or apposite, in view of the imminence of the Boer War, which proved to be a far greater test of the medical service. Abbott's advice when read at the War Office had the ring of authority: 'The Roentgen rays should always, if possible, be available at that hospital nearest the front in which the wounds can be first properly examined and dealt with. . . . The apparatus is of no use on the field where the detection of bullets can only be an incentive to premature exploration. The less wounds are tampered with before satisfactory surroundings are reached, the better. The modern bullet . . . . is practically aseptic and there is no urgency for removal. . . .'[2]

On the Turkish side, the team of the German Red Cross Society established its x-ray unit in the Yildiz Hospital, Constantinople. The apparatus, manufactured by Hirschmann of Berlin, consisted of a coil with a 40-cm spark gap, a Crookes tube and rechargeable accumulators. When the batteries failed to work satisfactorily, they were discarded and power was drawn from the hospital's own generating plant. The leader of the team employed an assistant, Dr. H. Küttner to use the apparatus. Küttner on his return to Germany published an account of his experiences in a leading surgical journal,[11] and his views were reported by a Berlin correspondent in the *British Medical Journal*.[12] Küttner believed that radiographs were indispensable in military surgery, and he recommended their introduction in all German reserve field hospitals.

THE TIRAH CAMPAIGN

In September 1897 the *British Medical Journal* reported: 'An x-ray apparatus was recently sent to Malakand. This is possibly the first time the apparatus has been used on field service with British troops.'[13] Readers of the *Journal* required no lesson in geography to understand. Tirah and Malakand were districts on the Indian border with Afghanistan, the legendary North-West Frontier, a region which the newspapers kept constantly before the eyes of the British public. For generations an uneasy peace had been maintained by a combination of force and diplomacy with the local tribesmen, the Afridis and Orakzanis. These war-like Mohammedans inhabited the strategic pathways into

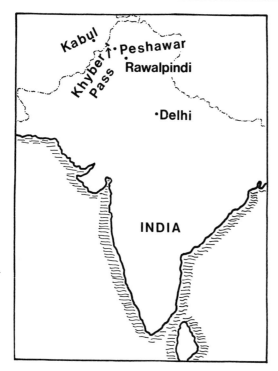

65. The Tirah Campaign, 1897

Afghanistan such as the Khyber Pass, and they were licensed by the British Army to protect travellers and guarantee the free passage of military transports.

Periodically the peace collapsed. In June 1897 there was a large-scale insurrection and fighting broke out all along the 500-mile part of the Frontier from Malakand to Tirah. The British authorities reacted swiftly, mobilising an army of 100,000 men into four field forces to punish the tribesmen and re-open the passes. One of these was the Tirah Expeditionary Force, an army consisting of 8,000 British and 30,000 Indian troops commanded by General Sir William Lockhart, who moved against the Afridis. Enormous logistic difficulties faced Lockhart's army, because the tribesmen inhabited roadless valleys and plateaux behind almost impassable mountains, which no European had ever penetrated before. The trek through the mountains took several months, but by October 1897 the army was encamped on the Tirah plateau. Within the next four months the tribesmen had been subdued and the peace restored.[14]

Twenty-three field hospitals were established on the Tirah plateau, and over 900 casualties were treated. The transfer of the wounded to the base hospitals at Rawalpindi over 100 miles away was a slow and complicated task. The first 40 miles was a journey by stretcher through hostile country down two mountain passes, then by bullock-drawn ambulance to the railhead, and the final leg by train to Rawalpindi. As a consequence of this slow transportation and the distances involved, surgeons treated wounds earlier and carried out more amputations than usual near the front line.

A novel feature of the medical arrangements in the field hospitals on the Tirah plateau was the use of x-rays. This occasion was their first use on the field of battle.[15] A regimental surgeon with the Coldstream Guards, W. C. Beevor, examined more than 200 cases on the Tirah plateau, and later he took additional x-rays in the hospital at Rawalpindi.

His experience established the value of the new diagnostic method and won over the Army medical establishment. Beevor's lecture at the United Services Institution on his return to London in May 1898 signalled the introduction of field x-ray units into the British Army.[1]

WALTER CALVERLEY BEEVOR, C.B. (Military, 1916), C.M.G., M.B., Ch.B. (Edinburgh) (1858–1927) was a well-to-do career army surgeon, the son of a Member of Parliament. At his own expense he purchased an x-ray apparatus, shipped it to India and used it during the Tirah hostilities – the first British military man to do so. Beevor's London lecture was probably the high-point of his career: the picture of the young batallion surgeon recounting his experiences on the edge of the Empire to the high and mighty at its vortex was not to be repeated. The Director-General of the Army Medical Department, Surgeon Major-General Jameson, took the chair, and the distinguished audience included another surgeon major-general and Dr. MacKenzie Davidson.

Beevor does not appear to have taken any further part in the development of radiology, and pursued his career as an army surgeon in the Boer War. He retired before the First World War, and was twice decorated for his services.[16]

Before he left for India in the middle of 1897, Beevor personally selected his x-ray equipment. A. E. Dean of Hatton Garden sold him the prototype model of his 'Portable or Field Service Type' of apparatus, which was subsequently supplied to the British Army (*see* 66). This equipment was made up of several sturdily-built wooden boxes housing respectively the induction coil, battery and fluorescent screen. Beevor had high praise for their design and robust manufacture; the ingenious tube-stand folded up and fitted into a special compartment. The fluorescent screen was coated with celamite to prevent scratching and it was housed for safety in an aluminium box. Dean also supplied Vulcanite cases for the three vacuum tubes, which were made by A. C. Cossor of Farringdon Street; miraculously all three survived the campaign intact.

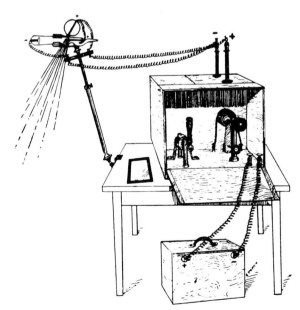

66. *A. E. Dean's portable military x-ray kit, 1898*

Parts of the apparatus proved less effective, and drew Beevor's criticism. The battery, a heavy and cumbersome object containing potassium bichromate and hydrochloric acid, gave endless trouble, and he condemned it as a source of power for use in future expeditions. The emulsion of the Eastman x-ray papers tended to melt in hot weather, and the Paget glass plates, of which he took three dozen, were more satisfactory.

Transporting the x-ray apparatus, including a supply of hydrochloric acid for the battery, posed a novel challenge in army logistics. After experiments with ox-carts, mule transport, and pack-bearers, Beevor chose to employ two *dhoolies* (Indian bearers) to carry each box of equipment suspended from a pole. All parts of his precious equipment were carried safely from the Bagh camp on the Tirah plateau down defiles into the Bara Valley below – a route of breath-taking beauty but containing precipitous paths, icy mountain rivers and hostile tribesmen – and thence to Peshawar and Rawalpindi.

Beevor's exploit fired the curiosity of the nation. He had taken his x-rays in the midst of a battle in some far-off place, and two of his patients were public figures – General Wodehouse and General Sir Ian Hamilton. The popular press as well as the medical journals gave the details. General Wodehouse's stoicism while having a bullet-wound in the leg probed under intense Afridi fire had already been reported in the newspapers.

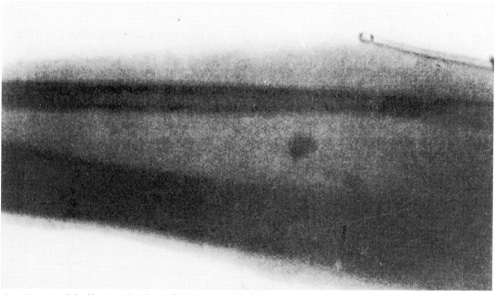

67. Retained bullet in the leg of General Wodehouse. The fragment lies in the calf muscles framed by the leg bones, the fibula above and the tibia below ; a safety-pin is visible in a bandage

The wound failed to heal, and Beevor photographed the leg some weeks later in Rawalpindi (*see* 67). His radiograph dramatically revealed the cause of the suppuration – a retained bullet fragment! Later the radiograph illustrated an article in *Strand Magazine* entitled 'The Röntgen Rays in Warfare'.[17] General Hamilton shattered the bones of a leg in a fall from his horse, and the *British Medical Journal* reported the details. The radiograph made after manipulation showed that the fractures had been perfectly reduced, 'and there will be no need now for his proceeding home'.[18]

Back in London, Beevor rose to the occasion presented him by his superiors' invitation to recount his experiences. After showing lantern slides of 15 patients to illustrate the value of radiography in managing battlefield casualties, he devoted the rest of his lecture to describing the problems of managing an x-ray unit at the Front Line. He described three particular aspects – the best type of apparatus, the safest means of transport, and the operational difficulties. His advice was simple. The ideal apparatus should be 'get-atable' – that is, constructed so that all components are accessible to the operator who must understand how they work. Secondly, the units must be mounted in robustly constructed boxes weighing no more than 80–100 lb and easily transportable. Mr. Dean's mobile kit had failed in only one respect, Beevor thought, namely that the bichromate battery was too heavy and the hydrochloric acid too dangerous to transport. At the conclusion, Surgeon Major-General Jameson rose to thank Beevor and compliment him on his lecture. He used the opportunity to review the Army's experience of the new diagnostic method, and by implication accepted radiology as a legitimate skill of the army surgeon, which his Department henceforth actively encouraged.

THE RIVER WAR

In 1898 a British-led army was dispatched from Cairo to liberate the Sudan from an Islamic fundamentalist group, the Mahdists, whom they fought and defeated at Omdurman on 1 September. The battle was the climax of a campaign which took two years to mount, and which itself finally established British control over the valley of the Nile. The details belong to the story of the European powers' scramble for African colonies a century ago, only the broad outlines are mentioned here.

For most of the 19th century the delta and upper reaches of the Nile, the modern states of Egypt and Sudan, remained a part of the Ottoman empire, ruled by the Sultan in Constantinople. However, Western influences in Cairo were strong and they increased after 1860: the Khedive freely employed Europeans in his service, including Englishmen as advisers and provincial governors. In 1882, when the old order collapsed, a British expeditionary force landed and fought a battle at Tel-el-Kebir, and seized control of Egypt. Coincidentally with this victory and unrelated to it, an Islamic revolt swept through the tribesmen of the upper provinces, and civil war reigned in the Sudan. In an attempt to restore a semblance of law, the British government appointed to Khartoum as Governor General – or rather, re-appointed, since he had previously held the post for the Khedive – a man of whom the world already knew and soon was to hear more, General 'Chinese' Gordon. He was an eccentric, Bible-reading general of the sort produced in the British Army in almost every generation. During his previous service in the Sudan he had familiarised himself with the one million square miles of the country from the back of a camel; and he had gained a reputation for energetic and incorruptible administration. The appointment would have been a good one if Gordon had obeyed his orders. The story of his defence of Khartoum and his fight to the finish; of how he refused to withdraw and thereby engineered his own martyrdom, forms part of the

Imperial catechism. The relief army, having fought its way painfully up-river, arrived beneath the ramparts of the city in January 1885 a few days after Gordon was killed, and the Mahdist soldiers chased it back to Egypt.

For ten years the Mahdist tyranny was left to run its cruel course, decimating the Sudanese and ravaging the land, because the treasury in Cairo was empty. Then, as the finances of the Egyptian government began to improve, political wills in Cairo and London coincided to send a punitive armada up the Nile to repossess the Sudan, perhaps to avenge Gordon's death. It was this mighty force, commanded by another eccentric military bachelor, General Herbert (later Lord) Kitchener, that began assembling in Cairo in 1896.

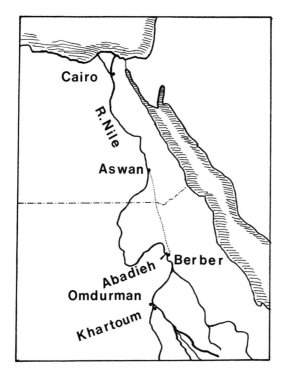

68. *The River War, 1898*

The plans for the expedition were laid slowly and thoroughly. Kitchener's force consisted of 20,000 men, mostly Egyptian soldiers, but it was an army led by British officers and equipped with modern weapons – 100 guns, Royal Naval gunboats, as well as thousands of camels and horses. Thomas Cook's local fleet of pleasure boats was requisitioned as water transports to ascend the Nile as far as the first cataract at Aswan. Beyond that point the force and its baggage left the River which winds its way in a great bend through the other cataracts, and struck out over the desert for the river settlement at Berber. Close to Berber, 1,250 miles upstream from Cairo, Kitchener in April 1898 encountered an advance force of the enemy and routed it; and here he established his forward base camp for the final assault on the Mahdists. The end came dramatically less than six months later within sight of Khartoum. Across the river at Omdurman – and in broad daylight, 50,000 Mahdist tribesmen hurled themselves at Kitchener's modern army. Armed with only spears and obsolete guns, they were no match, and in five hours it was all over. Walls of corpses covered the desert, the carnage was so great. Kitchener's casualties were slight. Winston Churchill, then a subaltern participating in the battle, observed that Omdurman was the last occasion in history in which a barbaric horde was to meet a modern army in battle.[19]

Among the many thousands of items of apparatus eventually despatched to the expedition, an x-ray set was sent out as an afterthought. The Army Medical Department, fortified by the experience by Surgeon-Major Beevor in India, ordered a similar portable field apparatus from A. E. Dean. But the decision came only after angry words had been uttered in the House of Commons. Kitchener's preliminary battle at Berber had already been fought, when a Member asked the Secretary of State for War a question about the supply of x-ray apparatus. The Financial Secretary of the War Office, St. John Brodrick, gave the Government's reply that the senior medical officer had reported no cases that would have benefited if the apparatus had been available, despite the claims of other doctors who disagreed with him. The Parliamentary exchange followed this curious reply precipitated the decision – imminent for months and finally reached soon after Beevor's lecture on 20 May – to provide x-ray equipment for the Sudan campaign.[20]

Charge of the apparatus was given to an army surgeon whose commitment to radiology was as transient as that of Beevor. He was Surgeon-Major Battersby, an Irishman who was introduced to x-rays by the Dublin pioneer, W. S. Haughton. Between July and October 1898, he examined about 60 casualties with x-rays at Abadieh near Berber on the upper Nile.

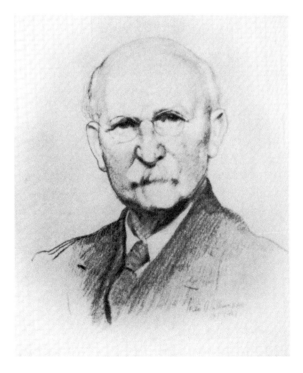

69. William Steele Haughton (1869–1951), the Dublin pioneer radiologist who trained several British Army experts to use x-rays

JOHN C. BATTERSBY, M.B., Ch.B. (Trinity College, Dublin, 1879) (died 1919) was one of the many Irish medical graduates who found their careers in the British Army. He joined upon qualifying and was present at the Battle of Tel-el-Kebir, being decorated by the Khedive.

Thus his knowledge of the terrain and climate of the Nile valley made him a suitable choice for the Sudan campaign.

   After his radiographic work at Abadieh and Omdurman and his lecture to the Röntgen Society in January 1899,[3] Battersby made no further contribution to radiology. Like Beevor, he disappeared into respectable professional anonymity, and retired before the First World War to his Irish estate.[21]

Battersby's x-ray equipment comprised the following items:

   One 10-inch coil specially wound and insulated by A. E. Dean. It was fitted in a sturdy oak box with condenser, commutator, interrupter, voltmeter, ammeter, fluorescent screen and two focus tubes.

   One 10-inch coil wound by Apps and housed in a teak case. A matching case held a condenser, commutator, and other items required to use it.

   One 6-inch coil (A. E. Dean).

   Four 10-inch focus tubes, each carefully packed in a wooden box (A. E. Dean), with each of the platinum wire terminals protected by a ferrule of thick rubber.

   One fluorescent screen, which was protected by a layer of celluloid, and a cross-thread localiser, which Dr. MacKenzie Davidson taught Battersby to use before he left London.

   A supply of glass plates with wooden holders, which were wrapped in dust-proof black bags.

   A bicycle fitted with a dynamo.

   Eight separate E.P.S. storage batteries.

   A copy of Dr. David Walsh's textbook, *The Röntgen Ray in Medical Work*.

Battersby recognised his main adversary to be the climate of the Sudan, and he laid careful plans to protect his equipment and to make it work in the heat. In the months of July, August and September the temperature hovers between 100 and 120 degrees in the shade, and the Nile waters are tepid; dust storms occur daily. He discovered before he left Cairo that the guttapercha (inspissated gum solution) used by Dean and Apps to insulate the wiring of the x-ray apparatus failed to withstand temperatures above 95 degrees and showed cracks in several places. By good fortune he came across an Italian electrical engineer installing telephones in the city, who obligingly provided a supply of heat-resistant cable. As a precaution Battersby had thick felt covers made for the outer boxes of the coils and batteries. By keeping the felt constantly wet with two-hourly applications of water on the overland journey between the River and Abadieh, when the equipment was exposed to fierce heat for several days, the temperature inside the coils was kept below 85 degrees and they reached Abadieh without mishap.

   Battersby's mud-hutted x-ray room on the bank of the Nile is a landmark in the history of radiology and of military medicine. Beevor's x-ray equipment had been his personal property, but the apparatus at Abadieh was issued by the War Office as regular medical supplies for the River War. Battersby's use of x-rays is a memorable event, not only for being the first occasion in the field by the Army Medical Department, but because he recorded the event with a camera. His four photographs are reproduced below (*see* 70–73). 'The Nile at Abadieh' is a panoramic shot, showing the x-ray hut close to the river bank, with a local native boat, a *gyassa* laden with commissariat stores. The other three photographs, taken up against the walls of the hut, illustrate the x-ray

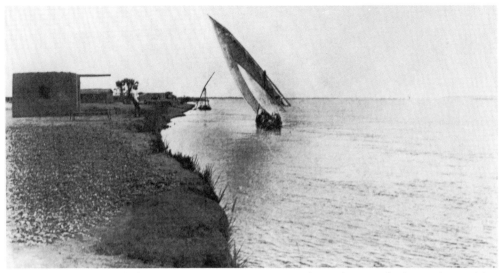

70. *The Nile at Abadieh, 1898. Surgeon-Major Battersby's photograph shows the mud hut on the river bank in which the x-ray work of the River War was carried out. See also 71–73*

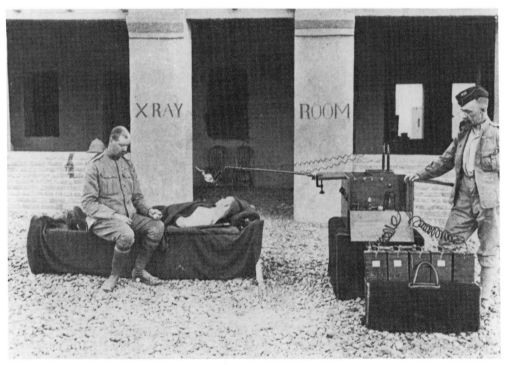

71. *Surgeon-Major Battersby and his orderly x-ray a patient's shoulder at Abadieh, using A. E. Dean's portable military x-ray kit. The orderly was probably Forbes Bruce, see 75*

unit in action. They were captioned: 'A method by which electricity was generated for charging storage batteries', 'Major Battersby and his orderly taking a radiograph', and 'Localising apparatus'.

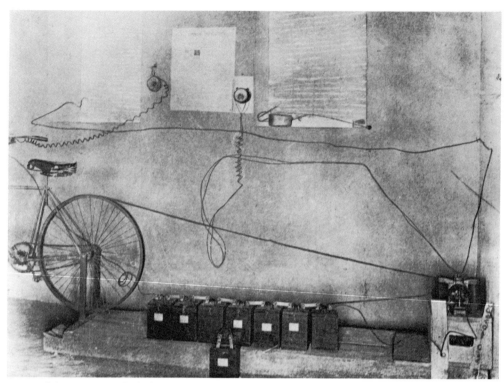

72. Pedal power at Abadieh. Surgeon-Major Battersby's solution to the problem of generating electricity: a bicycle mounted on a railway sleeper and pedalled by volunteers, was used to charge the batteries

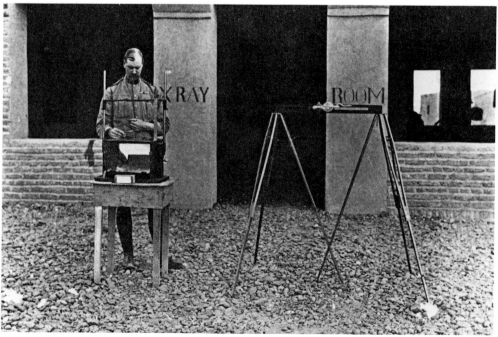

73. Surgeon-Major Battersby using the MacKenzie Davidson cross-thread localiser at Abadieh

The use of a soldier to generate electricity by pedalling a cycle attempted to solve a major problem of field radiology. It was an idea which won Battersby much praise – not least from Abbott and Beevor, whose own efforts to produce battlefield x-rays had been hampered by the lack of a reliable source of primary electricity. It was found that two cyclists were required, pedalling as hard as they could to overcome the resistance, and in a shade temperature of 110 degrees this activity had to be limited to 30 minutes each. Battersby found that the men were always willing to help with the x-ray apparatus, and there was no shortage of volunteers. The charge delivered to the batteries provided power to activate the induction coil and also to illuminate the desert with electric light. This was fortunate, since the heat dissolved their supply of 'specially-treated' candles. It should be mentioned that Battersby's own quartermaster, Forbes Bruce (see page 212), was less enthusiastic about the bicycle, the human generator which the soldiers dubbed the treadmill, and he took only the dynamo with him to South Africa, leaving the bicycle behind.

The other obstacles to radiography, the fierce sandstorms and the hot sun, were more difficult to combat, yet Battersby and his men improvised magnificently. They found that the sandstorms drove the dust into everything, and all sensitive equipment had to be wrapped up. The glass plates were particularly vulnerable since their wooden holders were not impervious, therefore each was kept in a cloth bag. The induction coils were securely protected, and Battersby sacrificed a flannel shirt to shield the dynamo from damage. The intense sunlight was another problem: it penetrated everywhere – under the fluoroscopic hood, into the development room, despite efforts at 'blacking out'. Consequently Battersby used the fluoroscopic screen only at night, and all the developing work was performed at 3.00 am, the darkest hour. This hour was also the coolest, the temperature in the mud-hutted dark room falling to 90–110 degrees, when photographic development could be achieved at a slightly slower rate.

After the battle of Omdurman, 121 British wounded were transferred to Abadieh for surgical treatment. Among these, there were 21 cases in which conventional surgical probing failed to find the bullet or to prove its absence. In 20 out of these 21, an accurate diagnosis was arrived at by means of x-rays; the last case was a man with a bullet in the chest who was too ill to examine. A senior surgeon reported:[3] 'The x-ray apparatus has been found of inestimable value in the treatment of the wounded. It has been applied to every case of gunshot wound in which the bullet was presumed to be lodged. . . . In many cases the x-rays prevented much suffering to the patient which would have been caused by probing, the use of the finger, or enlarging the wound in the ordinary search for the bullet, as the skiagraph at once indicated its exact position. . . . In more complicated cases, the MacKenzie method localised the exact position of the bullet, so that the surgeon was at once able to come to the conclusion if operative interference was judicious or otherwise.'

Battersby's entertaining description of his experiences, illustrated by lantern slides of the Abadieh department and several of his radiographs, was presented to the Röntgen Society on 10 January 1899. Less than seven months had passed since Surgeon-Major Beevor had made his passionate plea for x-rays on the battlefield, and the position had already altered. Battersby could report that most of the large British military hospitals at home and abroad now possessed the apparatus, and that the Director General encouraged his army surgeons to acquire the skills to operate it.

THE BOER WAR

One month after Kitchener's victory on the Nile, a war broke out at the other end of the Continent. The storm clouds had been gathering in South Africa for some time, and a showdown between the British government and the republican Boers had become inevitable. The nub of the dispute was the question, who was to own the mineral wealth of the country?

Gold was discovered in the Transvaal in 1884 but a decade passed before the world became aware of the full extent of the Witwatersrand deposits. A California-like rush resulted, and immigrants poured into South Africa. Soon lines were drawn between the original Boer farmers and the fortune-seekers, whom they called *uitlanders*. President Kruger and his countrymen, fearing to be swamped numerically, denied them the franchise. The *uitlanders'* leaders cleverly exploited this grievance against the Republican government, and they were abetted by Imperialists such as Cecil Rhodes and Alfred (later Lord) Milner, the High Commissioner, who were determined to bring the gold-mines under British control. When in 1899 efforts at conciliation broke down, the British Army prepared for war.

These preparations turned out to be hopelessly inadequate for what was eventually required; the limited campaign which the British public were told would be 'all over by Christmas (1899)' soon escalated into a full-scale war. In the opening months the British forces received a truer picture of their adversary when, in the short space of one week, Boer commandoes inflicted crushing defeats on three British armies and laid siege to Ladysmith, Kimberley, and Mafeking. 'Black Week' jolted the British public into realising that their troops were not fighting savages armed with spears. The Boer War was the first occasion since the Crimean campaign that British soldiers faced a white enemy with weapons as modern as their own, and who possessed the moral advantage of defending their country against invaders. It lasted two-and-a-half years and the victory had a pyrrhic ring. The peace, which delivered a devastated South Africa into the hands of the Boers' descendants, made even larger demands on the British taxpayer for reconstruction than the £200 million which the war had cost. Of nearly 500,000

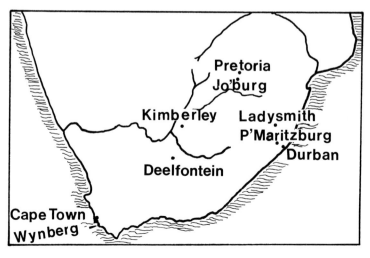

74. *The Boer War, 1899–1902*

British troops in South Africa, fewer than 6,000 were killed in battle and more than 16,000 died of disease. The Boers lost about 5,000 killed.

The medical arrangements grew as the war was prolonged. General military hospitals were established, each consisting of 500 beds and equipped for major surgery, to which soldiers were transferred from the field hospitals, usually within a day or two of being injured.[22] In army parlance, the general hospital was 'stationary' or 'fixed' – be it housed in barracks or tents – and the field hospital was 'movable', and the two hospitals served different purposes. The field hospital was the emergency dressing station, while the general hospital was the base hospital to which the injured soldier was evacuated for surgical treatment of his internal injuries.

For the first time in the British Army x-ray apparatus was provided for general hospitals as part of the essential equipment of the campaign. The principle was accepted that each general hospital, but not field hospitals would be equipped with portable x-ray equipment adequate to allow retained bullets to be localised and fractures to be diagnosed and corrected.

Each x-ray kit contained the following items:[23]

(a) 10-inch induction coil (Apps–Newton) with condenser, spring-hammer interrupter, rods and electrical cables – all packed in a teak case.
(b) Two 6-cell lithanode accumulators.
(c) Six focus tubes (Cox's 'Record') with tubestand – each packed in a box.
(d) MacKenzie Davidson cross-thread localiser with stand – in teak box.
(e) Nine dozen photographic glass plates (Edwards's cathodal XXX plates), photographic paper and chemicals.
(f) (Later on: $2\frac{1}{2}$ horsepower motorcycle engine and dynamo.)

The final item was supplied after the manufacturers were instructed to amplify the kits by providing a means of generating power for the batteries. The combination of a motorcycle engine and dynamo was successfully tested by the War Office before being accepted. A method was devised of fixing the engine and dynamo to an army bed frame, weighing under 200 lb and being easily detachable for carriage.

By the end of October 1899 four x-ray kits were being used in South Africa – two in Cape Town and two on the Natal front, and the War Office announced that six more kits were on the way.[23] Three weeks later Surgeon-General Jameson, Director General of the Army Medical Service, confirmed that a further three had been sent out, having been donated by private individuals. An expert able to repair the apparatus was also despatched.[24]

A key part of the plan to provide x-rays was Jameson's policy of allotting a surgeon to each general hospital who had been trained to take radiographs. He claimed to have officers on his staff who possessed sufficient experience of the new photography, and initially each allotted officer was ordered to devote all his time to x-ray work. In the *Official Account*, the following army surgeons were credited for their radiograpy: Brevet Lieutenant-Colonel M. W. Russell; Surgeon-Majors W. B. Day, H. E. Hale, D.S.O., and H. C. Thurston, C.M.G.; Surgeon-Captains G. E. F. Stammers, H. C. Hime, J. J. W. Prescott, D.S.O., A. F. Carlyon, J. T. Lenahan, and A. E. Weld. But there were other surgeon radiographers such as Colonel Charles Kilkelly and Dr. A. D. Bensusan and the civilians James Miller and John Hall-Edwards, who provided the best contemporary account of the use of x-rays in the Boer War, see below.

No. 1 General Hospital opened in the old military barracks at Wynberg, a suburb of Cape Town, on 18 October 1899, and it remained the medical headquarters of the British Army throughout the War. The first 95 casualties arrived by ship from the Natal front in mid-November, and a further 200 sick and wounded followed early in December. The army surgeon allotted to No. 1 General Hospital was Robert Fox Symons, the surgeon radiographer of the Graeco-Turkish war; his x-ray room was equipped and in use by the beginning of December.[24,25]

Of the other 13 general hospitals, five were near Cape Town, two were in Natal and six 'up-country', on the dry plateau called the Karoo or beyond the Orange River:

No. 2 – Wynberg Camp (moved to Pretoria in July 1900)
No. 3 – Rondebosch, Cape Peninsula (opened January 1900)
No. 4 – Natal
No. 5 – Woodstock, Cape Peninsula
No. 6 – Naauwpoort Junction (450 miles inland)
Nos. 7–10 – Bloemfontein
No. 11 – Kimberley
No. 12 – Rondebosch
No. 13 – Wynberg
No. 14 – Elandsfontein.[26]

The army surgeon radiographers did not last long. Pressure of circumstances in the first months of the War forced a change of policy. Because of the unexpectedly large number of sick and wounded admitted to the general hospitals, they were soon seconded to emergency duties, and other arrangements had to be made for radiography. Special 'skiagraphic experts', radiographic assistants, were hurriedly despatched from England – these included Henry Catlin, L. Sells, G. Paxton, and T. B. Eachus – and Quartermaster Forbes Bruce was transferred to Natal from the Citadel Hospital in Cairo. Henry Catlin, Dr. Barry Blacker's assistant at St. Thomas's Hospital, received high praise for his radiographic work in South Africa from the eminent surgeon, G. H. Makins.[27] Catlin contributed a perceptive account to *Archives of the Roentgen Ray* of his experience of examining nearly 400 patients with x-rays in the general hospitals at Cape Town and Bloemfontein.[28] His x-ray had no motorcycle engine or dynamo and, in places without a mains supply of electricity, the problem of recharging the batteries remained unsolved. Like Battersby in Cairo, Catlin had to improvise in Bloemfontein. Eventually he found a small oil engine in the railway yards, which when rigged up on trestles fulfilled the purpose. Of the MacKenzie Davidson localiser Catlin concluded that it was useful for bullets lodged in thicker parts of the body; 'but for such parts as the limbs and extremities, a lateral and an anteroposterior view were found more useful to the surgeon'.

Quartermaster Bruce reached Ladysmith, Natal on 16 October 1899.

LIEUTENANT AND QUARTERMASTER (later MAJOR) FORBES BRUCE (1859–1930) was the non-commissioned officer most involved in the introduction of radiography as a skill in the Army Medical Service.

He joined the Army as a private in 1879 and served for 30 years as a medical orderly and honorary officer. His interest in x-rays was aroused by Surgeon-Major Battersby in the Sudan, and in September 1899 he found himself attached to a base hospital in Cairo, when ordered to Natal. He wrote a lively account of the x-ray work in Ladysmith during the siege, which was read to members of the Röntgen Society in February 1901 (he was unable to attend the meeting).[29]

From the time that he returned from South Africa until he retired, Bruce was a practising radiographer. In the course of 1906 and 1907 he wrote a series of articles for the *Journal of the Royal Army Medical Corps* in which he described the different aspects of the radiographic process, e.g. electrical supply, coil and tubes, processing and chemicals, and localising apparatus.[30] These articles were expanded into an official handbook in 1907, *Hints Regarding the Management and Use of X-ray Apparatus*, which earned Bruce a military commendation for valuable services. At that time he was stationed in Dublin and collaborated in x-ray work with W. S. Haughton of Trinity College.[31] After retiring with the rank of captain in 1910, he was listed as 'former specialist in skiagraphy, R.A.M.C.'.[32]

Bruce arrived at Ladysmith with one of the Abadieh x-ray kits in his baggage. He brought all parts including the E.P.S. batteries and the dynamo – but not the bicycle. Unlike Surgeon-Major Battersby, he reserved his opinion over the success of pedal cycle x-ray power, and was determined to find another method of generating electricity. This he discovered on his journey between Durban and Pietermaritzburg: he noticed that the train was lighted by electricity and found out at the railway station that rechargeable wet batteries were used for the lamps. A word in the right ear at headquarters produced two batteries, and Bruce was able to reach Ladysmith with a complete working apparatus. Everything shipped from Cairo survived the voyage intact.

Bruce's x-ray kit was not the only one, or the first on the Natal front. The Military General Hospital in Pietermaritzburg was equipped with x-ray apparatus but no army expert could be found to make it work, and a local chemist, A. Allerston operated it. Another kit was available nearer the front line, and was hurriedly brought into use by Dr. Arthur Bensusan during the disaster at Colenso, some weeks after the Boers had cut off Ladysmith. A third kit was already in Ladysmith when Bruce arrived, in the charge of Lieutenant Alfred Weld, R.A.M.C., but the lithanode batteries had failed and the apparatus was useless. Bruce now worked under the charge of Surgeon-Major Westcott, the principal medical officer of the hospital.[33]

The municipal offices of the besieged town were converted into a hospital, the town hall serving as a ward and two small adjoining rooms being equipped for x-ray work. In one of these the council table, seven feet in length and sturdily built, doubled ideally as an examination couch for radiography and screening, and in the other Bruce established a dark room. Next door to the town hall he found a flour mill, and the manager allowed him to drive the dynamo from the millshaft by means of a pulley – and thus to solve the problem of recharging the accumulators. This arangement proved so successful that he was able to provide the surgeon with an electric light for the operating room at night.

The Boers started shelling on 'Black Monday' (30 October 1899), the day on which they cut off Ladysmith, and for a week shells dropped continuously near the town hall. Bruce wrote: 'Great caution had to be used in photographing the patients when shells were heard in the immediate vicinity, as they were sure to start, thinking the building would be hit. Exposures under these conditions had to be short. . . .'[29] Eventually he posted a lookout whenever he examined a patient to report on the firing of the guns, and there were fewer radiographic failures.

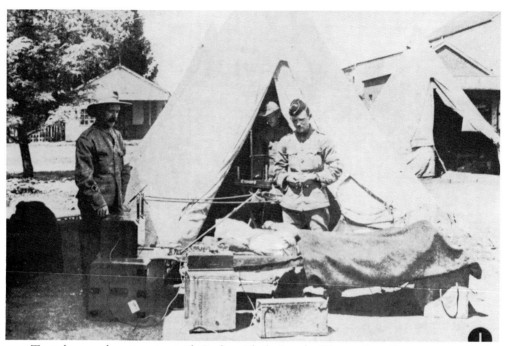

75. *Tented x-ray department outside Ladysmith during the Siege, 1899. Quartermaster Forbes*
Bruce assisted by a Colonial scout x-rays the wrist of a soldier

The fierce bombardment drove the hospital from the town centre, and it was evacuated to the open *veld* at Intombi Spruit. For several rain-drenched days Bruce protected
his precious apparatus under a railway truck tarpaulin, until a tent could be found
(*see* 75).[34]

As the scale of the War escalated and medical facilities expanded to receive the unexpectedly large number of casualties, the British public was obliged to take a hand in
providing more. Cruise ships and coastal packets were converted into hospital ships,
and civilian field hospitals, funded by public subscription, were rushed to South Africa.
Several of these were equipped with x-rays. The British Red Cross Society dispatched
a hospital ship, the *Princess of Wales* in December 1899 which was fitted with x-ray
apparatus donated by the Duke of Newcastle.[35] The Duke's gift included a second x-ray
kit – both supplied by Harry W. Cox Limited – for another ship, *Spartan*, and both
kits were despatched in the charge of Mr. John le Couteur, an enthusiastic London photographer with an interest in x-rays who had been present at Surgeon-Major Beevor's
lecture in May 1898.[36] Seven other vessels were converted for hospital service, including
Nubia, a 6,000-ton former Peninsula and Orient Liner which had space for 500 casualties.
Nubia plied between Natal and England, and Dr. Bensusan after Colenso had charge
of the x-ray apparatus. According to the *British Medical Journal*,[37] he manipulated it
with singular success.

The civilian field hospitals were the response of the British public to what they
believed to be inadequate medical arrangements in South Africa. Ever since the Crimean
disaster, the reproachful shadow of Florence Nightingale had hovered over the Army
Medical Department; periodically she accused them of incompetence and continually
she sought out deficiencies to put right. Aided by her prompting, the public came to

suspect that a poorer standard of care was given to its soldiers, and they responded generously to appeals aimed at betterment. The field hospitals were equipped with the latest kit, including x-ray apparatus. Only three of these hospitals will be described here:

1. *The Portland Hospital*, gifted by the Duke of Portland and 250 other subscribers, was the first civilian hospital to reach the Cape. It bivouacked at Rondebosch, near Cape Town and thereafter for three months the great tented hospital stood on the outskirts of Bloemfontein. A bell-tent was reserved for the x-ray work carried out by Surgeon-Major (later Colonel) Kilkelly of the Grenadier Guards. It received high praise from the surgeons who wrote: 'We may safely say that the usefulness of the Hospital would have been impaired considerably if it had gone out without the x-ray equipment.'[38]

2. *The Edinburgh and East of Scotland South African Hospital* was a small Scottish unit which landed at the Cape in April 1900 and was established at Norvals Pont, 500 miles up-country a month later; the first radiographs were made on 25 April. The x-ray apparatus was chosen on the advice of Dr. Milne Murray of Edinburgh Royal Infirmary, and operated by Dr. James Miller. Over 75 casualties were treated and 57 were examined by x-ray photographs or screening, the exposure times varying from 30 seconds (toes and fingers) to 30 minutes (trunk and hips). In all instances the radiographs eliminated the use of the 'telephone' probes to find retained bullets – a traumatic procedure if the wound had first to be re-opened.[39]

3. *Imperial Yeomanry Hospitals*. Deelfontein, the vast tented town outside De Aar on the Karoo 36 hours by train from Cape Town, was said to be the largest military hospital in South Africa, measuring a half-mile by a quarter-mile in area.[40] It was inhabited by 30 doctors, 60 nursing sisters, 300 assistants and 1,100 patients. The hospital had piped drinking water and sewage, a steam laundry, a telephone exchange and electric lights. The x-ray department was lavish – a large dark room supplied with running water and electricity and linked by telephone to the operating theatre, a large examination room with two assistants; all presided over by Dr. John Hall-Edwards.

DR. JOHN HALL-EDWARDS the Birmingham pioneer (see pages 39 and 114) became the publicist for military x-rays in Britain when the Boer War broke out. He wrote letters to *The Times* and the medical journals, pressed for more x-ray kits to be sent to South Africa, and plagued the War Office for employment.[41] His message was that military surgery was being rewritten in the light of Röntgen's discovery and the Army Medical Department had not yet awakened to the fact.

Rebuffed by the War Department, Hall-Edwards secured an appointment on the staff of the Imperial Yeomanry Hospitals and arrived at the Cape in March 1900. He spent 14 months in South Africa and wrote vivid and informative accounts of his experience and work at Deelfontein.[42] He also contributed an article to a photograph journal containing nine snapshot views of the camp.[43]

Hall-Edwards arrived at Deelfontein loaded with x-ray equipment – two complete kits donated by the ladies of Yorkshire and a businessman of Leamington Spa. It comprised:

2 induction coils (Dean 14-inch and Cox 12-inch)
15 Cox vacuum tubes

3 accumulators (two E.P.S., 1 eight-cell bichromate battery)
2 dynamos
A bicycle frame
Localising equipment (MacKenzie Davidson's couch and cross-thread localiser, Hall-Edwards's own device)
A portable developing tank
Chemicals, photographic plates and dark room supplies to last 12 months.

The one item that had been omitted, a reliable source of generating power, was to cause much vexation. The pedal bicycle, although a perfect arrangement in theory, was a practical failure because of the great effort required to operate it – as Quartermaster Bruce had found on the Nile. Moreover, Hall-Edwards's efforts to get the accumulators recharged in the electrical workshops at Cape Town or Kimberley proved fruitless. Each time that they were sent, they arrived back in a state of discharge. He thereupon secured a second-hand oil engine in Cape Town, a Clayton and Shuttleworth, and installed it in an engine house built on the edge of the camp behind a *koppie*. Two convalescent soldiers were found, formerly fitters in civilian life, who were familiar with the engine. They overhauled and installed it, and laid electrical cables to light the camp and supply the x-ray department.[40] Hall-Edwards was able to work his coil direct from the dynamo, and to dispense altogether with the accumulators.[39,42]

During the 14 months at Deelfontein, 280 patients were referred for x-ray examination, many on several occasions. Foreign body localisations invariably required three views, but the mathematical accuracy of the x-ray method dramatically influenced the success of surgical treatment. The senior surgeon, A. D. Fripp, C.B., told Hall-Edwards that the x-ray department was the most useful one in the hospital.

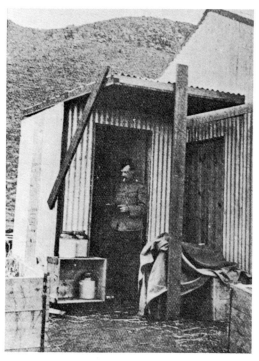

76. The temporary dark room at Deelfontein, 1900, with Dr. Hall-Edwards standing in the doorway

Fripp's view reflected the universal experience of surgeons in the Boer War, which finally established the x-ray as an essential part of the equipment of the military surgeon. Sir William MacCormac, one of the three eminent surgeons sent to South Africa during the War – Mr. (later Sir) Frederic Treves and Mr. W. D. Makins were the other two – wrote in *The Times* in May 1900: 'The Röntgen rays were used as a matter of course and nearly all the hospitals are now equipped with the apparatus for this method of diagnosis. It was always used previous to making exploration for a bullet. . . . An additional apparatus which not only determines the place of the bullet but also shows its depth from the surface, was proving of great value. The Boers also had the x-ray apparatus, I saw it working at the German Hospital at Jacobsdal.'[44]

ARMY X-RAY SCHOOL

In 1903 the Army established a school of radiography at the Royal Army Medical School at Netley, Southampton which is believed to have been the first of its kind in the world.[45] The School was housed in the impressive edifice facing Southampton Water, the Royal Victoria Hospital, which had been completed in 1863 after the Crimean War. The impetus came from Surgeon-Colonel Stevenson who had first included x-ray instruction in the army surgeons's curriculum at the end of 1896 after Sydney Rowland visited Netley and demonstrated the new method. Ironically, Stevenson was the officer obliged to defend the Army Medical Service against critics such as Hall-Edwards who claimed that the x-ray services in South Africa were inadequate.[46]

A civilian formerly a non-commissioned officer in the Royal Army Medical Corps, Mr. H. Henry, was the first tutor. He was answerable to the professor of military surgery and a member of the Surgical Department of the Hospital, and was given the title of Subordinate Employé. Whilst so employed, he wrote an article on film processing for army radiographers, and in 1922 he was one of the founders of the Society of Radiographers.[47] Henry was given a syllabus to teach, which was incorporated in the standing orders of the Royal Army Medical Corps. Successive professors of surgery adhered to Stevenson's policy of lecturing to officers on the rudiments of radiology and radiography. The professors did not lecture to the non-commissioned officers and men but examined them on completion of each course. The first examinations were held in the latter half of 1903 in order, according to the report in the *Archives of the Roentgen Ray*,[48] 'to test the efficiency of army surgeons in x-ray procedure. . . . Quartermasters were allowed to compete side-by-side with the surgeons.'

When the Royal Army Medical College left Southampton, the x-ray school followed – first to Savoy Hill, London, and then to the Queen Alexandra Military Hospital, Millbank. In 1910 A. J. Walton succeeded Henry and for the first time his post was designated Army X-ray Instructor. Walton remained at Millbank until he left the Army in 1922, except for service in France during the First World War. In the 1960s he reminisced:[49] 'I had had 5 years of practical experience (learning as you go) in Malta and took over (from Mr. Henry) after a course of instruction. I taught many nationalities: American, French and Portuguese. Up to the beginning of the 1914–18 war all pupils were required to be trained nurses (3 year course) . . .'

'In the post-war school we taught anatomy and physiology, ordinary photography, x-ray physics, radiographic positioning and particularly techniques for localisation of foreign bodies, radiotherapy, particularly for ringworm (of which there were many cases), the petrol engine, dynamos and motors, meters, rotary converters. At the request of Sir Archibald Reid details of this syllabus were in due course given to the Society of Radiographers. . . . . In fact, the first two or three Society's examinations were blueprints of the army examinations. . . .'

'Many hospitals used to write or telephone (to ask) if we had a trained man seeking employment. We had men leaving the service appointed from Aberdeen to Redruth, to large London hospitals, to places abroad, and some for the trade. . . .'

Walton himself went into civilian private practice in Taunton (as described in Chapter 9), and he was one of the founder members of the Society of Radiographers, serving as its vice-president.[50]

Sergeant Gibson succeeded Walton as Army X-ray Instructor, followed by W. Cairns and J. Levey, and all three men went on to complete careers of equal length in civilian radiography before retiring. Two post-war students later were distinguished civilian radiographers. Joseph Kenny, F.S.R. (1902–55) left the Army in 1925 and was successively superintendent radiographer of the Middlesex and King's College Hospital. Thomas Longmore, F.S.R., F.R.P.S. (1902–57) joined Kodak Limited in 1929 and became chief of the Company's medical sales laboratory and training school. His book, *Medical Radiography and Photography* was reprinted many times and sold in many countries. He edited the journal, *Radiography*, and served as President of the Society of Radiographers.[51]

The advent of the Army radiologist and specialist training came with the Cambridge diploma in radiology, which prompted the Army to invite radiologists to lecture in promotion courses after 1920. However, the Cambridge diploma and the College courses were not the first opportunity for Army oficers to study x-rays. In 1909 the Indian Medical Service established an X-ray Institute at Debra Dun which offered a specialist qualification in electrical science after a short course of lectures. The director of the Institute was an Army officer, Captain A. E. Walter, the author of an early textbook, *X-rays in General Practice* (1906). One of his most promising pupils was a 24-year-old Aberdonian surgeon, destined to return home to be the first specialist in radiology in the British Army – D. B. McGrigor.

BRIGADIER DALZIEL BUCHANAN MCGRIGOR, O.B.E., M.B., Ch.B. (Aberdeen, 1907), Hon. F.S.R. (1885–1958) was the Army's first specialist radiologist who, long beyond his retirement for a span of 25 years, continued to serve as an adviser.[45]

His first career covered the twelve years that he spent in India and with the Indian Expeditionary Force in France during the First World War; for which he received an O.B.E. McGrigor returned to England after the War to study radiology. Upon obtaining the Cambridge diploma, he was in 1921 appointed Specialist in Radiology to the Queen Alexandra Military Hospital, Millbank and Lecturer in Radiology in the Royal Army Medical College. He held these posts until he retired in 1927. During his work here he devised a method of localising foreign bodies of the eye which enjoyed popularity.[52] After retirement he remained active in London and was immediately appointed Secretary of the newly-established Army X-ray Advisory Committee, a body presided over by the consulting surgeon to the Army. On the outbreak of the Second World War this body was dissolved and the War Office decided to create a full-time adviser (later called Consultant) in radiology; Brigadier McGrigor was selected and served until 1945.

He forged close medical military ties with the United States Armed Forces, and was decorated with the American Order of Merit in 1946.

McGrigor's lifelong interests were the Army and radiology:

President, British Institute of Radiology, 1939–42
Honorary Fellow, Society of Radiographers, 1942
Joint winner of Röntgen Prize, 1946
Honorary Fellow, American College of Radiologists, 1952.

Chapter 11

RADIATION INJURY AND PROTECTION

TO THE RÖNTGENOLOGISTS AND RADIOLOGISTS OF ALL NATIONS
Doctors, Physicists, Chemists, Technical Workers, Laboratory Workers and
Hospital Sisters who gave their lives in the struggle against the diseases of mankind.
They were heroic leaders in the development of the successful and safe use of
X rays and radium in medicine. Immortal is the glory of the work of the dead.

Inscription on Martyrs' Memorial, Hamburg[1]

I am not a martyr to science, but a victim – a martyr knows what to expect.

Ernest Wilson (died 1911) of The London Hospital[2]

The most active and earnest of our workers were the worst victims.

J. H. Gardiner (1916)[3]

Within three months of Röntgen's *Preliminary Communication*, reports of the harmful effects of x-rays began to appear in the literature. None of the early experimenters with x-ray photography had taken measures to protect themselves or their patients from exposure, because there was no reason to expect adverse effects. The extent of radiation-induced injury to human tissues was not obvious immediately. Instead, the full picture was synthesized painfully from the anecdotal experiences of early workers in several countries over the course of five or more years.

The first biological effect of x-rays to be noticed by pioneer radiographers was irritation of the mucus membranes and the skin. Thomas Edison, the American inventor in March 1896 complained that his eyes were sore and red after prolonged experiments. On 18 April, Dr. L. G. Stevens reported the first British casualty in the *British Medical Journal*:[4] he described how he was consulted about a dermatitis by a gentleman who had been experimenting with x-ray fluoroscopy, and found a painful erythema of the upper and lower eyelids, alae nasi and prepuce; the man's hands and wrists showed signs of irritation and his lips were swollen. Before the year 1896 was out, radiation burns to the hands had been confirmed in many workers, and even more alarming ill-effects were becoming apparent.

Dr. David Walsh, of the Western Skin Hospital in London several months later encountered two patients with systemic reactions after exposure, which he described in the *Journal* as 'pointing to deep action of the focus tube rays'.[5] The first was a 49-year-old man who had been exposed to x-rays for several months and who had experienced several attacks of dermatitis. He developed a high fever, languor and sluggish pupils resembling the picture of sunstroke, as well as diarrhoea and vomiting. Walsh interpreted these signs as cerebral and gastric irritation. His second patient, a laboratory worker whose experiments involved two hours of x-ray exposure of the abdomen each day, complained of gastric symptoms – pain, tenderness, colic and diarrhoea. After a fortnight in the country the patient recovered, but when he resumed his experiments the symptoms recurred a few weeks later. After he had shielded his body from the x-ray tube by means of a sheet of lead, the symptoms finally disappeared. Walsh concluded that the x-rays produced a direct inflammatory reaction of the gastro-intestinal mucous membrane.

Other workers reported similar experiences. The London schoolboy Russell Reynolds found that the skin of his hands became red after using his x-ray tube for long periods. In an attempt to protect himself, he coated the cardboard box in which he kept it with lead paint.[6] At St. Thomas's Hospital in April 1897 a patient's head was exposed for 45 minutes in order to obtain a radiograph of the skull, and ten days later epilation of the temporal scalp occurred; the hair re-grew after three months. Subsequently another skull examination caused temporal epilation which led to blistering and a two-inch square ulcer which persisted for a month.[7]

During the next four years while the experiments which caused these effects continued, x-rays came to be applied deliberately to produce such effects – in other words, as a form of treatment. The rationale of this treatment was the biological action of the x-rays on human skin, which enabled Leopold Freund of Vienna to depilate a pigmented hairy naevus successfully in November 1896. Freund's case is viewed as the first authenticated successful application of radiotherapy, and his treatment heralded the birth of a new branch of medicine.[8] The apparent contradictions of exposing the skin to x-rays was immediately apparent, namely: (a) warts can be both destroyed and produced by the x-ray; (b) an ulcer can be healed and produced (x-ray burn); and (c) in the case of carcinoma, rodent ulcers may disappear under irradiation while epitheliomata may develop as a complication of prolonged exposure. Answers to these paradoxical reactions were eventually to be found in the accurate measurement of radiation dose, which is the scientific basis of radiotherapy. For two decades x-ray treatment was confined to lesions of the skin, until high-kilovoltage apparatus enabled deep therapy to be offered in the 1920s. Most of the pioneer radiologists made a living by treating scalp ringworm by epilation.

Röntgen himself was concerned only with the photographic action of his rays. When their biological effects became apparent, it was an Englishman, R. I. Bowles, who was the first to suggest that they were caused by x-radiation, rather than by any of the other possibilities suggested at that time.[9] The Röntgen Society in April 1898 nominated a committee to collect information about 'the alleged injurious effect of Roentgen rays'. A sheet of 13 medical and electrical questions was circulated with a view to determine if the injury was caused by the x-rays themselves or by the electrical field surrounding the tube, or by some other factor. Ernest Payne, the Brighton physicist, was the secretary, and Thomas Moore, F.R.C.S. and Dr. Barry Blacker were members.[10] Six months later Payne reported that the committee had received details of six cases of x-ray injury and they had been promised details of five more – sufficient material to discuss but not enough to report, he stated.[11] In December Payne and David Walsh presented their findings on x-ray dermatitis at the monthly meeting of the Society, but no report ever appeared. Controlled experiments performed by Kienböck with irradiated rats in 1900 and by Rollins in Boston shortly afterwards finally convinced scientists of the direct relationship between x-rays and the biological effects that followed prolonged exposure. Rollins warned: 'It is essential to prevent the escape of any ray not needed to make the radiograph or illuminate the screen'.[12,13]

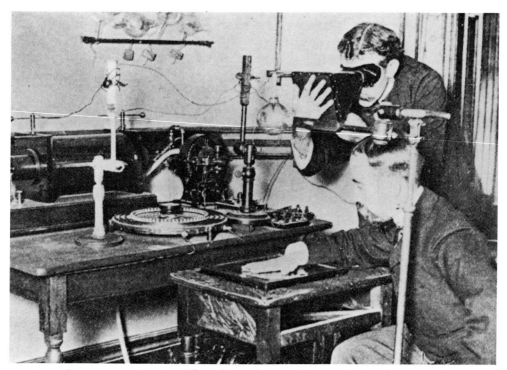

77. *An early x-ray examination. The radiographer uses his own hand, viewed in a fluoroscope, as a penetrometer in order to gauge the exposure required to x-ray the patient's hand*

By 1905 x-ray workers had begun to take precautions by protecting themselves. *The Journal of the Röntgen Society* in an early editorial note identified the operator, not his patient, as the person exposed to the greater risk.[14] The first measure was to abandon the operator's habit of using his own hand to judge the state of the tube prior to taking a radiograph. This precaution, as well as other measures, was willingly accepted because, although there was a latent period between the exposure and the development of dermatitis and irreversible lesions of the deeper tissues, illnesses and deaths due to x-irradiation were already being widely reported. Aprons, jackets, gloves and ray-proof goggles were recommended for all x-ray work. 'It is too late', wrote Deane Butcher,[15] 'to begin to adopt precautions when the hands begin to show signs of burning. The mischief is done, and is probably irreparable.'

Soon the principle of absorptive shielding began to emerge and various methods were devised for protecting the operator (and the patient) from the tube. But these developments were slow, and for many years the protection of many workers was rudimentary or non-existent, and injuries and deaths continued to result. The publicity given to several well known victims helped to hasten the introduction of official measures.

Dr. John Hall-Edwards who lost his remaining hand by amputation in 1908, described his disease in *Archives of the Roentgen Ray*:[16] 'The dermatitis commenced nine years back, and followed the usual course until three years ago, when I first noticed some loss of power in the middle, ring and little fingers of the left hand. This gradually increased until they became totally useless and immovable. The arm was carried in a sling. Amputation was ultimately rendered necessary by the extreme pain caused by a large epitheliomatous ulcer on the back of the hand . . .

'The condition of the bones was only ascertained after the decision to amputate. Beneath the ulcer they appeared to be normal but the terminal phalanges of each finger appeared to be breaking down. Small pieces of degenerated bone had separated from the shafts, and were lying in the surrounding soft-tissues. The second phalanx of the middle finger had a clear-cut hole which might have been cut out with a sharp-edged tool . . . The right hand, taken after amputation, showed only absorption of the spongy tissue of the terminal phalanges.' Hall-Edwards's paper, which had the aim of drawing attention to skeletal changes induced by x-rays, is a landmark in the English-language radiological literature. The author's plight, probably more than any other event in Britain, prompted the movement towards adequate protection.[17]

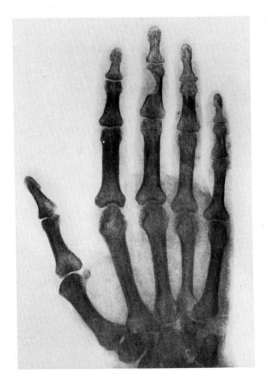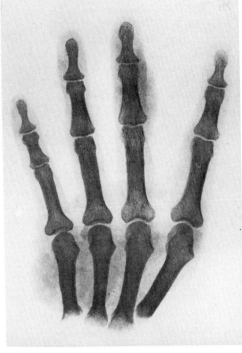

78. *Radiographs of the amputated left hand and wrist and right four fingers of Dr. John Hall-Edwards, which he published in 1908 to illustrate the effect on bone of prolonged x-ray exposure*

Within a year of Hall-Edwards's amputation, the injuries of two other x-ray pioneers were brought forcefully to public attention – Harry W. Cox and Ernest Wilson. Cox, the early manufacturer of x-ray apparatus in London, had his right arm amputated and was obliged to give up work in 1908 whilst still in his thirties. A public appeal for Cox and his family was launched in the *Daily Telegraph* by the Lord Mayor of London, Sir William Treloar, and a doctor wrote in the *British Medical Journal* of 22 January 1908 after visiting Cox, 'I have never witnessed a more pitiable case in any human being during my 33 years' professional career.'[18]

HAROLD WILLIAM COX (about 1870–1937) was a young electrical engineer in London when the discovery of x-rays was announced, and he immediately began to manufacture induction coils and vacuum tubes. Soon he supplied complete x-ray sets. For a decade his firm, Harry W. Cox Limited, maintained a leading position among the pioneer apparatus makers, largely as a result of his inventive ability. Early numbers of the *Archives of the Roentgen Ray* carried advertisements and descriptions of the apparatus which he manufactured or marketed, thus: an 18-inch induction coil; 'improved apparatus suggested by Dr. John Macintyre'; MacKenzie Davidson's motor-driven paddle mercury break; and mobile x-ray apparatus for military use.[19]

Cox soon paid the price for his early zeal. After 1901 he habitually wore a glove on his right hand to conceal an x-ray burn. The true nature of this lesion is said to have been at first unrecognised but soon his associates drew the correct conclusions. Dr. Reginald Morton of the London Hospital, when commenting on Dr. Hall-Edwards's injuries in 1908 recalled that 'after I saw the hands of Mr. Harry Cox in 1901, I kept out of the rays'.[20] Within three years pain appeared which remorselessly worsened, until his right arm was amputated and he was invalided from work in 1909. He survived for another 28 years in a state of semi-invalidism, undergoing countless operations. Cox is one of the British radiation victims whose names were added to the original 14 names on the Martyrs' Memorial in Hamburg.[21]

ERNEST E. WILSON (1871–1911) was the first of the four pioneer radiographers of the London Hospital to die of his radiation injuries, the others being Blackall (died 1920), Harnack (died 1942), and Suggars (died 1943).

Wilson was a young professional photographer in 1898 when he became Harnack's assistant at the London Hospital. In those days all patients were examined by fluoroscopy, and this procedure was carried out without protection to the operator who held the fluorescent screen for many hours a day and exposed his hands to the central beam of the rays. Wilson's case was as well documented and illustrated as Hall-Edwards's: shortly after his death his two colleagues at the London Hospital, Doctors Gilbert Scott and Reginald Morton, described the inexorable progression of his disease to their colleagues at meetings in London.[2,21,22]

Wilson within a few months of starting work at the London Hospital in 1898 developed a dermatitis of both hands. Two years later there were whitlows at the bases of his fingernails and the wounds, despite scraping and fomenting, never healed. Even at that early stage, it was noticed that the middle finger of his right hand was most severely affected, and in June 1904 the terminal phalanx was removed, followed by the middle phalanx 18 months later and the remaining stump in June 1906. The stump suppurated and failed to heal. Four years later it became painful and swollen, and enlarged axillary glands appeared; biopsy revealed cancerous changes. Wilson died in May 1911. *Archives of the Roentgen Ray* printed a remarkable series of 23 radiographs made by Wilson himself of his right middle finger, covering the six-year period from before the June 1904 amputation to the final operation in 1910. They present a complete picture of radiation osteonecrosis, complicated by osteomyelitis and malignant transformation.[2]

The response to these incidents and other evidence of radiation injury further prompted the use of protective coverings for the operator. The German and French radiologists were especially exercised by the discovery of Professor Heinrich Albers-Schönberg that the biological action of x-rays on the reproductive organs of animals may induce sterility. Soon, according to Deane Butcher,[15] the German Roentgen expert was 'encased from *Schnurrbart* to foot in a veritable suit of armour'. In Britain, protection against the rays took the form of enclosing the vacuum tube in a similar manner, in addition to the routine use of gloves and aprons after 1905.

For those who voluntarily sought a safe mode of practice, it was left to Dr. Hall-Edwards to write the rules:[17]

1. The room in which the apparatus is used must be large and well ventilated.
2. The tube must be enclosed in an opaque vessel or box, which should be provided with a hole through which the rays pass to the patient.
3. The hole in the tube-holder should be provided with an iris diaphragm or with a series of tubes which can be changed with ease.
4. A glass screen, or a wooden one lined with sheet-lead, and moving on castors, should be provided.
5. The switches should be placed in such a position that they can be worked from behind the screen.
6. Always keep as far away from the tube as possible when rays are being emitted.
7. Always keep behind the anti-cathode.
8. When using the fluorescent screen, use opaque gloves and lead-glass spectacles.
9. The fluorescent screen should be covered with a piece of thick lead-glass.
10. The tube should not be regulated whilst it is working.

At the London Hospital – early and long the scene of neglect – comprehensive protective measures were introduced in 1911 which a Belgian visitor considered to be near-perfect.[23] A. E. Dean of Hatton Garden encased each therapy tube in a lead-glass cupola impervious to x-rays, with only an aperture cut out to permit passage of the primary beam to the patient. Secondary radiation to the operator was prevented by shutting up the patient with the tube in a lead-walled cabin. The controls were so placed that the tube could only be regulated from outside the cabin.

Several events increased the need for protection after 1908. Tube output rose steeply when the Snook transformer was introduced and again when Coolidge's hot-cathode tube made its appearance in 1913; and these innovations heralded the modern era of high loadings and short exposure times. They rendered the apparatus more reliable and radiographs became easier to take – at the very moment when the greatly increased demands of the First World War overwhelmed existing x-ray facilities. An inexhaustible supply of radiographs was urgently needed to deal with the thousands of cases of fractures and retained bullets. Additional apparatus and emergency staff were quickly pressed into service by the War Office X-Ray Committee presided over by Dr. Archibald Reid, see Chapter 9. Much of the apparatus was primitive and dangerous, and many of the operators were untrained. Reid's committee was concerned with fulfilling demand, and not with protection; and soon there were protests.

The Röntgen Society took the lead (*see* 79). At the June 1915 meeting a discussion took place on protective devices for x-ray operators which was opened by Dr. (later

Professor) Sidney Russ.[24] Russ was concerned that many operators, particularly the novices recruited into x-ray work by the War, were likely to suffer injuries from hazards which had already been identified and could be avoided. At the conclusion of Russ's lecture, the meeting passed a resolution, proposed by Dr. C. R. C. Lyster, 'That the safety of operators should be secured by universal adoption of strict rules and that the Society should take steps to ensure this.' These rules were prepared, and they were issued in November 1915 as a broadsheet – the first British code of practice.

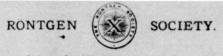

RONTGEN ✕ SOCIETY.

Recommendations for the Protection of X-ray Operators.

The harmful effects produced by X-rays are cumulative and do not generally appear until some weeks or months after the damage has been done. It is to be noted that X-rays of any degree of hardness are capable of producing ill effects, although it is commonly supposed that soft rays only are harmful.

It is undesirable that any X-ray treatment should be carried out except under the direction of a qualified medical practitioner experienced in X-ray work.

All X-ray tubes must be provided, when in use, with a protecting shield or cover which prevents the access of rays to the operators and which encloses the tube, leaving an adjustable opening only sufficiently large to allow the passage of a sheaf of rays of the size necessary for the work in hand. Even with this shielding the operator may not be completely protected in all cases (e.g., especially in screen work), and the use of movable screens, gloves and aprons is recommended.

Operators should be warned that shields obtainable commercially are often ineffective and tests of their opacity should be made.

Whenever possible the cubicle system should be used for X-ray treatment and the operator should be able to make all adjustments from a protected space.

When screen examination is required it is essential that the screen should be covered with thick lead glass of proved opacity and that the screen should be independently supported and not held in the hands of the operator. If the hands are so used they should be properly protected.

The hand or any portion of the body of the operator should never be used to test the hardness or quality of the X-ray tube ; any simple form of penetrometer can be easily arranged for this purpose.

November 1915

79. *The first British code of practice, 1915*

Eight months later the Society further stressed the dangers. During a further debate, concern was expressed over the state of x-ray installations in naval and military hospitals which, the speakers stated,[25] 'are defective in their means of protection and are in the hands of inexperienced x-ray workers who do not fully realise the attendant danger'. As a means of ensuring protection for patients and operators, they advised inspection by civilian experts. A more universal offer of practical help in checking exposure – also suggested by Dr. Russ – came from the Middlesex Hospital in 1918. Operators were invited to carry small photographic plates in lead-protected holders with circular exposure areas, which Russ and his team offered to supply and calibrate regularly. This was the first film badge service in Britain.[26,27]

Russ, one of the world's first biophysicists, continued to give attention to the injurious effects of x-rays for the rest of his life. In an article written in 1916, he emphasised that observance of the Röntgen Society's rules would largely eliminate the dangers of x-ray work. But he went on to point out that in addition to obvious effects such as dermatitis, there were 'hidden' biological dangers including the production of chronic blood changes.[28] These dangers he and his medical colleague, H. A. Colwell, later defined as: (a) injuries to the superficial tissues (usually the hands) which might become ulcerated or even cancerous; (b) prejudicial changes in the blood which might progress to fatal anaemia; and (c) derangements of internal organs, notably the reproductive organs.[29] More effective protection for the operator was clearly necessary, and their campaign for more attention to radiation protection was to bear fruit when the British X-Ray and Radium Protection Committee was established after the end of the War in response to public and professional disquiet.

But a harder blow had to be struck before minds concentrated on the subject. The Protection Committee was formed only after an occurrence which disturbed London radiologists so much that they called a meeting to take preventive action. In March 1921 Dr. Ironside Bruce, the respected radiographer of Charing Cross Hospital, died of aplastic anaemia, and his death was immediately and publicly attributed to radiation overexposure. Other British victims had followed Dr. Barry Blacker and Ernest Wilson to the grave in the previous two decades, and some of the more recent radiation deaths had been caused by a fatal blood disorder rather than chronic irritation of the skin; but Bruce's was the death that brought home the gravity of the risk to his colleagues, and the imperative need to tighten up their radiation precautions.[30]

A week later, on 29 March 1921, a letter appeared in *The Times* written by Robert Knox. It sought, apart from paying a fulsome tribute to the memory and work of his dead colleague, to calm the anxiety of the public about the safety of x-rays. A state of alarm erupted at that time, which threatened to force restrictions on the use of x-rays for examining patients. Knox's letter was one of the measures taken by responsible individuals to reduce passions. He knew practically all the British victims, he wrote, and spoke for all in saying that not one of them would have wished to curtail the medical use of x-rays because of personal danger. It was imperative that nothing should be done to retard the development of radiotherapy, in spite of the hazards to workers posed by the administration of radium and the new high-penetration x-rays.

The way forward, he suggested, was to adopt more stringent protective measures, including the regular inspection of all hospital departments by acknowledged experts. The Röntgen Society's wartime code of practice and other advice had to be acted upon, and the medical profession intended to provide the leadership. Knox announced the appointment of a standing committee consisting of radiologists, physiologists and physicists to investigate and report on the following:

(1) The changes induced in tissues by x-rays, and particularly on the blood changes.
(2) The properties of the x-rays and the best means of controlling their actions.
(3) The equipment of x-ray and electrical departments with a special view to the protective measures employed.
(4) Recommendations for the guidance of the assistants in these departments, particularly dealing with the hours of work and the need for fresh air and change.

THE BRITISH X-RAY AND RADIUM PROTECTION COMMITTEE (1921–52)

The British X-Ray and Radium Protection Committee came into being a few weeks later. It comprised the following:

CHAIRMAN
Sir Humphry Rolleston – Regius Professor of Physic in the University of Cambridge, Past President of the Royal College of Physicians

MEMBERS
Nominated by the British Institute of Radiology:
Robert Knox (The Cancer Hospital, Fulham) and
Sir Archibald Reid (St. Thomas's Hospital)
Nominated by the Royal Society of Medicine:
Stanley Melville (St. George's Hospital) and
S. Gilbert Scott (The London Hospital)
Nominated by the Röntgen Society:
Cuthbert Andrews and G. Harrison Orton (St. Mary's Hospital)
Nominated by The Institute of Physics:
Professor Sidney Russ (Middlesex Hospital)
Nominated by the Radium Institute, London:
J. C. Mottram
Nominated by the National Physical Laboratory:
G. W. C. Kaye

HONORARY SECRETARIES
Stanley Melville and Professor Sidney Russ

The members gave their services voluntarily and always paid their own way. Rolleston paid for the printing of the first report from his own pocket, and on several occasions the other members contributed to expenses. Yet, when this body was finally disbanded in 1952 their work was taken over by the Medical Research Council and the Ministry of Health, and radiation monitoring and protection became a State concern; and from them came the seeds out of which grew many national committees and eventually the International Commission on Radiological Protection (see below). Throughout the 31 years, they performed work of great economic as well as scientific benefit to the country and they won the respect of industry, science and medicine – in the words of Sir Ernest Rock Carling, the last chairman, the Protection Committee's record was a typically illogical and satisfactory British story.[31]

The instigator and moving force was Professor Sidney Russ, who in 1921 had only recently been promoted to the Joel Chair of Medical Physics at the Middlesex Hospital. He had witnessed the terminal suffering and deaths of his colleagues, Reginald Mann (1916) and Cecil Lyster (1920): indeed, Lyster was himself active in promoting the Protection Committee up to his death.[32] The other physicist, Dr. G. W. C. Kaye, provided the Protection Committee with teeth: as one of the heads of the National Physical

Laboratory, he was responsible for the physical measurement of equipment and the inspection of hospitals – in other words, for ensuring that the Protection Committee's recommendations were carried out. According to Kaye,[1] it was Stanley Melville who took the initiative in April 1921 to seek nominations from the various radiological and scientific bodies to establish the Protection Committee, and most of the London enthusiasts of the embryo British Institute of Radiology were among the original ten members. Knox in his letter in *The Times* coupled the work of the Protection Committee with that of the Institute, since he saw radiation protection as a function of the Institute. J. C. Mottram was the haematologist at the Radium Institute, who was one of the first to describe the blood changes induced in radium workers. Cuthbert Andrews with his extrovert manner frequently had a leavening effect on proceedings, and he provided an engaging account of the Protection Committee's early years.[33] The central figure was the chairman, Sir Humphry Rolleston, a white knight of British medicine in the 1920s and the spokesman of many medical organisations.

SIR HUMPHRY DAVY ROLLESTON, Bt., G.C.V.O., K.C.B., M.D., F.R.C.P. (1862–1944) was the most honoured physician of his day, the great clinician of St. George's Hospital, whom his colleague, Stanley Melville persuaded to preside over the Protection Committee.[34] Rolleston was introduced to x-rays during the Boer War, when he served as physician to the Imperial Yeomanry Hospital in Pretoria, and his fascination with the new diagnostic method did not diminish.[35] He was to chair the Protection Committee for 21 years, and his election led also to other associations with the young radiological profession.

In 1922–3 he was elected President of the Röntgen Society, in 1924–7 President of the British Association of Radiologists and Physiotherapists, and from 1927 to 1929 he served as the first President of the resurrected British Institute of Radiology. It was no secret that the radiologists, unable to reconcile their differences with the physicists over amalgamation, turned to an exalted medical figure, Rolleston, to lead them into it. Rolleston was Physician-In-Ordinary to King George V and Past President of the Royal College of Physicians, and in 1925 he succeeded Sir Clifford Allbutt as Regius Professor of Physic at Cambridge.[36] A. E. Barclay who was a party to this amalgamation which was destined to give substance to the radiological profession, wrote after Rolleston's death: 'Radiologists owe much to this great man who laboured so unselfishly to establish a branch of medicine in which himself took no active part.'[34]

PROFESSOR SIDNEY RUSS, C.B.E., D.Sc. (1879–1963) is credited with sowing the seed of a radiation protection committee, in the paper on protective devices for radiation workers which he read to the Röntgen Society in 1915. However, Russ himself believed that the public outcry caused by the deaths of several radiologists was the event which was responsible.[24] He shares with Kaye and C. E. S. Phillips the honour of being the pioneer hospital physicists, whose contribution transcended radiation protection; all three men helped to mould the fabric of the radiological profession.

A product of University College, London, and of Rutherford's Manchester laboratory, Sydney Russ was attracted to Hospital work by the possibilities of the medical applications of radio-activity. He joined the Middlesex Hospital as Beit Memorial Fellow in 1910 and served the hospital and medical school for the next 36 years as hospital physicist (1913–9) and professor of medical physics (1920–46).[37] Russ's association with the Middlesex Hospital ranks with that of F. L. Hopwood at St. Bartholomew's Hospital, as the first career hospital physicists in Britain.[38]

Russ remained joint secretary (successively with Stanley Melville, Harrison Orton and D. W. Smithers) for the whole life of the Protection Committee. Cuthbert Andrews, the other long-surviving member, recalled that Russ and Kaye were the most vocal, presenting 'well-mannered arguments, and neither amenable to criticism or opposition, (being) contemptuous and outspoken of other ideas and theories'.[39]

Russ was best known to radiologists as a teacher of physics in London. In 1917 he was one of the eleven persons present at MacKenzie Davidson's home, at the meeting which inaugurated radiological teaching in Britain, and he was responsible with Professor Crowther for writing the physics syllabus of the Cambridge Diploma course. The Part 1 course moved to the Middlesex Hospital in 1921 and he and his colleagues continued to teach the students there until the course ceased in 1942.[40] He wrote a textbook, *Physics for Medical Students*, in 1927,[41] and two books in partnership with his Middlesex Hospital colleague, Hector Colwell – *Radium, X-Rays and the Living Cell*, and *X-Ray and Radium Injuries, Prevention and Treatment*.[29] He was:

> Co-editor (with Robert Knox and E. P. Cumberbatch) of *Archives of Radiology and Electrology* (1915–23)
> President, Röntgen Society, 1919–20
> Founder, Hospital Physicists' Association
> Scientific Secretary, National Radium Commission.

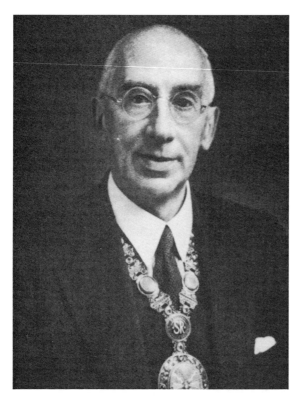

80. *Dr. G. W. C. Kaye*

GEORGE WILLIAM CLARKSON KAYE, O.B.E., D.Sc., F.R.S. (1880–1941), the distinguished pioneer medical physicist, was a Londoner who studied at the Royal College of Science and the Cavendish Laboratory, Cambridge, where he was personal assistant to Professor (later Sir) J. J. Thomson. His work during the First World War was rewarded with the O.B.E. and led to an appointment in the War Office which brought him into contact with the application of radium to medicine. In 1922 at the age of 42 he was appointed Superintendent of the Physics Department of the National Physical Laboratory, Teddington, a post which he held until his death. His introduction to hospital medical physics came with an invitation from Sidney Russ to join the Protection Committee.

Kaye's brilliant intellect and energetic, cautious approach suited him for the task of pursuing the ideal of radiological protection. This he did by devising practical methods for protecting x-ray workers which he persuaded the Protection Committee to define as standards, as well as by inspecting departments and rooms to ensure that these standards were maintained.[41] At the National Physical Laboratory he established a section to measure the content of radium applicators and to test x-ray tubes and electrical equipment according to the Protection Committee's recommendations.[42]

Kaye also ranks with Butcher, Gardiner and Knox as one of the foremost British radiological editors. He was associated with four journals:

> *The Journal of the Röntgen Society*, 1919–23
> *British Journal of Radiology (Röntgen Society Section)*, 1923–7
> *British Journal of Radiology* (New Series), 1928–32
> *Radiography*, 1935–41.

He served as the president of three radiological bodies and played a leading part in the creation of the Society of Radiographers, of which he later was President:[43]

> President, Röntgen Society, 1917–8
> President, British Institute of Radiology, 1929–30
> President, Society of Radiographers, 1941.

He wrote several books dealing with physics and x-rays including *X-Rays* (1923) and *Roentgenology* (1929), and delivered most of the prized radiological memorial lectures. The best remembered of these were his presidential address in 1929 entitled 'Radiology, Medieval and Modern', and the Stanley Melville Memorial Lecture in 1940, 'The Story of Protection'.[1]

Dr. Kaye in the course of delivering his lecture in 1940 digressed to sketch the x-ray scene which confronted the Protection Committee in 1921, as well as to describe their difficulties to specify and standardise protective measures.[1] 'The need was great, for the conditions in the majority of x-ray departments were thoroughly unsatisfactory in those days. I well recall many departments where it was possible to see the bones of the hand on a portable fluorescent screen almost everywhere in the x-ray room ... The absence of an accepted physical unit of quality or radiation was an obstacle; and the best the Committee could do was to try to translate into specific recommendations a sort of grand average of the protective measures which could be gleaned from the working conditions of a number of experienced radiologists who had escaped injury and still enjoyed normal health.'

The Protection Committee set to work with a will. They recognised three sources of danger – namely, undue exposure to x-rays, high-voltage risks from exposed electrical conductors, and undue exposure to toxic gases produced by coronal discharge. Without measurement techniques or any background knowledge of radiobiology, they applied their energy to defining pragmatically sensible precautions for the x-ray operator, e.g. lead shielding thicknesses for x-ray tubes, hours of work, periodic blood checks. Between April and June 1921 they met regularly at The Royal Society of Medicine, 1 Wimpole Street. Working speedily and at high pressure, they issued their series of protective recommendations as a 'Preliminary Report' in June for publication in the July number of *The Journal of the Röntgen Society*:[44]

X-RAY AND RADIUM PROTECTION.

THE X-ray and Radium Protection Committee, representing various radiological and other scientific bodies in this country, has issued a preliminary report which sets out present knowledge in regard to equipment, ventilation and working conditions of X-ray and radium departments.

The committee proposes to investigate experimentally a number of points which have arisen. Offers of assistance are invited by the committee, and should be sent to the Hon. Secretaries, from whom copies of the preliminary report may be had on application.

The Committee is constituted as follows :—

Chairman : Sir Humphry Rolleston, K.C.B. *Members :* Sir Archibald Reid, K.B.E., C.M.G., St. Thomas's Hospital ; Dr. Robert Knox, King's College Hospital ; Dr. G. Harrison Orton, St. Mary's Hospital ; Dr. S. Gilbert Scott, London Hospital ; Dr. J. C. Mottram, Pathologist, Radium Institute ; Dr. G. W. C. Kaye, O.B.E., National Physical Laboratory ; Mr. Cuthbert Andrews, *Hon. Secretaries :* Dr. Stanley Melville, St. George's Hospital ; Prof. S. Russ, the Middlesex Hospital. *Address :* Care of Royal Society of Medicine, 1, Wimpole Street, W.1.

X-RAY AND RADIUM PROTECTION COMMITTEE. PRELIMINARY REPORT.

INTRODUCTION.

The danger of over-exposure to X-rays and radium can be avoided by the provision of efficient protection and suitable working conditions.

The known effects on the operator to be guarded against are :—

(1) Visible injuries to the superficial tissues which may result in permanent damage.

(2) Derangements of internal organs and changes in the blood. These are especially important as their early manifestation is often unrecognised.

GENERAL RECOMMENDATIONS.

It is the duty of those in charge of X-ray and Radium departments to ensure efficient protection and suitable working conditions for the *personnel*.

The following precautions are recommended :—

(1) Not more than seven working hours a day.

(2) Sundays and two half-days off duty each week, to be spent as much as possible out of doors.

(3) An annual holiday of one month or two separate fortnights.

Sisters and nurses, employed as whole-time workers in X-ray and Radium departments, should not be called upon for any other hospital service.

PROTECTIVE MEASURES.

It cannot be insisted upon too strongly that a primary precaution in all X-ray work is to surround the X-ray bulb itself as completely as possible with adequate protective material, except for an aperture as small as possible for the work in hand.

The protective measures recommended are dealt with under the following sections :—

I. X-rays for diagnostic purposes.
II. X-rays for superficial therapy.
III. X-rays for deep therapy.
IV. X-rays for industrial and research purposes.
V. Electrical precautions in X-ray departments.
VI. Ventilation of X-ray departments.
VII. Radium therapy.

It must be clearly understood that the protective measures recommended for these various purposes are not necessarily interchangeable ; for instance, to use for deep therapy the measures intended for superficial therapy would probably subject the worker to serious injury.

I. X-rays for Diagnostic Purposes.

(1) *Screen Examinations.*

(*a*) The X-ray bulb to be enclosed as completely as possible with protective material equivalent to not less than 2 mms. of lead. The material of the diaphragm to be equivalent to not less than 2 mms. of lead.

(*b*) The fluorescent screen to be fitted with lead glass equivalent to not less than 1 mm. of lead and to be large enough to cover the area irradiated when the diaphragm is opened to its widest. (Practical difficulties militate at present against the recommendation of a greater degree of protection).

(*c*) A travelling protective screen, of material equivalent to not less than 2 mms. of lead, should be employed between the operator and the X-ray box.

(*d*) Protective gloves to be of lead rubber (or the like) equivalent to not less than $\frac{1}{2}$ mm. of lead and to be lined with leather or other suitable material. (As practical difficulties militate at present against the recommendation of a greater degree of protection, all manipulations during screen examination should be reduced to a minimum).

(*e*) A minimum output of radiation should be used with the bulb as far from the screen as is consistent with the efficiency of the work in hand. Screen work to be as expeditious as possible.

(2) *Radiographic Examinations " Overhead " Equipment.*

(*a*) The X-ray bulb to be enclosed as completely as possible with protective material equivalent to not less than 2 mms. of lead.

(*b*) The operator to stand behind a protective screen of material equivalent to not less than 2 mms. of lead.

II. X-rays for Superficial Therapy.

It is difficult to define the line of demarcation between superficial and deep therapy.

For this reason it is recommended that, in the reorganization of existing or the equipment of new, X-ray departments, small cubicles should not be adopted, but that the precautionary measures suggested for deep therapy should be followed.

The definition of superficial therapy is considered to cover sets of apparatus giving a maximum of 100,000 volts (15 cm. spark-gap between points ; 5 cm. spark-gap between spheres of diameter 5 cms.).

Cubicle System.

Where the cubicle system is already in existence it is recommended that :

(1) The cubicle should be well lighted and ventilated, preferably provided with an exhaust electric fan in an outside wall or ventilation shaft. The controls of the X-ray apparatus to be outside the cubicle.

(2) The walls of the cubicle to be of material equivalent to not less than 2 mms. of lead. Windows to be of lead glass of equivalent thickness.

(3) The X-ray bulb to be enclosed as completely as possible with protective material equivalent to not less than 2 mms. of lead.

III. X-rays for Deep Therapy.

This section refers to sets of apparatus giving voltages above 100,000.

(1) Small cubicles are not recommended.

(2) A large, lofty, well-ventilated and lighted room to be provided.

(3) The X-ray bulb to be enclosed as completely as possible with protective material equivalent to not less than 3 mms. of lead.

(4) A separate enclosure to be provided for the operator, situated as far as possible from the X-ray bulb. All controls to be within this enclosure, the walls and windows of which to be of material equivalent to not less than 3 mms. of lead.

IV. X-rays for Industrial and Research Purposes.

The preceding recommendations for voltages above and below 100,000 will probably apply to the majority of conditions under which X-rays are used for industrial and research purposes.

V. Electrical Precautions in X-ray Departments.

The following recommendations are made :—

(1) Wooden, cork or rubber floors should be provided ; existing concrete floors should be covered with one of the above materials.

(2) Stout metal tubes or rods should, wherever possible, be used instead of wires for conductors. Thickly insulated wire is preferable to bare wire. Slack or looped wires are to be avoided.

(3) All metal parts of the apparatus and room to be efficiently earthed.

(4) All main and supply switches should be very distinctly indicated. Wherever possible double-pole switches should be used in preference to single-pole. Fuses no heavier than necessary for the purpose in hand should be used. Unemployed leads to the high-tension generator should not be permitted.

VI. Ventilation of X-ray Departments.

(1) It is strongly recommended that the X-ray department should not be below the ground level.

(2) The importance of adequate ventilation in both operating and dark-rooms is supreme. Artificial ventilation is recommended in most cases. With very high potentials coronal discharges are difficult to avoid and these produce ozone and nitrous fumes, both of which are prejudicial to the operator. Dark-rooms should be capable of being readily opened up to sunshine and fresh air when not in use. The walls and ceilings of dark-rooms are best painted some more cheerful hue than black.

VII. Radium Therapy.

The following protective measures are recommended for the handling of quantities of radium up to one gram. :—

(1) In order to avoid injury to the fingers the radium, whether in the form of applicators of radium salt or in the form of emanation tubes, should be always manipulated with forceps or similar instruments and it should be carried from place to place in long-handled boxes lined on all sides with 1 cm. of lead.

(2) In order to avoid penetrating rays of radium all manipulations should be carried out as rapidly as possible and the operator should not remain in the vicinity of radium for longer than is necessary.

The radium when not in use should be stored in an enclosure the wall thickness of which should be equivalent to not less than 8 cms. of lead.

(3) In the handling of emanation all manipulations should, as far as possible, be carried out during its relatively inactive state. In manipulations where emanation is likely to come into direct contact with the fingers thin rubber gloves should be worn. The escape of emanation should be very carefully guarded against and the room in which it is prepared should be provided with an exhaust electric fan.

EXISTING FACILITIES FOR ENSURING SAFETY OF OPERATORS.

The Governing Bodies of many institutions where radiological work is carried on may wish to have further guarantees of the general safety of the conditions under which their *personnel* work.

(1) Although the Committee believe that an adequate degree of safety would result if the recommendations now put forward were acted upon, they would point out that this is entirely dependent upon the loyal co-operation of the *personnel* in following the precautionary measures outlined for their benefit.

(2) The Committee would also point out that the National Physical Laboratory, Teddington, is prepared to carry out exact measurements upon X-ray protective materials, and to arrange for periodic inspection of existing installations on the lines of the present recommendations.

(4) Further, in view of the varying susceptibilities of workers to radiation the Committee recommend that wherever possible periodic tests, *e.g.*, every three months, be made upon the blood of the *personnel*, so that any changes which occur may be recognised at an early stage. In the present state of our knowledge it is difficult to decide when small variations from the normal blood-count become significant.

June, 1921.

The Preliminary Report was the first set of recommendations to be issued by any country, and so gave the lead to the world in radiation protection. The American Roentgen Ray Protection Committee although founded six months earlier than the British Protection Committee, only published its findings in September 1922, more than one year after the Preliminary Report appeared. The most immediate effect of the Preliminary Report was the involvement of the National Physical Laboratory in inspections of hospital departments – a step which became the source of the Protection Committee's authority. The experience of Dr. Kaye and his assistants who carried out the tests and made the reports formed the basis of their next report ('Revised Report No. 1 and No. 2') which was issued in December 1923.[45] In the single-page leaflet of 'Report No. 2' consisting of only five clauses, no specific guidelines were laid down, instead it recommended that all questions be referred to the National Physical Laboratory; the name 'N.P.L.' appeared seven times in thirteen sentences.[46]

The Protection Committee continued to revise their advise and issue reports:

Third Revised Report	–	May 1927[47]
Fourth Revised Report	–	1934
Fifth Revised Report	–	1938
Sixth Revised Report	–	1943
Seventh Revised Report	–	1048

With the Third and Fourth publications the Recommendations became more definite and exact figures and tables were provided for the guidance of x-ray workers, and the dominance of the National Physical Laboratory appeared to be less evident, although Dr. Kaye's benevolent influence on the Protection Committee was undiminished. The Fifth Report was more precise and the Recommendations were even more detailed and extended their scope to include film storage, electromedical apparatus and ultraviolet therapy.[1]

Certain radiologists and equipment makers strongly criticised the Recommendations, especially during the early years of the Protection Committee, claiming that they were unnecessarily drastic. The Committee's efforts to provide adequate protection against stray radiation were deprecated as heavy, clumsy and costly. Many a radiologist complained that the Recommendations restricted him too much in his work. But presently the heavy lead protection was superseded by safer-to-use devices such as the self-protected x-ray tube, in which the full thickness of lead protection laid down by the Protection Committee was incorporated in the tube itself. Certain of the original Recommendations were relaxed a little. Further technical improvements followed, such as shock-proof tubes, insulated high-tension cables and transformers immersed in oil. The mid-1930s saw the beginning of the end of x-ray tubes enclosed in glass globes with naked high-tension wires and Snook rectifiers. The objections to protective measures had been overcome: patients no longer suffered skin burns or depilation and all operators wore aprons and gloves.[48] The Protection Committee's seeds had borne fruit in abundance and their critics were silenced.

Government agencies as well as the National Physical Laboratory sanctioned the authority of the Protection Committee by enforcing its Recommendations. The Ministry of Health and the Ministry of Pensions lent early and continual support, and the Medical Research Council in later years gave financial help. In 1926 an Inter-Services Advisory X-Ray Committee was formed which compelled military hospitals to conform to civilian practice, and ensured that in 1939 the three defence services entered the Second World War with safe apparatus and equipment – an interesting reversal of the conditions which obtained at the outbreak of the First World War. The x-ray operators themselves supported the work of the Protection Committee with very few exceptions. The Protection Committee for its part realised that the safe use of x-rays and radium depended to a large extent on the cooperation of the operators, and on their skill and care. It was significant that the Protection Committee was established almost in the same year as proficiency qualifications were introduced for radiologists and radiographers; both the D.M.R.E. and M.S.R. boards aiming at adequate training, examinations and professional status. Protection was a matter of major concern to all three bodies.

International collaboration between radiologists was inaugurated at the First International Congress of Radiology in London in 1925. Recommendations from both the British and the American Protection Committees were considered by the delegates, but the discussions were inconclusive. Three years later in Stockholm at the Second Congress, an International X-Ray and Radium Protection Committee (IXRPC) was established, with a committee representing six nations, Doctors Stanley Melville and G. W. C. Kaye acting as joint secretaries. As a basis for the international regulations Dr. Kaye successfully proposed adoption of the Third Revised Report (1927) of the

British Protection Committee. His proposal was accepted with a few minor modifications,[49] and these recommendations have been revised triennially since, on the occasions of successive international congresses.

THE MARTYRS' MEMORIAL, HAMBURG

'Spare a thought' – wrote G. W. C. Kaye in 1940[1] – 'for those x-ray pioneers who, undaunted by long and sometimes unbearable suffering which drugs might utterly fail to relieve and which was, perhaps, followed by mutilating operations or a cruel death, continued to apply themselves indefatigably to perfect the use of Röntgen's discovery for the benefit of humanity. Their martyrdom prepared the way which rendered the present use of x-rays free from danger.'

In 1936 the German Röntgen Society at the suggestion of Professor Hans Meyer of Bremen erected a monument to the x-ray and radium martyrs of all nations. The monument stands beside the radiological department of St. George's Hospital, Hamburg – the hospital of Heinrich Albers-Schönberg, the celebrated pioneer who succumbed to his radiation injuries in 1921. It takes the form of a rectangular column of sandstone surmounted by a laurel wreath, and at the front bears the inscription recorded at the head of this chapter. The sides and back of the column are inscribed with the names of x-ray and radium workers of many nationalities who died before 1936.

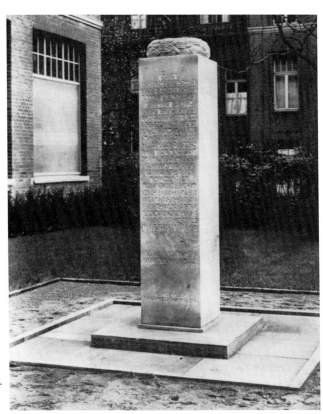

81. The Martyrs' Memorial, erected in 1936 in the grounds of St. George's Hospital, Hamburg

A total of 169 deaths was originally recorded, including 14 British, and Professor Meyer compiled a brief biography of each martyr which was published in a special number of the German radiological journal, *Strahlentherapie*, and then reprinted as a book, *Ehrenbuch der Röntgenologen und Radiologen aller Nationen*.[21,50]

The 169 original martyrs came from 15 countries:

Germany	20	Austria	6
Belgium	4	Russia	2
Denmark	5	Switzerland	6
Finland	1	Spain	4
France	47	Czechoslovakia	5
Great Britain	14	Hungary	6
Italy	9	U.S.A.	39
Dutch East Indies	1		

The 14 British names include 12 radiologists and two radiographers:

Reginald G. Blackall – page 81	George Alexander Pirie – see below
Barry Blacken (*sic*) – page 88	J. R. Riddell – page 119
William Ironside Bruce – page 99	J. W. L. Spence – page 126
William Hope Fowler – page 126	Dawson Turner – page 125
John Hall-Edwards – page 114	Hugh Walsham – page 86
C. R. C. Lyster – page 97	John Chisholm Williams – page 108
Stanley Melville – page 109	Ernest E. Wilson – page 224

GEORGE ALEXANDER PIRIE, M.S., M.D.(Edinburgh) (1863–1928) was the pioneer radiologist in Dundee who was disabled by radiation injuries after 20 years of practice, and he died of them. The son of a Dundee doctor, he joined the family practice in 1898 after studying medicine at St. Andrew's and Edinburgh Universities. He was the first doctor in Dundee to specialise in x-ray work and devoted the last 30 years of his life to diagnostic radiology. From 1908 to his death he served as the medical electrician to the Dundee Royal Infirmary. He published several articles in the radiological journals between 1908 and 1915 including his early experience of chest radiography and the use of bismuth for examining the oesophagus and colon in 30 patients.[51]

Pirie early suffered from radiodermatitis of his hands which led inexorably to finger amputations, axillary lymphadenopathy and death from cancer in 1928. Disabled by 1925, the citizens of Dundee made him a gift of £1,200 and he received the bronze plaque of the Carnegie Hero Fund, which carried an annual pension of £200. His radiographer was William Waddell (died 1953), who joined him in Dundee after service in the First World War.[52]

A further 28 British names were added to the Martyr's Memorial in the mid-1950s, largely through the efforts of Dr. F. G. Spear of the Strangeways Research Laboratory, Cambridge, who was concerned 'that they may not be forgotten'.[53] They were:

H. J. B. Aimer – page 68	H. W. Jenneson – page 239
N. E. Aldridge – page 140	R. F. Mann – page 97
W. L. St. J. Alton – page 240	A. C. Mooney
H. E. Bateman – page 239	J. P. O'Connor – page 240
F. R. Butt – page 71	G. Harrison Orton – page 102
Ellen Clark – page 97	A. A. Parsons – page 239
W. A. Colwell – page 239	E. Payne – page 150

DR. HINTON ERNEST BATEMAN (1864–1954) qualified from St. Bartholomew's Hospital in 1883 and settled in York, a city which he never left. He was a pioneer in radiology who was severely burnt and underwent countless operations including amputation of his left arm at the age of nearly 90 years.[21]

WALTER AUGUSTUS COLWELL (1864–1929) worked for the chemists, Allen and Hanburys in London when Röntgen's discovery became known, and he was thereafter employed to run a radiographic service for general practitioners. In 1906 he went into independent private practice in Mandeville Place and later Welbeck Street, and for 20 years provided a high-quality and remarkably successful service for doctors. Severe dermatitis of both hands led to more than 20 operations and the amputation of several fingers, and death from axillary metastases.[54]

Colwell had a son, Dr. Hector Augustus Colwell, who was a well-known radiologist in London and the author of several textbooks, *X-Ray and Radium Injuries* (with Sidney Russ), *Radium, X-Rays and the Living Cell* (with Sidney Russ), and *An Essay on the History of Electrotherapy and Diagnosis* (1922).

HERBERT WILLIAM JENNESON (1880–1946) joined the Hull Royal Infirmary as a radiographic assistant in 1902, having previously used an x-ray apparatus in the Boer War while serving in the Army. Later he worked in Bridlington Hospital. Jenneson's radiation injuries appeared in about 1920 – multiple epitheliomata of both hands, and he lost five fingers by amputation. Axillary glands were excised in 1939 but he succumbed to disseminated cancer some years later.[21]

ARTHUR AUGUSTUS PARSONS, M.S.R. (1877–1928) was an early London radiographer. He was appointed to the staff of the Westminster Hospital in 1902, having previously had experience of x-ray work. By 1918 his fingers were ulcerated, and some years later a finger of his right hand was amputated. Malignant degeneration occurred, and he died of spinal-cord metastases. He was a founder member of the Society of Radiographers.[21]

ELLIS PEARSON, L.R.C.P., F.R.C.S.(Edinburgh, 1898) (1869–1954) was a general practitioner in Bideford for 40 years after 1902, serving for over 20 years as H.M. Coroner of North Devon. He was born and studied medicine in Liverpool, and at the turn of the century he received part of his surgical training at the Royal Southern Hospital under Mr. (later Sir) Robert Jones, acquiring the rudiments of radiography from Dr. Thurstan Holland. He continued to practise radiography for the rest of his life. At the age of 79 years three fingers of his right hand and the middle finger of his left hand were amputated, and some years later he succumbed to malignant degeneration of his radiation injuries.[21]

Five of the British martyrs were injured by radium. Dr. William Alton (1880–1954) was the first chemist of the Radium Institute in London, being responsible for the assay of radium salts for medical purposes. In the 1930s he lost several fingers by amputation and he died of an aplastic anaemia. E. Lowndes Glew (1895–1948), the son of F. Harrison

Glew (see page 65), was Alton's assistant, and died of radiation-induced myelomatosis. Another of Alton's assistants was George Randall (1912–54), who was employed in the laboratory to fill ampoules with radium. After numerous operations to his fingers and his hands, he succumbed to malignant changes and fatal lung metastases. Similar injuries overtook James O'Connor (1905–50) who was the curator of radium in the Radium Institute of Manchester (later the Christie Hospital and Holt Radium Institute).

The eloquent words of Dr. Antoine Béclère, the celebrated French pioneer, at the unveiling ceremony of the Martyrs' Memorial on 4 April 1936 are an appropriate conclusion to this chapter:[1] 'I come to bow with reverence before this monument which was piously erected to the victims of x-rays and radium. I come to salute their memory, and honour their sufferings, their sacrifices and their premature deaths. I come also to pay homage to the generous thought of which this monument is the expression . . .

'All these victims acquitted their task, humble or exalted, and with the same devotion. All have acquired equal merit, all have equal right to honour. These noble martyrs did not speak the same language, did not belong to the same country, they were of different races and religions. Forgive me, I am wrong – they were all of the same race, the race of brave people; they were all faithful to the same religion, the religion of duty. They were all devoted to the mission of fighting, at the peril of their lives, the same enemies, illness and suffering, with the aid of the marvellous weapon which Röntgen gave to medicine, without fear that this weapon was double-edged and, wielded, as it was, without the precautions now in use, would one day wound and kill them.

'The great name and the celebrated discovery of Röntgen form part of your national inheritance of which you are naturally proud. You might, without incurring criticism, have reserved this monument for the victims of German nationality alone. You did not desire this, and so the names of those who in all civilised countries have devoted and sacrificed their lives to a common ideal, are here fraternally united in a common homage.'

REFERENCES AND NOTES

Chapter One – THE GREAT DISCOVERY

1. THOMPSON, S. P. Presidential Address to the Röntgen Society, 5 November 1897. Archives of the Roentgen Ray, *2*, 23–31, 1897–8.
2. DAVIDSON, J. M. Röntgen or X-rays. British Medical Journal, *1*, 1190, 1902.
3. DAMPIER, W. C. *The History of Science*, 3rd edition, London: Cambridge University Press, 1942.
4. SCHALL, W. E. Series and parallel. Radiography, *12*, 1–6, 1946.
5. KAYE, G. W. C. Radiology, medieval and modern. British Journal of Radiology, *2*, 3–28, 1929; and Röntgen and his forerunners. Radiography, *27*, 406–412, 1961.
6. CRANE, A. W. The research trail of the X-ray. Radiology, *23*, 131–148, 1934.
7. *Dictionary of National Biography, 1912–21*, 136–137. Oxford University Press, London, 1927.
8. RAMSEY, L. J. Some notable early contributors to radiography – Thompson, Jackson and Campbell Swinton. Radiography, *46*, 289–297, 1890.
9. *Dictionary of National Biography, 1931–40*, 469–470. Oxford University Press, London, 1849.
10. UNDERWOOD, E. A. Wilhelm Conrad Röntgen (1845–1923) and the early development of radiology. Proceedings of the Royal Society of Medicine, *38*, 697–706, 1945.
11. JOLY, J. Report of Dublin University Experimental Association meeting in February 1896. The Lancet, *1*, 457, 1896.
12. LONGMORE, T. A. Something old, something new. Radiography, *19*, 71–85, 1953.
13. VAN WYLICK, W. A. H. W. C. Roentgen and the early days of X-rays. Medicamundi, *16*, 1–8, 1971.
14. GLASSER, O. *Wilhelm Conrad Röntgen and the Early History of the Roentgen Rays*. London: John Bale, Sons and Danielsson, 1933.
15. BRAILSFORD, J. F. Roentgen's discovery of X-rays. Their application to medicine and surgery. British Journal of Radiology, *19*, 453–461, 1946.
16. DAM, H. J. W. The new marvel in photography. McClure's Magazine, *6*, 403 et seqq., 1896.
17. SCHALL, W. E. Letter to the editor. British Journal of Radiology, *24*, 26, 1951.
18. RÖNTGEN, W. C. Ueber eine neue Art von Strahlen. (Vorläufige Mitteilung). Sitzungsberichte der physikalisch-medizinischen Gesellschaft zu Würzburg, 1896.
19. RÖNTGEN, W. C. Ueber eine neue Art von Strahlen. (Zweite Mitteilung). Ibid., N.S. *30*, 11–19, 1896.
20. RÖNTGEN, W. C. Weitere Beobachtungen uber die Eigenschaften der X-Strahlen. (Dritte Mitteilung). Annalen der Physik und Chemie, *26*, 576–592, 1897. This paper, dated 10 March 1897, was translated as 'Further Observations on the Properties of X-rays' in Archives of the Roentgen Ray, *3*, 80–88, 1898–9.
21. MEREDITH, W. J. 'What Manchester thinks . . .' British Journal of Radiology, *41*, 2–11, 1968.

Chapter Two – THE NEWS RECEIVED

1. UNDERWOOD, E. A. Wilhelm Conrad Röntgen (1845–1923) and the early development of radiology. Proceedings of the Royal Society of Medicine, *38*, 697–706, 1945.
2. GLASSER, O. *Wilhelm Conrad Röntgen and the Early History of the Roentgen Rays*. London: John Bale, Sons and Danielsson, 1933.

3. SCHUSTER, N. H. Early days of Roentgen photography in Britain. British Medical Journal, *2*, 1164–1166, 1962.

4. THOMSON, J. J. The Röntgen rays. Nature, *5*, 302–306, 1896.

5. HOLLAND, C. T. X-rays in 1896. British Journal of Radiology, *11*, 1–24, 1938; and ANDREWS, C. Half a century of shadows. Radiography, *22*, 250–254, 1956.

6. STEINER, R. E. The President's speech. British Journal of Radiology, *45*, 878–880, 1972. These verses first appeared in Photography in February 1896 under the title *X-actly So.*

7. JUPE, M. Early days of radiology in Britain. Clinical Radiology, *12*, 147–154, 1961; and RAMSEY, L. J. Radiography and monarchy. Radiography, *44*, 134–141, 1978.

8. WILD, C. H. J. High tension generators in 1898 and 1908. Radiography, *23*, 91–94, 1957.

9. British Journal of Photography, *43*, 26 et seqq., 1896.

10. British Journal of Photography, *43*, 434 et seqq., 1896.

11. British Journal of Photography, *43*, 177 et seqq., 1896.

12. RÖNTGEN, W. C. On a new kind of rays. Nature, *53*, 274–276, 1896.

13. DAVIES, H. W. Three score years and ten. British Journal of Radiology, *38*, 641–652, 1965.

14. The Lancet, *1*, 112, 1896.

15. The new photography. The Lancet, *1*, 179, 1896.

16. The new photography. The Lancet, *1*, 245–246, 1896.

17. SCHUSTER, A. On the new kind of radiation. British Medical Journal, *1*, 172–173, 1896.

18. The new photography. British Medical Journal, *1*, 289–290, 1896.

19. ROWLAND, S. Report on the application of the new photography to medicine and surgery. British Medical Journal, 1896. Parts I–XIII appeared on successive weeks between 8 February (361) and 6 June (1411).

20. British Medical Journal, *1*, 532, 1896.

21. Obituary notice, The Lancet, *1*, 552, 1917.

22. British Medical Journal, *1*, 620, 1896.

23. British Medical Journal, *1*, 559, 1896.

24. British Medical Journal, *1*, 493, 1896.

25. British Medical Journal, *1*, 749, 1896.

26. British Medical Journal, *1*, 750, 1896.

27. British Medical Journal, *1*, 807, 1896.

28. British Medical Journal, *1*, 1225, 1896.

29. SWINTON, A. A. C. The new shadow photography, The Photographic Journal, *20*, 150 et seqq., 1896.

30. Southport Visitor, 26 March 1896, quoted by Mould, R. F. *A History of X-rays and Radium.* Sutton; IPC Business Press, 1980.

31. WARD, H. S. The Journal of the Röntgen Society, *3*, 11, 1906–7; and ROBERTS, E. A. The new photography. Radiography, *21*, 169–171, 1955.

32. BARCLAY, A. E. The old order changes. British Journal of Radiology, *22*, 300–302, 1943.

33. British Medical Journal, *1*, 494, 1896, quoted by JUPE, M. Early days of radiology in Britain. British Journal of Radiology, *12*, 147–154, 1961.

34. British Medical Journal, *1*, 532, 1896.

35. British Medical Journal, *1*, 875–876, 1896; and HALE-WHITE, W. Letter to the editor. The Lancet, *2*, 1370, 1930.

36. BOWERS, B. *X-rays.* H.M.S.O., 1970.

37. British Medical Journal, *1*, 677–678, 1896.

Chapter Three – THE FIRST EXPERIMENTERS

1. SWINTON, A. A. C. Some early radiograms. The Journal of the Röntgen Society, *2*, 11–12, 1905–6.

2. GRIGG, E. R. N. *The Trail of the Invisible Light.* Springfield, Illinois: Charles C. Thomas, 1964.

3. RAMSEY, L. J. Some notable early contributors to radiography – Thompson, Jackson and Campbell Swinton. Radiography, *46*, 289–297, 1980.

4. SWINTON, A. A. C. *Autobiographical and Other Writings.* London: Longmans, Green & Co., 1930; and BRIDGEWATER, T. H. *A. A. Campbell Swinton FRS 1863–1930.* London: Royal Television Society, 1982.

5. The Times, 17 January, 1896.

6. SWINTON, A. A. C. Professor Röntgen's discovery. Nature, *53*, 276–277, 1896.

7. The Lancet, *1*, 245, 1896.

8. The Lancet, *1*, 326, 1896.

9. MAYNEORD, M. V. Radiological physics, a retrospect. British Journal of Radiology, *46*, 754–756, 1973.

10. Obituary notice, British Journal of Radiology, *18*, 400, 1945.

11. ANDREWS, C. Half a century of shadows. Radiography, *22*, 250–254, 1956.

12. British Institute of Radiology Collection: The C. E. S. Phillips Papers.

13. BOAG, J. W. Looking both ways. British Journal of Radiology, *50*, 84–92, 1977.

14. PHILLIPS, C. E. S. *Bibliography of X-ray Literature and Research, 1896–1897.* London: 'The Electrician' Printing and Publishing Co., 1897; and Archives of the Roentgen Rays, *2*, 33, 1897–8.

15. BISHOP, P. J. Sixty years of radiology. British Journal of Radiology, *46*, 833–836, 1973.

16. REYNOLDS, R. J. Sixty years of radiology. British Journal of Radiology, *29*, 238–245, 1956.

17. REYNOLDS, J. and REYNOLDS R. J. A $13\frac{1}{4}$ inch spark induction coil. English Mechanic and World of Science, No. 1716, 598–599, 1898.

18. FINZI, N. S. The early days of radiology. Clinical Radiology, *12*, 143–146, 1961.

19. Obituary notice. British Journal of Radiology, *38*, 71, 1965.

20. ALLSOPP, C. B. Russell Reynolds: pioneer of radiology. Medical and Biographical Illustration, *16*, 44–47, 1966.

21. REYNOLDS, R. J. The early history of radiology in Britain. Clinical Radiology, *12*, 136–142, 1961.

22. STEAD, G. 1895 and all that. British Journal of Radiology, *32*, 425–431, 1959.

23. THOMPSON, J. S. and THOMPSON, H. G. *Silvanus Phillips Thompson, His Life and Letters.* London: Fisher and Unwin, 1920.

24. British Medical Journal, *1*, 875–876, 1896.

25. SCOTT, J. The birth of radiology in Scotland. Radiography, *17*, 46–49, 1951.

26. *Dictionary of National Biography 1901–11, 508–517.* London: Oxford University Press, 1920.

27. *Dictionary of National Biography, 1901–11, 1, 297–298.* London: Oxford University Press, 1920.

28. JUPE, M. Early days of radiology in Britain. Clinical Radiology, *12*, 147–154, 1961.

29. DAVIES, H. Three score years and ten. British Journal of Radiology, *38*, 641–652, 1965.

30. Glasgow Medical Journal, *23*, 17–24, 1885.

31. BOTTOMLEY, J. F. On Röntgen's rays. Nature, *53*, 268–269, 1896. The letter from Lord Kelvin to Professor Röntgen dated 17 January 1896 is in the collection of the British Institute of Radiology.

32. MACINTYRE, J. Early X-ray photographs. The Journal of the Röntgen Society, *3*, 137–138, 1906–7.

33. MACINTYRE, J. and ADAM, J. British Medical Journal, *1*, 750, 1896.

34. ARDRAN, G. M. Cineradiology. British Journal of Radiology, *46*, 885–888, 1973.

35. MACINTYRE, J. X-ray records for the cinematograph. Archives of Clinical Skiagraphy, *1*, 37, 1896–7.

36. MACINTYRE, J. Letter 'X-rays: Instantaneous photography and experiments upon the heart and other soft tissues'. The Lancet, *1*, 1455, 1896.

37. MACINTYRE, J. Roentgen rays in laryngeal surgery. British Medical Journal, *1*, 1094, 1896.

38. SCHUSTER, N. Early days of Roentgen photography in Britain. British Medical Journal, *2*, 1164–1168, 1962; and Radiographic history made in Lancashire. Manchester Medical Gazette, *47*, 18–20, 1968.

39. MEREDITH, W. J. 'What Manchester thinks . . .' British Journal of Radiology, *41*, 2–11, 1968.

40. SCHUSTER, A. On Röntgen's rays. Nature, *53*, 268, 1896.

41. British Medical Journal, *1*, 621, 1896; and SCHUSTER, LADY. Letter to The Times, 5 February, 1932.

42. *Dictionary of National Biography, 1931–40*, 791–793. London: Oxford University Press, 1949.

43. HOLLAND, C. T. X-rays in 1896. Liverpool Medico-Chirurgical Journal, *45*, 61–76, 1937.

44. JONES, R. and LODGE, O. The discovery of a bullet lost in the wrist by means of the Roentgen rays. The Lancet, *1*, 476–477, 1896.

45. *Dictionary of National Biography 1931–40*, 498–500. London: Oxford University Press, 1949.

46. *Dictionary of National Biography 1931–40*, 541–543. London: Oxford University Press, 1949.

47. LODGE, O. Lectures to medical practitioners on physics applied to medicine. Archives of the Roentgen Ray, *8*, 159–164, 186–194, 211–220, 1903–4; and *9*, 4–11, 38–45, 54–64, 1904–5.

48. Obituary notice, British Journal of Radiology, *13*, 319, 1940.

49. Obituary notice, British Journal of Radiology, *14*, 94–95, 1941.

50. BRAILSFORD, J. F. Roentgen's discovery of X-rays. Their application to medicine and surgery. British Journal of Radiology, *19*, 453–461, 1946.

51. REYNOLDS, H. Mr. John Hall-Edwards, L.R.C.P., F.R.P.S. The Moseley Society Journal, *3*, 1–6, 1896.

52. Obituary notice, British Medical Journal, *2*, 363, 1926.

53. Southport Visitor, 15 February 1896; and CLAYTON, J. H. Needle in Hand: Removal. British Medical Journal, *1*, 749, 1896.

54. British Medical Journal, *1*, 735, 1896.

55. HALL-EDWARDS, J. F. Radiography popularly described. The Photographic Review, 91–97, 1896.

56. British Medical Journal, *1*, 749, 1896.

57. TURNER, D. Medico-Chirurgical Society of Edinburgh meeting of 5 February 1896. The Lancet, *1*, 425, 1896.

58. Obituary notice, British Journal of Radiology, *2*, 330, 1929.

59. Report on The Royal Infirmary of Edinburgh. Radiography, *29*, 11–19, 1963.

60. GLASSER, O. *Wilhelm Conrad Röntgen and the Early History of the Roentgen Rays.* London: John Bale, Sons and Danielsson Ltd., 1933.

61. HARTLEY, J. B. The diagnosis and delineation of cancer. British Journal of Radiology, *38*, 321–327, 1965.

62. SOUTTAR, H. S. Team work in the treatment of cancer. British Journal of Radiology, *17*, 229–234, 1944.

63. DAVIDSON, J. M. The position of a broken needle in the foot determined by means of Roentgen's rays. British Medical Journal, *1*, 558–559, 1896.

64. LODGE, T. Developmental defects of the cranial vault. British Journal of Radiology, *48*, 421–434, 1975.

65. WARD, H. S. Marvels of the new light. Notes on the Rontgen rays, The Windsor Magazine, *3*, 372 et seqq., 1896; and Obituary notice, British Journal of Radiology, *4*, 338, 1931.

66. Editorial, The new photography. The Lancet, *1*, 875, 1896.

67. Archives of the Roentgen Ray, *11*, 188–193, 1906–7.

68. Nature, *55*, 12, 1896.

69. The Journal of the Röntgen Society, *3*, 26, 1906–7.

70. Obituary notice, British Journal of Radiology, *28*, 209, 1955.

Chapter Four – EARLY APPARATUS AND THE MAKERS

1. GROVER, H. W. Reflections on early X-ray engineering. British Journal of Radiology, *46*, 757–761, 1973.

2. WRIGHT, R. S. Letter to the editor. British Journal of Radiology, *1*, 441, 1928.

3. GLASSER, O. *Wilhelm Conrad Röntgen and the Early History of the Roentgen Rays*. London: John Bale, Sons and Danielsson, 1933.

4. LEMP, H. Some interesting history on the X-ray rectifying switch. In A. J. Bruwer (editor): *Classic Descriptions in Diagnostic Roentgenology*. Springfield, Illinois: Charles C. Thomas, 1964.

5. Archives of the Roentgen Ray, *5*, 13, 1900–1.

6. Archives of the Roentgen Ray, *3*, 12–13, 1898–9, and *8*, 14, 1903–4.

7. Archives of the Roentgen Ray, *14*, 338, 1909–10.

8. Archives of the Roentgen Ray, *3*, 95–105, 1898–9.

9. Archives of the Roentgen Ray, *10*, end-page advertisement, 1905–6.

10. BURNSIDE, E. E. The Wappler interrupter. The Journal of the Röntgen Society, *6*, 50–51, 1910.

11. Archives of the Roentgen Ray, *3*, 59–60, 1898–9.

12. WILD, C. H. J. High tension generators in 1898 and 1908. Radiography, *23*, 91–94, 1957.

13. MORTON, E. R. The relative value of various types of high-tension transformers (including coil) used for the production of X-rays. Archives of the Roentgen Ray, *15*, 192–197, 1910–1.

14. GRIGG, E. R. N. *The Trail of the Invisible Light*. Springfield, Illinois: Charles C. Thomas, 1964.

15. SNOOK, H. C. A new Roentgen generator. Archives of the Roentgen Ray, *13*, 186–188, 1908–9.

16. WRIGHT, R. S. The new Snook Röntgen apparatus. The Journal of the Röntgen Society, *5*, 95–99, 1909.

17. Archives of the Roentgen Ray, *14*, 160, 1909–10.

18. HONDIUS BOLDINGH, W. Technical evolution of roentgenology. Medicamundi, *16*, 9–17, 1971.

19. GARDINER, J. H. The origin, history and development of the X-ray tube. The Journal of the Röntgen Society, *5*, 66–80, 1905.

20. REYNOLDS, R. J. Sixty years of radiology. British Journal of Radiology, *29*, 238–245, 1956; and The early history of radiology in Britain. Clinical Radiology, *12*, 136–142, 1961.

21. FINZI, N. S. The early days of radiology. Clinical Radiology, *12*, 143–146, 1961.

22. Archives of the Roentgen Ray, *3*, 59–60, 1898–9.

23. Archives of the Roentgen Ray, *8*, 14, 1903–4.

24. WILD, C. H. J. Tubes at the turn of the century. Radiography, *23*, 129–132, 1957.

25. RODMAN, G. H. The historical collection of X-ray tubes. The Journal of the Röntgen Society, *5*, 85–87, 1909.

26. MOULD, R. F. The British Institute of Radiology historical collection of X-ray tubes, lantern slides, journals and books. British Institute of Radiology Bulletin, *5*, 3–10, 1979.

27. The Journal of the Röntgen Society, *7*, 22, 1911.

28. Obituary notice, British Journal of Radiology, *48*, 1050, 1975.

29. COOLIDGE, W. D. A powerful Röntgen ray tube with a pure electron discharge. The Physical Review, *2* (N.S.), 409–430, 1913; and Archives of the Roentgen Ray, *18*, 359–368, 1913–4.

30. British Medical Journal, *1*, 431–434, 1896.

31. PHILLIPS, C. E. S. An automatic vacuum pump. The Journal of the Röntgen Society, *1*, 53–58, 1904–5.

32. OWEN, E. A. Fifty years of X-ray production and measurement in medical radiology. British Journal of Radiology, *18*, 369–376, 1945.

33. Proceedings of the Royal Society of Medicine, *9*, Electro-Therapeutical Section 134–141, 1915–6.

34. Archives of the Roentgen Ray, *19*, 159–160 and 196–197, 1914–5.

35. TUNNICLIFFE, E. J. The British X-ray industry: a brief historical review. British Journal of Radiology, *46*, 861–871, 1973.

36. SHANKS, S. C. Radiology in the twenties. British Journal of Radiology, *46*, 766–767, 1973.

37. British Journal of Radiology, *2*, N.S., 1, 1929.

38. RAMSEY, L. J. Radiography and monarchy. Radiography, *44*, 137–141, 1978.

39. Illustrated London News, 1142, 15 December 1928.

40. Obituary notice, Radiography, *34*, 35, 1968.

41. Some X-ray appliances. Archives of the Roentgen Ray, *3*, 32–33, 1898–9.

42. Obituary notice, British Medical Journal, *1*, 468, 1919.

43. Archives of the Roentgen Ray, *7*, 100, 1902–3.

44. WILD, C. H. J. Radiographic technique and X-ray protection 1898–1908. Radiography, *23*, 193–197, 1957.

45. Archives of the Roentgen Ray, *10*, 289, 1905–6.

46. REID, A. D. The technique of skiagraphy. Archives of the Roentgen Ray, *16*, 70–73, 1909–10.

47. BUCKY, G. A grating-diaphragm to cut off secondary rays from the object. Archives of the Roentgen Ray, *18*, 6–9, 1913–4.

48. RAMSEY, L. J. Luminescence and intensifying screens in the early days of radiography. Radiography, *42*, 245–253, 1976.

49. FUCHS, A. W. Evolution of Roentgen film. American Journal of Roentgenology, *75*, 30–48, 1956.

50. SALVIONI, E. Investigations on Röntgen rays. Nature, *53*, 424–425, 1896.

51. Archives of Clinical Skiagraphy, *1*, 7–8, 1896–7.

52. Nature, *53*, 470, 1896.

53. RÖNTGEN, W. C. On a new kind of rays. Nature, *53*, 274–276, 1896.

54. BRUWER, A. J. (editor), *Classic Descriptions in Diagnostic Roentgenology*. Springfield, Illinois: Charles C. Thomas, 1964.

55. MEES, C. E. K. *From Dry Plates to Ektachrome Film. A Story of Photographic Research.* New York: Ziff-Davis Publishing Company, 1961.

56. GAUNTLETT, M. D. *A History of Kodak Limited to 1977*. Harrow: Privately printed, 1978.

57. SWINTON, A. A. C. The action of the Röntgen rays upon photographic film. Nature, *53*, 613, 1896.

58. WRIGHT, R. S. Letter to the editor. The Journal of the Röntgen Society, *5*, 103, 1909.

59. Obituary notice, British Journal of Radiology, *13*, 122, 1940.

60. Obituary notice, British Journal of Radiology, *34*, 820, 1961.

61. *Ehrenbuch der Röntgenologen und Radiologen aller Nationen. Grossbritannien.* Munich: Urban & Schwarzenberg, 1959.

62. Radiography, *14*, 116, 1948.

63. Obituary notice, British Journal of Radiology, *50*, 768, 1977.

64. ANDREWS, C. Sixty years of radiology – X-ray apparatus. British Journal of Radiology, *29*, 249–252, 1956.

65. Obituary notice, British Journal of Radiology, *22*, 610, 1949.

66. The Journal of the Röntgen Society, *3*, 44–46 and 139, 1906–7.

67. Obituary notice, British Journal of Radiology, *47*, 68, 1974.

68. Archives of the Roentgen Ray, *6*, 3, 1901–2.

69. Archives of Radiology and Electrotherapy, *21*, 199, 1916–17.

70. SHANKS, S. C. Radiology in the twenties. British Journal of Radiology, *46*, 766–767, 1973.

71. The Journal of the Röntgen Society, *5*, 20, 1909.

72. Archives of the Roentgen Ray, *3*, 114–115, 1898–9.

73. WARD, H. S. Marvels of the new light. Notes on the Röntgen rays. The Windsor Magazine, *3*, 372 et seqq., 1896.

74. The Journal of the Röntgen Society, *5*, 84, 1909.

75. Archives of the Roentgen Ray, *3*, 2–13 and 59–60, 1898–9; and *5*, 61–68, 1900–1.

76. DAVIES, H. W. Three score years and ten. British Journal of Radiology, *38*, 641–652, 1965.

77. Obituary notice, Radiography, *32*, 68, 1966.

78. ANDREWS, C. Half a century of shadows. Radiography, *22*, 250–254, 1956.

79. Obituary notices, Radiography, *38*, 156, 1972; and British Journal of Radiology, *46*, 837, 1973.

80. Obituary notice, British Journal of Radiology, *43*, 912, 1970.

81. Obituary notice, British Journal of Radiology, *16*, 198, 1943.

Chapter Five – EARLY X-RAY DEPARTMENTS – I: THE MILLER, THE LONDON, ST. BAR-
THOLOMEW'S, ST. THOMAS'S AND GUY'S HOSPITALS

1. SIMMONS, G. A. The constitution and organization of the X-ray department of a general hospital. British Medical Journal, *1*, 535–537, 1910.
2. Special article. The 'X' rays at the Miller Hospital, Greenwich Road. The Kentish Mercury, 4 October 1901.
3. Obituary notice, The Kentish Mercury, 14 September 1900.
4. Archives of the Roentgen Ray, *2*, 50–54, 1897–8.
5. Obituary notice, British Medical Journal, *2*, 870, 1900.
6. Archives of the Roentgen Ray, *5*, 35, 1900–1.
7. Archives of the Roentgen Ray, *2*, 13–16, 1897–8.
8. Archives of the Roentgen Ray, *4*, 103, 1899–1900.
9. Archives of the Roentgen Ray, *6*, 40, 1901–2.
10. Obituary notice, The Kentish Mercury, 16 March 1906.
11. Archives of the Roentgen Ray, *3*, 48, 1898–9.
12. Archives of the Roentgen Ray, *2*, 61, 1897–8.
13. REYNOLDS, R. J. The early history of radiology in Britain. Clinical Radiology, *12*, 136–142, 1961.
14. Editorial comment, The Journal of Physical Therapeutics, *1*, 1, 1900.
15. Obituary notice, British Medical Journal, *1*, 800, 1930.
16. DAVIDSON, J. M. and HEDLEY, W. S. A method of precise localisation and measurement by means of Roentgen rays. The Lancet, *2*, 1001, 1897.
17. BARCLAY, A. E. Early days of X-rays at the London Hospital. London Hospital Gazette, 170–173, September 1947.
18. Archives of the Roentgen Ray, *2*, 62, 1897–8.
19. SEQUEIRA, J. H. and MORTON, E. R. The light, X-ray and electrical departments at The London Hospital. Archives of the Roentgen Ray, *10*, 270–274, 1905–6.
20. BARNARD, T. W. Illustrated notes from the early days of radiography. Radiography, *33*, 234–238, 1967.
21. BATTEN, G. Men, booms, steady progress. Proceedings of the Royal Society of Medicine, *20*, Electrotherapeutical Section 31–42, 1926; and British Journal of Radiology, *32*, 26–33, 1927.
22. SPEAR, F. G. Radiation martyrs. British Journal of Radiology, *29*, 273, 1956.
23. MACLEOD, J. M. H. Further remarks on the treatment of ringworm of the scalp by the X-rays. British Medical Journal, *2*, 619–620, 1905.
24. Obituary notice, British Journal of Radiology, *17*, 82, 1944.
25. Obituary notices, British Medical Journal, *1*, 691, 1941; and British Journal of Radiology, *14*, 214, 1941.
26. JONES, H. L. The Electrical Department, St. Bartholomew's Hospital. Archives of the Roentgen Ray, *10*, 108–111, 1905–6.
27. BURROWS, H. J. Pioneer radiology at Barts. The Barts Journal, to be published in 1986.
28. Obituary notices. Archives of Radiology and Electrotherapy, *20*, 61, 1915–6; and British Medical Journal, *1*, 664 and 700, 1915.
29. Archives of the Roentgen Ray, *4*, 102, 1899–1900; and Archives of the Roentgen Ray, *11*, 170, 1906–7.
30. COSTA, J. R. Notes and impressions of Europe. Archives of the Roentgen Ray, *13*, 296–298, 1908–9.
31. COHEN OF BIRKENHEAD, LORD. The physician's debt to radiology. British Journal of Radiology, *31*, 170–173, 1958.
32. Obituary notice, British Journal of Radiology, *29*, 227–228, 1924.
33. Archives of the Roentgen Ray, *4*, 36 and 85, 1899–1900; and *7*, 114–115, 1902–3.
34. McLAREN, J. W. An historic X-ray. St. Thomas's Hospital Gazette, *42*, 7–8, 1944.
35. Report of a meeting of Medical and Physical Society on 13 February 1896. Cited by McLaren, see Reference 5-34.

36. The new X-ray department. St. Thomas' Hospital Gazette, *7*, 94–96, 1897; reprinted in Radiography, *30*, 213–214, 1964.

37. Obituary notice, Archives of the Roentgen Ray, *7*, 50, 1902–3; and BRUWER, A. J. Letter to the editor. Radiography, *31*, 226, 1965.

38. Archives of the Roentgen Ray, *5*, 35, 1900–1.

39. KAYE, G. W. C. The story of protection. Radiography, *6*, 41–60, 1940.

40. Obituary notice, Radiography, *24*, 44, 1958.

41. REID, A. D. History of the X-ray department at St. Thomas' Hospital. Proceedings of the Royal Society of Medicine, *7*, Electro-Therapeutical Section 23–25, 1913–4.

42. GOULDESBOROUGH, C. Summary of work in the X-ray department at St. Thomas' Hospital for the year 1913. Proceedings of the Royal Society of Medicine, *7*, Electro-Therapeutical Section 25–28, 1913–4.

43. The Roentgen rays. Guy's Hospital Gazette, 187, 1896.

44. Guy's Hospital Gazette, 185, 1897.

45. Skiagraphy in the Hospital. Guy's Hospital Gazette, 202, 1897.

46. J.T.D. How to take a Skiagram. Guy's Hospital Gazette, 496–498, 1897.

47. ALLSOPP, C. B. The development of radiology. Guy's Hospital Gazette, 457–463, 1964.

48. KIRKMAN, A. H. B. and SHENTON, E. W. H. The Roentgen rays as a means of diagnosis. Guy's Hospital Gazette, 462–464, 1899.

49. SHENTON, E. W. H. Notes on the setting up and working of an X-ray installation. Guy's Hospital Reports, *55*, 69–82, 1901.

50. Archives of the Roentgen Ray, *7*, 100, 1902–3.

51. SHENTON, E. W. H. The diagnosis of renal calculi in Guy's Hospital. Archives of the Roentgen Ray, *8*, 26–33, 1903–4; and Archives of the Roentgen Ray, *11*, 298–300, 1906–7 (The Lancet, 15 September 1906).

52. Journal of Physical Therapeutics, *3*, 110–112, 1902.

53. Obituary notice, British Medical Journal, *2*, 1273–4, 1955.

54. SHENTON, E. W. H. A system of radiography. Archives of the Roentgen Ray, *6*, 62–70, 1901–2.

55. Archives of the Roentgen Ray, *4*, 18, 1899–1900.

56. Medical Electrology and Radiology, *8*, 119–121, 1907.

57. *Medical Who's Who*, 1918.

58. JORDAN, A. C. X-ray examinations for the physician. Archives of the Roentgen Ray, *14*, 70–75, 1909–10.

59. Archives of the Roentgen Ray, *16*, 116–117, 1911–2.

Chapter Six – EARLY X-RAY DEPARTMENTS – II: OTHER LONDON HOSPITALS

1. Editorial, Archives of the Roentgen Ray, *16*, 241, 1911–2.

2. COSTA, J. R. Notes and impressions of Europe. Archives of the Roentgen Ray, *13*, 296–298, 1908–9.

3. Medical Electrology and Radiology, *6*, 3–5, 102–103 and 135–144, 1905.

4. REID, A. D. The technique of skiagraphy. Archives of the Roentgen Ray, *16*, 70–73, 1910–1.

5. GRAHAM-HODGSON, H. The radiography of the paranasal sinuses. British Journal of Radiology, *4*, 421–431, 1930.

6. Obituary notices, British Medical Journal, *2*, 740, 1960; and British Journal of Radiology, *33*, 708, 1960.

7. THOMSON, H. C. *The Story of the Middlesex Hospital Medical School 1835–1935*. London: John Murray, 1935; and Radiography, *25*, 111–117, 1959.

8. *Ehrenbuch der Röntgenologen und Radiologen aller Nationem. Grossbritannien,* Munich: Urban & Schwarzenberg, 1959.

9. LYSTER, C. R. C. The treatment of disease by different forms of rays. Archives of the Middlesex Hospital, *1*, 87–100, 1903.

10. Obituary notice, British Journal of Radiology, *24*, 273–275, 1920.

11. OLIVER, R. Seventy-five years of radiation protection. British Journal of Radiology, *46*, 854–860, 1973.

12. Radiography, *3*, 115, 1937; and *25*, 111–117, 1959.

13. Obituary notice, Radiography, *21*, 75, 1955.

14. Obituary notices, The Lancet, *1*, 633, 1919; and British Journal of Radiology, *17*, 229, 1919.

15. Archives of the Roentgen Ray, *2*, 14, 1897–8.

16. DAVIDSON, J. M. A method of localization by means of X-rays. Archives of the Roentgen Ray, *2*, 64–68, 1897–8.

17. Archives of the Roentgen Ray, *5*, 35, 1899–1900.

18. DAVIDSON, J. M. Stereoscopic radiography. Archives of Radiology and Electrotherapy, *23*, 340–346, 1918–9.

19. Obituary notice, Archives of Radiology and Electrotherapy, *23*, 337–340, 1918–9.

20. Obituary notice, British Medical Journal, *1*, 480, 1921.

21. The Journal of the Röntgen Society, *4*, 22, 1907–8; and Archives of the Roentgen Ray, *12*, 89, 1907–8.

22. SHANKS, S. C. Radiology in the twenties. British Journal of Radiology, *46*, 766–767, 1973.

23. ROWLAND, S. Archives of Skiagraphy, *1*, 13, 1896–7.

24. Obituary notice, British Journal of Radiology, *5*, 853–858, 1932.

25. Medical Electrology and Radiology, *8*, 119–121, 1907.

26. Medical Electrology and Radiology, *7*, 153–161, 1906; The Journal of the Röntgen Society, *3*, 83–86, 1906–7.

27. The Lancet, *2*, 1621, 1896.

28. SIMMONS, G. A. The constitution and organization of the X-ray department of a general hospital. British Medical Journal, *1*, 535–537, 1910.

29. Archives of the Roentgen Ray, *12*, 238–248, 1907–8; and Medical Electrology and Radiology, *8*, 238, 1907.

30. Obituary notice, British Journal of Radiology, *20*, 297, 1947.

31. FINZI, N. S. Sixty years of radiology – radiotherapy. British Journal of Radiology, *29*, 245–249, 1956.

32. ORTON, G. H. The X-ray diagnosis of renal and uteral calculi. Archives of the Roentgen Ray, *12*, 238–248, 1907–8.

33. Obituary notice, British Journal of Radiology, *20*, 441, 1947.

34. ANDREWS, C. Half a century of shadows. Radiography, *22*, 250–254, 1956; and Obituary notice, British Journal of Radiology, *7*, 256–262, 1934; and Obituary notice, British Medical Journal, *1*, 693–654, 1934.

35. Archives of the Roentgen Ray, *7*, 50, 1902–3.

36. MELVILLE, S. Presidential address to the British Institute of Radiology, *7*, 3–8, 1934.

37. Archives of the Roentgen Ray, *15*, 31, 1910–1; Radiography, *20*, 177–178, 1954.

38. BLAIR, L. G. The role of radiography in the diagnosis and treatment of diseases of the chest. Radiography, *14*, 103–109, 1948.

39. The Electrical Institute of the Cancer Hospital, Fulham. Archives of the Roentgen Ray, *17*, 248–253, 1912–3.

40. Appreciation, British Journal of Radiology, *1*, 104–107, 1927; and SCOTT, J. Looking back. Radiography, *36*, 206–209, 1970.

41. WILLIAMS, C. X-rays in the treatment of carcinoma and sarcoma. Medical Electrology and Radiology, *7*, 70–77, 1906; and X-rays in the treatment of cancer. Archives of the Roentgen Ray, *11*, 134–142, 1906–7.

42. Medical Electrology and Radiology, *7*, 93–94; and *113*, 1906.

43. Archives of the Roentgen Ray, *13*, 221, 1908–9.

44. WATSON, W. 1895 and all that. Radiography, *27*, 305–315, 1961.

45. Obituary notice, British Journal of Radiology, *28*, 163, 1955.

Chapter Seven – EARLY X-RAY DEPARTMENTS – III: HOSPITALS IN THE PROVINCES AND BEYOND

1. BARCLAY, A. E. The organisation and equipment of an X-ray department. The Journal of the Röntgen Society, *19*, 55–74, 1923.
2. Obituary notice, British Medical Journal, *2*, 363, 1926.
3. Archives of the Roentgen Ray, *12*, 302, 1907–8; and *13*, 87–88, 1908–9.
4. Archives of the Roentgen Ray, *13*, 44, 1908–9.
5. Archives of the Roentgen Ray, *13*, 243–250, 1908–9.
6. Obituary notice, The Lancet, *2*, 410, 1926.
7. BRAILSFORD, J. F. Tuberculosis and radiography. Radiography, *23*, 157–161, 1957.
8. Radiography, *26*, 231–233, 1960.
9. Radiography, *28*, 389–390, 1962.
10. Obituary notices, British Journal of Radiology, *34*, 269, 1961; and British Medical Journal, *1*, 433, 1961.
11. The new method in hospital practice. British Medical Journal, *1*, 1412, 1896.
12. SMITH, C. Medical radiology: its practical application 1895–1914. In CHECKLAND, O. and LAMB, M. (editors): *Health Care and Social History. The Glasgow Case.* Aberdeen: Aberdeen University Press, 1982.
13. MACINTYRE, J. The application of the Röntgen rays in the medical and surgical departments of the Royal Infirmary, Glasgow. Glasgow Hospital Reports, *1*, 290–320, 1898.
14. SCOTT, J. The birth of radiology in Scotland. Radiography, *17*, 46–49, 1951.
15. MACINTYRE, J. The Electrical Pavilion, Glasgow Royal Infirmary. Archives of the Roentgen Ray, *7*, 101–102, 1902–3.
16. RAMSAY, A. M. Penetrating wounds of the eye, complicated by the presence of a foreign body in the eyeball. Glasgow Hospital Reports, *3*, 386–396, 1900.
17. Obituary notice, British Medical Journal, *1*, 445–446, 1928.
18. JUPE, M. Early days in radiology in Britain. Clinical Radiology, *12*, 147–154, 1961.
19. Archives of the Roentgen Ray, *5*, 13, 1900–1.
20. MACQUEEN, L. and KERR, A. B. *The Western Infirmary 1874–1974*. Glasgow: Horn, 1974.
21. Obituary notices, British Medical Journal, *2*, 90–91, 1935; and British Journal of Radiology, *8*, 598–9, 1935.
22. JONES, R. and LODGE, O. The discovery of a bullet lost in the wrist by means of the Roentgen rays. The Lancet, *1*, 476–477, 1896.
23. HOLLAND, C. T. X-rays in 1896. Liverpool Medico-Chirurgical Journal, *45*, 61–76, 1937.
24. HOLLAND, C. T. Presidential address. The Journal of the Röntgen Society, *1*, 25–38, 1904–5.
25. HOLLAND, C. T. X-rays at the Liverpool hospitals. Archives of the Roentgen Ray, *7*, 112–114, 1902–3.
26. Archives of the Roentgen Ray, *12*, 271–272, 1907–8.
27. WHITAKER, P. H. The birth and growth of radiology. Transactions of the Liverpool Medical Institution 21–35, 1961.
28. Archives of the Roentgen Ray, *4*, 79, 1899–1900.
29. MARSDEN, P. H. On radiography applied to the dental surgeon. Archives of the Roentgen Ray, *6*, 54–57, 1901–2.
30. Obituary notice, British Journal of Radiology, *1*, 24–25, 1927.
31. Archives of the Roentgen Ray, *16*, 328, 1911–2.
32. BARCLAY, A. E. Early days of radiology in Manchester. The Manchester University Medical School Gazette, *1*, 114–121, 1948.
33. Obituary notice, British Journal of Radiology, *14*, 94–95, 1941.
34. Obituary notice, British Medical Journal, *2*, 211–212, 1946.
35. TURNER, D. Some reflections based upon the work done in the Electrical Department of the Royal Infirmary, Edinburgh. Archives of the Roentgen Ray, *13*, 82–83, 1908–9.
36. TURNER, A. L. *Story of a Great Hospital, the Royal Infirmary of Edinburgh, 1728–1929*. Edinburgh: James Thin, The Mercat Press, 1979.

37. Obituary notice, British Journal of Radiology, *2*, 330, 1929.
38. Obituary notice, British Journal of Radiology, *2*, 284, 1929.
39. KAYE, G. W. C. The story of protection. Radiography, *6*, 41–60, 1940.
40. Obituary notice, British Journal of Radiology, *6*, 691–694, 1933.
41. BARCLAY, A. E. Passing of the Cambridge diploma. British Journal of Radiology, *15*, 351–354, 1942.
42. Report of Meeting, British Journal of Radiology, *3*, 565–566, 1930.
43. FAWCITT, R. Opportunity knocks at the door. British Journal of Radiology, *24*, 57–66, 1951.
44. British Journal of Radiology, *24*, 580, 1951.
45. Edinburgh Royal Infirmary X-ray Department. Radiography, *29*, 11, 1963.
46. MORISON, J. Edinburgh Royal Infirmary Radiological Department. British Journal of Radiology, *31*, 516–517, 1926.
47. Radiography, *38*, 66–67, 1972.
48. BARCLAY, A. E. The old order changes. British Journal of Radiology, *22*, 300–308, 1949.
49. ENGLAND, I. A. Northern lights – Manchester's outstanding contribution. Radiography, *37*, 27–38, 1971.
50. McGRIGOR, D. B. A personal tribute to Dr. A. E. Barclay. British Journal of Radiology, *22*, 298–299, 1949.
51. Obituary notices, Radiography, *15*, 121, 1949; British Journal of Radiology, *22*, 295–297, 1949.
52. BYTHELL, W. J. S. The X-ray evidence of early pulmonary tuberculosis in young children. Proceedings of the Royal Society of Medicine, *6*, Electrotherapeutical Section 73–79, 1912–3; and The radiographic appearance of bone tumours, benign and malignant. Proceedings of the Royal Society of Medicine, *7*, Electrotherapeutical Section 63–72, 1913–4.
53. Personal information from Professor Ian Isherwood.
54. ANDREWS, C. Sixty years of radiology. British Journal of Radiology, *29*, 249–252, 1956.
55. BARCLAY, A. E. The value of X-ray diagnosis in the digestive system. Archives of the Roentgen Ray, *13*, 310–312, 1908–9.
56. Obituary notice, British Journal of Radiology, *12*, 383, 1939.
57. Obituary notice, British Journal of Radiology, *12*, 318, 1939.
58. Obituary notices, The Lancet, *1*, 1185, 1939; and British Journal of Radiology, *12*, 383–385, 1939.
59. TWINING E. W. The radiology of the chest. British Journal of Radiology, *4*, 658–679, 1930.
60. TWINING, E. W. Tomography by means of a simple attachment to the Potter-Bucky couch. British Journal of Radiology, *10*, 332–347, 1937.
61. LYSHOLM, E. Experiences of venticulography of tumours below the tentorium. British Journal of Radiology, *19*, 437–452, 1946.
62. Archives of the Roentgen Ray, *3*, 40–41, 1898–9.
63. British Medical Journal, *1*, 1225, 1896.
64. WARRICK. C. K. Notes on the history of the Department of Radiology of the Royal Victoria Infirmary, Newcastle upon Tyne. Radiography, *43*, 190–194, 1977.
65. Obituary notice, British Journal of Radiology, *2*, 95, 1929.
66. Obituary notices, British Medical Journal, *1*, 442, 1950; and The Lancet, *1*, 331, 1950.
67. Obituary notice, Radiography, *23*, 337, 1957.
68. Medical Electrology and Radiology, *4*, 222–228, 1903; and *5*, 450–469, 1904.
69. GAMLEN, H. E. A simple, rapid and accurate method for localisation of foreign bodies so as to indicate to surgeons the position of the patients when skiagraphed. Archives of Radiology and Electrotherapy, *21*, 175–177, 1916–7.
70. Obituary notice, British Journal of Radiology, *17*, 12, 1944.
71. Obituary notice, Radiography, *19*, 135, 1953.
72. Obituary notices, British Journal of Radiology, *50*, 155, 1977; and British Medical Journal, *2*, 705, 1976.

73. WATSON, D. M. *Proud Heritage. A History of the Royal South Hants Hospital 1838–1971.* Southampton: G. F. Wilson, 1979.

74. ZORAB, E. C. *Plus ça change.* Southampton Medical Gazette, *1*, 5–7, 1975; and Minute Book of the Southampton Medical Society.

75. Proceedings of the Royal Society of Medicine, *6*, Electrotherapeutical Section 157–158, 1912–3.

76. Obituary notices, The Times, 17 June 1933; British Journal of Radiology, *6*, 504, 1933; and The Lancet, *1*, 1367, 1933.

77. Proceedings of the Royal Society of Medicine, *7*, Electrotherapeutical Section 5–24, 1913–4.

78. PORTER, D. C. The new photography. Ulster Medical Journal, *31*, 117–127, 1962.

79. MARSHALL, R. *Fifty Years on the Grosvenor Road. An Account of the Rise and Progress of the Royal Victoria Hospital, Belfast during the Years 1903–1953.*

80. RANKIN, J. C. Report on the X-ray treatment of lupus at the Royal Victoria Hospital, Belfast. Archives of the Roentgen Ray, *10*, 40–42, 1905–6.

81. RANKIN, J. C. Treatment of malignant diseases by X-rays. Archives of the Roentgen Ray, *10*, 302–303, 1905–6.

82. LEMAN, R. M. Fifty years – a radiographic retrospect. Radiography, *33*, 101–107, 1967.

83. LEMAN, R. M. General technique for radiography of the joints. British Journal of Radiology, *5*, 501–512, 1932; and report in Radiography, *25*, 155, 1959.

84. Obituary notice, British Journal of Radiology, *14*, 63–64, 1941.

85. Obituary notice, British Medical Journal, *2*, 650, 1972.

Chapter Eight – RADIOLOGICAL JOURNALS BEFORE 1930

1. ALLSOPP, C. B. Nothing new? British Journal of Radiology, *37*, 325–333, 1964.

2. JUPE, M. Early days of radiology in Britain. Clinical Radiology, *12*, 147–154, 1961.

3. Archives of the Roentgen Ray, *3*, 45, 1898–9.

4. Obituary notices, British Medical Journal, *1*, 375, 1917; and The Lancet, *1*, 552, 1917.

5. BISHOP, P. J. The evolution of the British Journal of Radiology. British Journal of Radiology, *46*, 833–836, 1973.

6. HEDLEY, W. S. Roentgen rays. A survey, present and retrospective. Archives of the Roentgen Ray, *2*, 6–12, 1897–8.

7. Archives of the Roentgen Ray, *2*, 14, 1897–8.

8. Archives of the Roentgen Ray, *2*, 31–32, 1897–8; and REYNOLDS, R. J. The early history of radiology in Britain. Clinical Radiology, *12*, 136–142, 1961.

9. Archives of the Roentgen Ray, *4*, 14, 1899–1900; and DAVIES, H. W. Three score years and ten. British Journal of Radiology, *38*, 641–652, 1965.

10. The Journal of the Röntgen Society, *4*, 75–84, 1907–8.

11. Obituary notice, British Medical Journal, *2*, 725, 1940.

12. Archives of the Roentgen Ray, *5*, 10, 1900–1.

13. Archives of the Roentgen Ray, *8*, 23–24, 1903–4.

14. Archives of the Roentgen Ray, *9*, 37, 1904–5.

15. The Journal of the Röntgen Society, *1*, 18, 1904–5.

16. Archives of the Roentgen Ray, *13*, 169, 1908–9.

17. Archives of the Roentgen Ray, *13*, 225, 1908–9.

18. Obituary notice, The Journal of the Röntgen Society, *15*, 55–56, 1919.

19. FINZI, N. S. The early days of radiology. Clinical Radiology, *12*, 143–146, 1961.

20. Medical Electrology and Radiology, *6*, 243–246, 1906.

21. Archives of the Roentgen Ray, *14*, 371, 1909–10.

22. Archives of the Roentgen Ray, *19*, 119, 1914–5.

23. Archives of the Roentgen Ray, *19*, 239–240, 1914–5.

24. Archives of the Roentgen Ray, *19*, 275–276, 1914–5.

25. Archives of the Roentgen Ray, *20*, 1–2, 1915–6.

26. Archives of the Roentgen Ray, *25*, 152, 1920–1.

27. Archives of the Roentgen Ray, *23*, 1–2, 1918–9.

28. SHENTON, E. W. H. The Journal of Physical Therapeutics, *3*, 110–112, 1902; and WALSHAM, H., The Journal of Physical Therapeutics, *3*, 161–168, 1902.

29. Medical Electrology and Radiology, *8*, 239, 1907.

30. The Journal of the Röntgen Society, *1*, 1, 1904–5.

31. The Journal of the Röntgen Society, *5*, 66–80, 1909.

32. ROBERTS, R. E. Our heritage. British Journal of Radiology, *11*, 38–45, 1938.

33. Obituary notice, British Journal of Radiology, *19*, 348, 1946.

34. The Journal of the Röntgen Society, *3*, 137–138, 1906–7.

35. The Journal of the Röntgen Society, *3*, 134–135, 1906–7.

36. Proceedings of the Royal Society of Medicine, *1*, Electro-Therapeutical Section 35–54, 1907–8.

37. Proceedings of the Royal Society of Medicine, *6*, Electro-Therapeutical Section 69–86, 1912–3.

38. Proceedings of the Royal Society of Medicine, *2*, Electro-Therapeutical Section 53–68, 1908–9.

39. Proceedings of the Royal Society of Medicine, *3*, Electro-Therapeutical Section 109–124, 1908–9.

40. Proceedings of the Royal Society of Medicine, *4*, Electro-Therapeutical Section 13–30, 1910–1.

41. Proceedings of the Royal Society of Medicine, *6*, Electro-Therapeutical Section 117–154, 1912–3.

42. Proceedings of the Royal Society of Medicine, *5*, Electro-Therapeutical Section 1–8, 1911–2.

43. Proceedings of the Royal Society of Medicine, *7*, Electro-Therapeutical Section 5–22, 1913–4; and *8*, 66–69, 1914–5.

44. BENNETT, W. H. The use of the X-rays in the diagnosis of appendicitis and other abdominal conditions. The Lancet, *1*, 1461–1465, 1908.

45. Proceedings of the Royal Society of Medicine, *1*, Electro-Therapeutical Section 15–34, 1907–8.

46. Proceedings of the Royal Society of Medicine, *2*, Electro-Therapeutical Section 105–106, 1908–9.

47. Proceedings of the Royal Society of Medicine, *3*, Electro-Therapeutical Section 141–147, 1909–10.

48. Proceedings of the Royal Society of Medicine, *4*, Electro-Therapeutical Section 31–32, 1910–1.

49. Proceedings of the Royal Society of Medicine, *7*, Electro-Therapeutical Section 79–86, 1913–4.

50. Proceedings of the Royal Society of Medicine, *9*, Electro-Therapeutical Section 55–59, 1915–6.

51. Proceedings of the Royal Society of Medicine, *1*, Electro-Therapeutical Section 55–64, 1907–8.

52. Proceedings of the Royal Society of Medicine, *3*, Electro-Therapeutical Section 53–72, 1909–10.

53. Proceedings of the Royal Society of Medicine, *3*, Electro-Therapeutical Section 125–138, 1909–10.

54. Proceedings of the Royal Society of Medicine, *4*, Electro-Therapeutical Section 47–69, 1910–1.

55. Proceedings of the Royal Society of Medicine, *2*, Electro-Therapeutical Section 11–34, 1908–9.

56. Proceedings of the Royal Society of Medicine, *8*, Electro-Therapeutical Section 1–18, 1914–5.

57. British Journal of Radiology (Röntgen Society Section), *20*, 1–2, 1924.

58. British Journal of Radiology (B.A.R.P. Section), *29*, 1–2, 1924.

59. BARCLAY, A. E. The history and future of British radiology. British Journal of Radiology (Röntgen Society Section), *21*, 3–20, 1925.

Chapter Nine – SOCIETIES, SECTIONS, AND THE INSTITUTE

1. BARCLAY, A. E. The jubilee of the Röntgen Society. British Journal of Radiology, *20*, 221–222, 1947.
2. BARCLAY, A. E. The dangers of specialisation in medicine. British Journal of Radiology, *4*, 60–82, 1930.
3. Archives of Skiagraphy, *1*, 37, 1896–7.
4. WALSH, D. Cited by Barclay, see Reference 9-1.
5. DAVIES, H. W. Three score years and ten. British Journal of Radiology, *38*, 641–652, 1965.
6. REYNOLDS, R. J. The early history of radiology in Britain. Clinical Radiology, *12*, 136–142, 1961.
7. JUPE, M. Early days of radiology in Britain. Clinical Radiology, *12*, 147–154, 1961.
8. HALE-WHITE, W. Letter to the editor. The Lancet, *2*, 1370, 1930.
9. RUSS, S. Silvanus Thompson Memorial Lecture. British Journal of Radiology, *17*, 261–264, 1944.
10. SPEAR, F. G. The National Radium Commission in retrospect. British Journal of Radiology, *22*, 617–626, 1949.
11. PORTER, G. Molecules in microtime. British Journal of Radiology, *42*, 801–804, 1969.
12. RAMSEY, L. J. Some notable early contributors to radiography – Thompson, Jackson and Campbell Swinton. Radiography, *46*, 289–297, 1980.
13. THOMPSON, J. S. and H. G. *Silvanus Phillips Thompson, his Life and Letters*. London: Fisher Unwin, 1920.
14. Archives of the Roentgen Ray, *2*, 5–6, 1897–8.
15. Archives of the Roentgen Ray, *3*, 46–49, 898–9.
16. *Dictionary of National Biography 1912–1921*, pp 392–394. London: Oxford University Press, 1927.
17. Obituary notices, The Journal of the Röntgen Society, *9*, 1, 1913; and British Medical Journal, *2*, 1426, 1912.
18. Archives of the Roentgen Ray, *2*, 21–30, 1897–8.
19. VEZEY, J. J. The Röntgen Society: its past work and future prospects. The Journal of the Röntgen Society, *1*, 2–8, 1904–5.
20. BATTEN, G. B. Men, booms, steady progress. British Journal of Radiology (B.I.R. Section), *32*, 26–34, 1927.
21. BARCLAY, A. E. The history and future of British radiology. British Journal of Radiology, (Röntgen Society Section), *21*, 3–20, 1925.
22. Obituary notice, The Journal of the Röntgen Society, *3*, 91, 1906–7.
23. RODMAN, G. H. The historical collection of X-ray tubes. The Journal of the Röntgen Society, *5*, 85–87, 1909.
24. Obituary notice, British Journal of Radiology, *6*, 436, 1933.
25. Obituary notice, British Journal of Radiology, *15*, 242, 1942.
26. The Journal of Physical Therapeutics, *3*, 90, 1902.
27. Medical Electrology and Radiology, *5*, 28–36, 1904.
28. Medical Electrology and Radiology, *6*, 219–224, 1905.
29. Medical Electrology and Radiology, *8*, 191, 1907.
30. Proceedings of the Royal Society of Medicine, *1*, 1–14, 1907–8.
31. British Journal of Radiology, *5*, 520, 1932.
32. Archives of the Roentgen Ray, *17*, 125–126, 1912–3.
33. Medical Electrology and Radiology, *4*, 81–82, 1903.
34. Archives of the Roentgen Ray, *8*, 23, 1903–4.
35. Archives of the Roentgen Ray, *9*, 84–85, 1904–5.
36. Archives of the Roentgen Ray, *12*, 90–102, 1907–8; and The Journal of the Röntgen Society, *6*, 123–126, 1910.
37. Archives of Radiology and Electrotherapy, *23*, 1–4, 1918–9.
38. BARCLAY, A. E. The passing of the Cambridge Diploma. British Journal of Radiology, *15*, 351–354, 1942.

39. HOLLAND. C. T. Presidential address to the Röntgen Society. Archives of Radiology and Electrotherapy, *21*, 397–403, 1916–7.
40. Archives of Radiology and Electrotherapy, *20*, 41–42, 1915–6.
41. Archives of the Roentgen Ray, *16*, 328, 1911–2.
42. DAVIDSON, J. M. Stereoscopic radiography. Archives of Radiology and Electrotherapy, *23*, 340–346, 1918–9.
43. Obituary notice, Archives of Radiology and Electrotherapy, *23*, 340–346, 1918–9.
44. ROLLESTON, H. Presidential address to the British Institute of Radiology, British Journal of Radiology, *1*, 1–7, 1928.
45. Letter to the editor. The Lancet, *1*, 1920; and Archives of Radiology and Electrotherapy, *24*, 306–307, 1919–20.
46. ORTON, H. The necessity for education in radiology and electrotherapeutics. Archives of Radiology and Electrotherapy, *22*, 284–288, 1917–8.
47. The British Association of Radiology and Physiotherapy. Archives of Radiology and Electrotherapy, *23*, 1–4, 1918–9.
48. Obituary notice, British Medical Journal, *1*, 494, 1927.
49. Obituary notice, British Journal of Radiology, *22*, 295–299, 1949.
50. Obituary notice, Radiography, *15*, 121, 1949.
51. British Journal of Radiology, *24*, 331, 1951.
52. Obituary notices, British Medical Journal, *1*, 173, 1924; and British Journal of Radiology, *29*, 33–34, 1924.
53. Obituary notice of C. E. S. Phillips, British Journal of Radiology, *18*, 400, 1945.
54. ANDREWS, C. Half a century of shadows. Radiography, *22*, 250–254, 1956.
55. The Journal of the Röntgen Society, *3*, 139, 1906–7.
56. Archives of Radiology and Electrotherapy, *19*, 445, 1914–5.
57. Obituary notice, British Journal of Radiology, *1*, 344–348, 1928.
58. SPEAR, F. G. Questioning the answers. British Journal of Radiology, *35*, 77–89, 1962.
59. Obituary notice, British Journal of Radiology, *24*, 225, 1951.
60. BARCLAY, A. E. Presidential address to the British Institute of Radiology. British Journal of Radiology, *5*, 10–20, 1932.
61. British Journal of Radiology, *4*, 365–366, 1931.
62. British Journal of Radiology, *4*, 404, 1931.
63. British Journal of Radiology, *5*, 78, 1932.
64. KINLOCH, J. The Society and the College of Radiographers – 60 years on. Radiography, *46*, 271–287, 1980.
65. WINCH, C. L. Presidential address to the Society of Radiographers. British Journal of Radiology, *3*, 488–492, 1930.
66. SCOTT, J. Looking back. Radiography, *36*, 206–209, 1970.
67. Archives of Radiology and Electrotherapy, *23*, 201–205, 1918–9.
68. MOODIE, I. *50 Years of History*. London: The Society of Radiographers, 1970.

Chapter Ten – X-RAYS ON THE BATTLEFIELD

1. BEEVOR, W. C. The working of the Roentgen ray in warfare. Journal of the Royal United Service Institution, *42*, 1152–1170, 1898.
2. ABBOTT, F. C. Surgery in the Graeco-Turkish War. The Lancet, *1*, 80–83, 152–156, 1899.
3. BATTERSBY, J. C. The present position of the Roentgen rays in military surgery. Archives of the Roentgen Ray, *3*, 74–80, 1898–9; reprinted as The Roentgen rays in military surgery. British Medical Journal, *1*, 112–114, 1899.
4. ROWLAND, S. The value of the new photography in military surgery. British Medical Journal, *1*, 1059, 1896; and Archives of Clinical Skiagraphy, *1*, 18, 1896–7.

5. STEVENSON, W. F. Notes on Cox's new platinum contact breaker, for use with spark coils. Journal of the Royal Army Medical Corps, *4*, 421–423, 1905.

6. STEVENSON, W. F. Notes on experiences of the Boer War. Journal of the Royal Army Medical Corps, *1*, 83–91, 1903.

7. ALVARO, G. I vantaggi practici della scoperta di Röntgen in chirurgia. Giornale medico del regio esercito, *44*, 385–394, 1896.

8. BURROWS, E. H. The first use of X-rays in war. British Journal of Radiology, *45*, 393–394, 1972; and REYNOLDS, L. The history of the use of the Roentgen ray in warfare. American Journal of Roentgenology, *54*, 649–672, 1945.

9. Obituary notice, British Medical Journal, *2*, 923, 1938.

10. Obituary notices, British Journal of Radiology, *5*, 568, 1932; and The Lancet, *2*, 48, 1932.

11. KÜTTNER, H. Ueber die Bedeutung der Röntgenstrahlen für die Kriegschirurgie; nach Erfahrungen im griechisch-türkischen Krieg 1897. Beitrage zur klinische Chirurgie, *20*, 167–230, 1898.

12. British Medical Journal, *1*, 339, 1898; and Archives of the Roentgen Ray, *3*, 1–2, 1898–9.

13. British Medical Journal, *2*, 666, 1897.

14. HUTCHINSON, H. D. *The Campaign in Tirah, 1897–1898. An Account of the Expedition against the Orakzanis and Afridis under General Sir William Lockhart.* London: Macmillan, 1898.

15. CANTLIE, N. *A History of the Army Medical Department.* Edinburgh: Churchill Livingstone, 1974.

16. Obituary notice, British Medical Journal, *1*, 357, 1927.

17. Strand Magazine, *17*, 777–783, 1899.

18. British Medical Journal, *2*, 1742, 1897.

19. Churchill, W. S. *The River War: an Account of the Reconquest of the Soudan.* London: Longman, 1899.

20. Archives of the Roentgen Ray, *3*, 1–2, 1898–9; and MELVILLE, S. X-ray protection. British Journal of Radiology, *5*, 180, 1932; and REYNOLDS, R. J. Sixty years of radiology. British Journal of Radiology, *29*, 238–245, 1956.

21. Obituary notice, British Journal of Radiology, *1*, 533, 1919.

22. STEVENSON, W. F. (editor). *Report on the Surgical Cases noted in the South African War, 1899–1902.* London: Harrison, 1905.

23. Roentgen ray apparatus for South Africa. British Medical Journal, *2*, 1322, 1899.

24. British Medical Journal, *2*, 1487, 1899.

25. The Lancet, *2*, 1545, 1899.

26. Information from Colonel (Retired) A. V. Tennucci, Curator of Royal Army Medical Corps Historical Museum, Aldershot.

27. MAKINS, G. H. *Surgical Experiences in South Africa 1899–1900.* London: Smith, Elder, 1901.

28. CATLIN, H. X-rays at the War. Archives of the Roentgen Ray, *5*, 48–50, 1900–1.

29. BRUCE, F. Experiences of X-ray work during the siege of Ladysmith. Archives of the Roentgen Ray, *5*, 69–74, 1900–1; reprinted in Journal of the Royal Army Medical Corps, *1*, 92–100, 1903.

30. Journal of the Royal Army Medical Corps, *6*, 403–407, 507–511, 646–652, 1906; and *7*, 17–21, 163–171, 266–270, 380–383, 1907.

31. Journal of the Royal Army Medical Corps, *4*, 421–423, 1905.

32. Archives of the Roentgen Ray, *16*, 55–61, 1911–2.

33. BENSUSAN, A. D. *Silver Images – History of Photography in Africa.* Cape Town: Howard Timmins, 1966; and STOKES, W. A visit to the general hospital, Ladysmith. British Medical Journal, *1*, 1495, 1900.

34. KISCH, H. and TUGMAN, H. St. J. *The Siege of Ladysmith in 120 Pictures.* London: Newnes, 1900.

35. British Medical Journal, *2*, 1452, 1899; and The Lancet, *2*, 1545, 1899.

36. British Medical Journal, *2*, 1489, 1899.

37. British Medical Journal, *2*, 1495, 1900.

38. *A Civilian Hospital, being an Account of the Work of the Portland Hospital and of Experience*

of Wounds and Sickness in South Africa, 1900. London: John Murray, 1901.

39. WALLACE, D. and BOYD, F. D. (editors): *Report of the Work of the Edinburgh and East of Scotland South African Hospital.* Edinburgh: Oliver and Boyd, 1901.

40. FRY, C. M. An old soldier remembers. The Argus (Cape Town), 3 October 1970.

41. HALL-EDWARDS, J. The Roentgen rays in military surgery. British Medical Journal, *2*, 1391, 1899.

42. HALL-EDWARDS, J. The War in South Africa. The Lancet, *1*, 130–131, 1901; and The Roentgen rays in South Africa. The Lancet, *1*, 1755–1756, 1901; and Bullets and their billets. Archives of the Roentgen Ray, *6*, 31–39, 1901–2; and Report of the X-ray department. In Countess Howe (editor): *The Imperial Yeomanry Hospitals in South Africa, 1900–1902, 3,* 90–104. London: Arthur L. Humphreys, 1902.

43. HALL-EDWARDS, J. Photographic experiences in South Africa with the Imperial Yeomanry Hospital. The Amateur Photographer, *31*, 311–314, 1900.

44. Archives of the Roentgen Ray, *4*, 84, 1899–1900.

45. McGRIGOR, D. B. Radiology (In arduis fidelis) 1898–1948. Journal of the Royal Army Medical Corps, *90*, 334–338, 1948.

46. Letter to the editor, The Lancet, *1*, 213, 1900.

47. HENRY, H. Hints for beginners on the development, etc, of X-ray negatives. Journal of the Royal Army Medical Corps, *4*, 418–420, 1905.

48. Archives of the Roentgen Ray, *8*, 45, 1903–4.

49. WALTON, A. J. Early days recalled. Radiography, *32*, 131, 1966; and Early techniques recalled. Radiography, *33*, 134, 1967.

50. Radiography, *38*, 159, 1972.

51. Obituary notice, Radiography, *24*, 44, 1958.

52. McGRIGOR, D. B. A simple apparatus and method for readily detecting the exact location of radio-opaque foreign bodies in the eye or orbital region by radiography. British Journal of Radiology, *2*, 136–148, 1929.

Chapter Eleven – RADIATION INJURY AND PROTECTION

1. KAYE, G. W. C. The story of protection. Radiography, *6*, 41–60, 1940.

2. SCOTT, S. G. Notes on a case of X-ray dermatitis with a fatal termination. Archives of the Roentgen Ray, *15*, 443–444, 1910–1.

3. GARDINER, J. H. Presidential address. The Journal of the Röntgen Society, *12*, 1–10, 1916.

4. British Medical Journal, *1*, 997–998, 1896.

5. WALSH, D. Deep tissue traumatism from Roentgen ray exposure. British Medical Journal, *2*, 272–273, 1897.

6. REYNOLDS, R. J. Sixty years of radiology. British Journal of Radiology, *29*, 238–245, 1956.

7. JUPE, M. Early days of radiology in Britain. Clinical Radiology *12*, 147–154, 1961.

8. FINZI, N. S. The early days of radiology. Clinical Radiology, *12*, 143–146, 1961.

9. BOWLES, R. I. Pathological and therapeutic value of the Roentgen rays. The Lancet, *1*, 655–656, 1896.

10. Archives of the Roentgen Ray, *2*, 82–83 and 92, 1897–8.

11. Archives of the Roentgen Ray, *3*, 46, 1898–9.

12. KIENBÖCK, R. Die Einwirkung des Röntgenlichtes auf die Haut. Münchener medizinische Wochenschrift, *47*, 1581–1582, 1900.

13. ARDRAN, G. M. The Society and protection. Radiography, *37*, 157–165, 1971.

14. The Journal of the Röntgen Society, *1*, 47, 1904–5.

15. BUTCHER, W. D. Protection in X-ray work. Archives of the Roentgen Ray, *10*, 38–39, 1905–6.

16. HALL-EDWARDS, J. The effects upon bone due to prolonged exposure to the X-rays. Archives of the Roentgen Ray, *13*, 144, 1908–9.

17. HALL-EDWARDS, J. On X-ray dermatitis and its prevention. Archives of the Roentgen Ray, *13*, 243–248, 1908–9.

18. Archives of the Roentgen Ray, *14*, 304, 1909–10; and British Medical Journal, *1*, 236, 1910.

19. Archives of the Roentgen Ray, *3*, 59–60, 1898–9; *7*, 22 and 68, 1902–3; and *8*, 12, 1903–4.

20. Proceedings of the Royal Society of Medicine, *2*, Electrotherapeutical Section 11–34, 1908–9.

21. *Ehrenbuch der Röntgenologen und Radiologen aller Nationen. Grossbritannien*, Munich: Urban & Schwarzenberg, 1959.

22. MORTON, E. R. Some bony changes in a case of chronic X-ray dermatitis. British Medical Journal, *2*, 541–543, 1910.

23. Measures of protection against the X-rays at the London Hospital. Archives of the Roentgen Ray, *16*, 343, 1911–2.

24. RUSS, S. On protective devices for X-ray operators. The Journal of the Röntgen Society, *11*, 110–113, 1915.

25. Archives of Radiology and Electrotherapy, *21*, 64, 1916–7.

26. OLIVER, R. Seventy-five years of radiation protection. British Journal of Radiology, *46*, 854–860, 1973.

27. RUSS, S. and LYSTER, R. C. A biological basis for protection against X-rays. The Journal of the Röntgen Society, *14*, 87–93, 1918.

28. RUSS, S. Injurious effects of X-radiation. The Journal of the Röntgen Society, *12*, 38–56, 1916.

29. COLWELL, H. A. and RUSS, S. *X-Ray and Radium Injuries*. London: Oxford University Press, 1934.

30. RUSS, S. The British X-Ray and Radium Protection Committee – a personal retrospect. British Journal of Radiology, *26*, 554–555, 1953.

31. ROCK CARLING, E. The British X-Ray and Radium Protection Committee – *Vale*. British Journal of Radiology, *26*, 557, 1953.

32. SPEAR, F. G. The British X-ray and Radium Protection Committee – the first years. British Journal of Radiology, *26*, 553–554, 1953.

33. ANDREWS, C. The British X-Ray and Radium Committee – the first years. British Journal of Radiology, *26*, 555–557, 1953.

34. Obituary notice, British Journal of Radiology, *17*, 326, 1944.

35. HOWE, Countess (editor). *The Imperial Yeomanry Hospitals in South Africa, 1900–1902*, volume 3, London: Arthur L. Humphreys, 1902.

36. Obituary notice, British Medical Journal, *2*, 452–453, 1944.

37. Obituary notice, British Journal of Radiology, *36*, 702, 1963.

38. COHEN, M. Seventy-five years of radiological physics. British Journal of Radiology, *46*, 841–853, 1973.

39. Obituary notice, British Journal of Radiology, *36*, 862, 1963.

40. STEAD, G. The place of physics in the training of the medical radiologist. British Journal of Radiology, *21*, 373–379, 1948.

41. Obituary notice, American Journal of Roentgenology, *46*, 553–555, 1941.

42. Obituary notice, British Journal of Radiology, *14*, 242–243, 1941.

43. ANDREWS, C. Half a century of shadows. Radiography, *22*, 250–254, 1956.

44. British X-Ray and Radium Protection Committee. Preliminary Report. The Journal of the Röntgen Society, *17*, 100–103, 1921.

45 British X-Ray and Radium Protection Committee. Revised Report No. 1 and 2. The Journal of the Röntgen Society, *20*, 27–34, 1924.

46. KAYE, G. W. C. Radiology and physics. Proceedings of the Royal Society of Medicine, *15*, Electro-Therapeutical Section 33–44, 1921–2.

47. British X-Ray and Radium Protection Committee. Third Revised Report, May 1927. British Journal of Radiology, *32*, 330–336, 1927.

48. ARDRAN, G.M. The Society and X-ray protection. Radiography, *37*, 157–165, 1971.

49. International X-Ray Protection Committee. International recommendations for X-ray and radium protection. British Journal of Radiology, *1*, 358–363, 1928.

50. LOHMÜLLER, F. Prof. Hans Meyer, Bremen, zu seinem 60. Geburtstag. Strahlentherapie, *60*, 5–8, 1937.

51. PIRIE, G. A. Routine examination of the chest. Archives of the Roentgen Ray, *12*, 260–1,

1907–8; and Notes on the value of bismuth in the X-ray examination of the oesophagus and colon (30 cases). Proceedings of the Royal Society of Medicine, *2*, Electro-Therapeutical Section 69–78, 1908–9.

52. Obituary notice, Radiography, *19*, 68, 1953.
53. SPEAR, F. G. Radiation martyrs. British Journal of Radiology, *29*, 273, 1956.
54. Obituary notice, British Journal of Radiology, *2*, 578, 1929.

PICTURE SOURCES

1 Science Museum, London.
2 Ramsey, L. J. Radiography, *46*, 293, 1980.
3 British Institute of Radiology.
4 Glasser, O. *Wilhelm Conrad Röntgen und die Geschichte der Röntgenstrahlen*, 2e Auflage. Berlin: Springer-Verlag, 1959, page 6.
5 Punch, *110*, 45, 1896.
6 British Medical Journal, *1*, 557, 1896.
7 Royal College of Radiologists.
8 Robbins, E. A. Radiography, *21*, 169, 1955.
9 Ramsey, L. J. Radiography, *42*, 249, 1976.
10 T. H. Bridgewater.
11 Ward, W. S. The Windsor Magazine, *3*, 383, April 1896.
12 Left – Science Museum, London.
12 Right – T. H. Bridgewater.
13 Dr. J. D. Duncan.
14 British Institute of Radiology.
15 Ramsey, L. J. Radiography, *42*, 248, 1976.
16 British Institute of Radiology.
17 City of Birmingham Public Libraries Department.
18 Ward, W. S. The Windsor Magazine, *3*, 379, April 1896.
19 Siemens.
20 Left – British Institute of Radiology.
20 Right – Wright, R. S. The Journal of the Röntgen Society, *5*, 96, 1909.
21, 22 British Institute of Radiology.
23 British Journal of Radiology, *1*, 251, 1927.
24 Illustrated London News, 15 December 1928.
25 Archives of the Roentgen Ray, *3*, 32, 1898–9.
26 Davies, H. British Journal of Radiology, *38*, 645, 1965.
27 Walsh, D. *The Röntgen Rays in Medical Work*, 4th edition. London: Ballière, Tindall and Cox, 1907, page 37.
28 Reid, A. Archives of the Roentgen Ray, *14*, 72, 1911–12.
29 Rowland, S. Archives of Clinical Skiagraphy, *1*, 8, 1896–7.
30 Royal College of Radiologists.
31 Kodak News, February 1897.
32 Royal College of Radiologists.

33, 34 Grover, H. W. British Journal of Radiology, *46*, 759, 1973.

35 Ward, W. S. The Windsor Magazine, *3*, 375, April 1896.

36 Greenwich District Hospital Archives by courtesy of Dr. Maxwell J. Wright.

37 Barnard, T. W. Radiography, *33*, 235, 1967.

38 Sequiera, J. H. and Morton, E. R. Archives of the Roentgen Ray, *10*, 274, 1905–6.

39 Colwell, H. A. *An Essay on the History of Electrotherapy and Diagnosis.* London: William Heinemann (Medical Books), 1922.

40 Jordan, A. C. Archives of the Roentgen Ray, *14*, CCCXX(7), 1909–10.

41 British Journal of Radiology, *5*, 853, 1932.

42 Simmons, G. A. British Medical Journal, *1*, 536, 1910.

43 Kaye, G. W. C. Radiography, *6*, 43, 1940.

44 Archives of the Roentgen Ray, *17*, 267, 1912–13.

45 Watson, W. Radiography, *27*, 306, 1961.

46 Reynolds, H. The Moseley Journal, *3*, 1, 1896.

47 Macintyre, J. Archives of the Roentgen Ray, *7*, CLVIII(5 and 7), 1902–3.

48 Left – Whitaker, P. H. Transactions of the Liverpool Medical Institution, *29*, 1961.

48 Right – British Journal of Radiology, *14*, 94, 1941.

49 British Journal of Radiology, *22*, 295, 1949.

50 Barclay, A. E. The Manchester University Medical School Gazette, *1*, 114, 1948.

51 Barclay, A. E. The Journal of the Röntgen Society, *19*, 65, 1923.

52 Warrick, C. K. Radiography, *43*, 193, 1977.

53 Leman, R. M. Radiography, *33*, 102, 1967.

54–59 British Institute of Radiology.

60 British Journal of Radiology, *29*, 35, 1924.

61 British Institute of Radiology.

62 Southern Newspapers, Southampton.

63 The author.

64 National Maritime Museum, Greenwich.

65 The author.

66 Wild, C. H. J. Radiography, *23*, 194, 1957.

67 Strand Magazine, *17*, 777, 1899.

68 The author.

69 Pencil sketch by Sean O'Sullivan by courtesy of Mr. J. B. Prendiville, F.R.C.S.I.

70–73 Battersby, J. C. Archives of the Roentgen Ray, *3*, LVII (a and b) and LVIII (a and b), 1898–9.

74 The author.

75 Kisch, H. and Tugman, H. St. J. *The Siege of Ladysmith in 120 Pictures.* London: Newnes, 1900.

76 Hall-Edwards, J. The Amateur Photographer, *31*, 314, 1900.

77 Scott, J. Radiography, *26*, 98, 1960.

78 Hall-Edwards, J. Archives of the Roentgen Ray, *13*, CCCI (1 and 2), 1908–9.

79 Oliver, R. British Journal of Radiology, *46*, 855, 1973.

80 Kaye, G. W. C. Radiography, *27*, 406, 1961.

81 Kaye, G. W. C. Radiography, *6*, 59, 1940.

INDEX